The EACVI Handbook of Cardiovascular CT

T0258088

EUROPEAN SOCIETY OF CARDIOLOGY PUBLICATIONS

The EACVI Handbook of Cardiovascular CT

Editors

Oliver Gaemperli
HeartClinic Zurich AG, Hirslanden Hospital, Zurich, Switzerland

Pal Maurovich-Horvat
Medical Imaging Centre, Semmelweis University, Budapest, Hungary

Koen Nieman
Stanford University School of Medicine, Division of Cardiovascular
Medicine and Department of Radiology, Stanford, CA, USA

Gianluca Pontone
Department of Perioperative Cardiology and Cardiovascular
Imaging, Centro Cardiologico Monzino IRCCS, Milan, Italy

Francesca Pugliese
Queen Mary University of London and St Bartholomew's Hospital,
London, UK

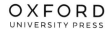

OXFORD
UNIVERSITY PRESS

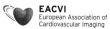

EACVI
European Association of
Cardiovascular Imaging

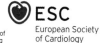

ESC
European Society
of Cardiology

Great Clarendon Street, Oxford, OX2 6DP,
United Kingdom

Oxford University Press is a department of the University of Oxford.
It furthers the University's objective of excellence in research, scholarship,
and education by publishing worldwide. Oxford is a registered trade mark of
Oxford University Press in the UK and in certain other countries

First Edition published in 2023

Published in the United States of America by Oxford University Press
198 Madison Avenue, New York, NY 10016, United States of America

British Library Cataloguing in Publication Data
Data available

Library of Congress Control Number: 2022941528

ISBN 978–0–19–288445–9

DOI: 10.1093/med/9780192884459.001.0001

Printed in Great Britain by
Bell & Bain Ltd., Glasgow

Preface

Since the introduction of computed tomography (CT) in 1969 by Sir Godfrey Hounsfield, this technology has evolved at a breathtaking pace to become a cornerstone of non-invasive imaging in clinical practice. A giant leap was realized with the introduction of multislice CT scanners with short rotation times and the necessary spatial and temporal resolution to resolve the smallest, moving parts of cardiac anatomy: the coronary arteries. Supported by further technological refinements, clinical trial evidence, and guideline recommendations, cardiac CT, and, foremost, coronary CT angiography (CCTA), has been embraced as an indispensable non-invasive cardiac imaging modality and an important first-line test for coronary artery disease. Recently, the potential of cardiac CT has become evident in the diagnosis and guidance of treatment in a variety of other cardiac pathologies beyond coronary artery disease, including valvular disease, atrial fibrillation and other arrhythmias, endocarditis, cardiac masses, cardiomyopathies, and others.

On these grounds, the European Association of Cardiovascular Imaging (EACVI) has declared that one of their foremost priorities is to facilitate education and training in cardiovascular CT through teaching courses, congresses, and a structured certification programme (see Chapter 4.1). This handbook represents an important step towards the dissemination of skills and knowledge in cardiovascular CT. It is conceived as a concise and practical companion, to benefit students, trainees, or advanced users (cardiologists, radiologists, cardiac surgeons, and technicians) in their everyday practice. Four broad sections cover the technical aspects and physical background, coronary indications (e.g. CCTA, atherosclerosis imaging, stents and bypasses, and functional CT imaging), non-coronary indications (CT for valve disease, infective endocarditis, CT of the left atrium, congenital heart disease, cardiac masses, extracardiac findings, etc.), and, finally, training and competence in cardiac CT. The handbook features short chapters, enriched with plenty of illustrations, tables, and condensed summaries, which facilitate rapid and intuitive access. We believe that among the many textbooks available, our handbook fills an important gap, and hope that it will find its way into the pockets of many practitioners' lab coats.

The recent COVID-19 pandemic has placed tremendous strain on healthcare systems worldwide. The disease has not only caused a large toll of casualties, but also exhausted medical resources to an unprecedented level. CT has become a central imaging tool in patients with COVID throughout the entire course of their disease and associated conditions. High-resolution CT of the pulmonary parenchyma can visualize the typical ground-glass and reticular opacities of COVID pneumonia and allow for rapid diagnosis and risk stratification. In the least ill patients, expedited discharge from the overcrowded Emergency Room is facilitated by CT. Beyond pulmonary involvement, a vast number of complications can affect the cardiovascular system and can be readily assessed with CT, including thromboembolic complications and pericardial and pleural effusions. Patients with acute chest pain and inconclusive electrocardiograms can be rapidly and safely investigated with cardiac CT, thus avoiding invasive coronary angiography, which poses a higher infection risk for medical personnel. In addition, using cardiac CT instead of transoesophageal echocardiography in ruling out left atrial appendage thrombus before atrial fibrillation ablation proved to be invaluable during the pandemic. Indeed, the COVID-19 pandemic has reinforced interest in CT as a robust, rapid, and reliable imaging technology, and has emphasized the need for appropriate education and training. We sincerely hope that this handbook will contribute to improving the skills and knowledge of the large number of healthcare providers fighting every day at the forefront of the global pandemic.

Oliver Gaemperli
Pal Maurovich-Horvat
Koen Nieman
Gianluca Pontone
Francesca Pugliese

Contents

Contributors

Thomas Allmendinger
Siemens Healthcare GmbH, Computed
Tomography, Forchheim, Germany
Chapters 1.2 and 1.5

Murat Arslan
Erasmus Medical Center, Department
of Cardiology, Rotterdam,
the Netherlands
Chapter 2.9

Andrea Baggiano
Department of Perioperative
Cardiology and Cardiovascular Imaging,
Centro Cardiologico Monzino IRCCS,
Milan, Italy
Chapters 3.6, 3.8, and 4.1

Sujana Balla
University of California San Francisco
Fresno, Fresno, CA, USA
Chapter 2.7

Andrea Bartykowszki
Heart and Vascular Center,
Semmelweis University,
Budapest, Hungary
Chapter 2.10

Anna Beattie
The Newcastle Upon Tyne Hospitals
NHS Foundation Trust, Newcastle
upon Tyne, UK
Chapter 1.7

Dominik C. Benz
University Heart Center, University
Hospital Zurich, Zurich, Switzerland
Chapters 3.11 and 3.14

Ricardo Budde
Erasmus Medical Center, Department
of Radiology and Nuclear Medicine,
Rotterdam, the Netherlands
Chapter 1.11

Csilla Celeng
Department of Radiology, University
Medical Center Utrecht, Utrecht,
the Netherlands
Chapters 2.2 and 3.1

Andrew Chang
Stanford University School of Medicine,
Division of Cardiovascular Medicine,
Department of Medicine, Stanford,
CA, USA
Chapter 2.8

Admir Dedic
Northwest Clinics, Department of
Cardiology, Alkmaar, the Netherlands
Chapter 2.9

Oliver Gaemperli
HeartClinic Zurich AG, Hirslanden
Hospital, Zurich, Switzerland
Chapter 1.8

Tessa Genders
Stanford University School of Medicine,
Division of Cardiovascular Medicine,
Stanford, CA, USA
Chapter 2.3

Andreas A. Giannopoulos
Department of Cardiology, University
Heart Center Zurich and Department
of Nuclear Medicine, University
Hospital Zurich, Zurich, Switzerland
Chapters 3.10 and 3.12

Marco Guglielmo
Department of Cardiovascular Imaging,
Centro Cardiologico Monzino IRCCS,
Milan, Italy
Chapters 3.4, 3.5, and 3.7

Ulrike Haberland
Siemens Healthcare GmbH, Computed
Tomography, Forchheim, Germany
Chapters 1.2 and 1.5

Jens D. Hove
Department of Cardiology,
Copenhagen University
Hospital – Amager and Hvidovre,
Denmark; Department of Clinical
Medicine, University of Copenhagen,
Denmark
Chapter 1.3

Mihály Károlyi
Institute of Diagnostic and
Interventional Radiology,
University Hospital Zurich, Zurich,
Switzerland
Chapters 1.4 and 1.9

Jamal Khan
Department of Cardiology, University
Hospitals of Coventry & Warwickshire
NHS Trust, Coventry, UK
Chapter 1.6

Martina de Knegt
Barts Heart Centre, Centre for
Advanced Cardiovascular Imaging,
William Harvey Research Institute,
Queen Mary University of London,
London, UK
Chapter 1.3

Márton Kolossváry
Cardiovascular Imaging Research
Center, Massachusetts General
Hospital, Harvard Medical School,
Boston, MA, USA
Chapters 2.6 and 3.16

Bibi Martens
Cardiovascular Research Institute
Maastricht (CARIM), Maastricht
University, and Department of
Radiology and Nuclear Medicine,
Maastricht University Medical Center,
Maastricht, the Netherlands
Chapter 1.10

Mohamed Marwan
Cardiology Department, University
Hospital Erlangen, Erlangen, Germany
Chapter 1.9

Domenico Mastrodicasa
Stanford University School of Medicine,
Department of Radiology, Center for
Academic Medicine, Palo Alto, CA, USA
Chapter 2.4

Pál Maurovich-Horvat
Medical Imaging Centre, Semmelweis
University, Budapest, Hungary
Chapter 2.2

Michael Messerli
Department of Nuclear Medicine,
University Hospital Zurich/University
of Zurich, Zurich, Switzerland
Chapters 3.9 and 3.15

Casper Mihl
Cardiovascular Research Institute
Maastricht (CARIM), Maastricht
University, and Department of
Radiology and Nuclear Medicine,
Maastricht University Medical Center,
Maastricht, the Netherlands
Chapter 1.10

Sarah Moharem-Elgamal
Liverpool Heart and Chest Hospital,
Liverpool, UK; National Heart Institute,
Giza, Egypt
Chapters 1.6, 1.11, and 3.13

Giuseppe Muscogiuri
School of Medicine and Surgery,
University of Milano-Bicocca, Milan,
Italy; Department of Radiology, IRCCS
Istituto Auxologico Italiano, San Luca
Hospital, Milan, Italy
Chapters 3.2 and 3.3

Koen Nieman
Stanford University School of
Medicine, Division of Cardiovascular
Medicine and Department of
Radiology, Stanford, CA, USA
Chapters 2.5, 2.7, and 2.8

Gianluca Pontone
Department of Perioperative Cardiology
and Cardiovascular Imaging, Centro
Cardiologico Monzino IRCCS, Milan, Italy
Chapter 2.5

Francesca Pugliese
Queen Mary University of London and
St Bartholomew's Hospital, London, UK
Chapters 1.1, 1.5, 1.6, and 1.7

Ronak Rajani
Guy's and St Thomas' NHS Foundation
Trust and King's College London,
London, UK
Chapter 1.4

Ian Rogers
Stanford University School of Medicine,
Division of Cardiovascular Medicine,
Department of Medicine, Stanford,
CA, USA
Chapter 2.8

Alexia Rossi
Department of Nuclear Medicine,
University Hospital Zurich; and Center
for Molecular Cardiology, University of
Zurich, Zurich, Switzerland
Chapter 1.3

Marcel van Straten
Erasmus Medical Center, University
Medical Center, Department of
Radiology and Nuclear Medicine,
Rotterdam, the Netherlands
Chapter 1.1

Bálint Szilveszter
Semmelweis University Heart and
Vascular Center, Budapest, Hungary
Chapter 2.2

Richard A.P. Takx
Amsterdam University Medical Center,
Department of Radiology and Nuclear
Medicine, Amsterdam, the Netherlands
Chapters 2.2 and 3.1

Sebastian Vandermolen
Barts Heart Centre, London, UK
Chapter 1.1

Martin Willemink
Stanford University School of Medicine,
Department of Radiology, Stanford,
CA, USA
Chapter 2.1

Contributors

xiii

Abbreviations

AC	alternating current
ACHD	adult congenital heart disease
ACS	acute coronary syndrome
AF	atrial fibrillation
AHA	American Heart Association
AI	artificial intelligence
ALARA	as low as reasonably achievable
ALCAPA	anomalous LMCA from the pulmonary artery
AR	aortic regurgitation
ARCAPA	anomalous RCA from the pulmonary artery
AS	aortic stenosis
ASD	atrial septal defect
BAV	bicuspid aortic valve
BMI	body mass index
bpm	beats per minute
BSA	body surface area
CA	catheter ablation
CAA	coronary artery anomaly
CABG	coronary artery bypass grafting
CAC-DRS	Coronary Artery Calcium Data and Reporting System
CAD	coronary artery disease
CAD-RADS	Coronary Artery Disease – Reporting and Data System
CAV	cardiac allograft vasculopathy
CCT	cardiac CT
CCTA	coronary CT angiography
CDRIE	cardiac device-related infective endocarditis
CIN	contrast-induced nephropathy
CM	contrast media
CMR	cardiac magnetic resonance
cMPR	curved multiplanar reconstruction
CS	coronary sinus

CTA	CT angiography
DC	direct current
EACVI	European Association of Cardiovascular Imaging
ECF	extracardiac finding
ECG	electrocardiogram
ECV	extracellular volume
ED	Emergency Department
EDV	end diastole
EF	ejection fraction
ESC	European Society of Cardiology
ESV	end systole
FBP	filtered back projection
FFR	fractional flow reserve
FoV	field of view
GCV	great cardiac vein
GFR	glomerular filtration rate
HR	heart rate
HTX	heart transplantation
HU	Hounsfield unit
ICA	invasive coronary angiography
ICRP	International Commission on Radiological Protection
IDR	iodine delivery rate
IE	infective endocarditis
IMA	internal mammary artery
IMH	intramural haematoma
IV	intravenous(ly)
IVC	inferior vena cava
keV	kiloelectron volts
kV	kilovoltage
LAA	left atrial appendage
LAD	left anterior descending artery
LCA	left coronary artery
LCX	left circumflex artery
LMA	left main artery
LMCA	left main coronary artery
LNT	linear no-threshold
lp/cm	line-pairs per cm

LR	likelihood ratio
LV	left ventricle
LVOT	left ventricle outflow tract
mA	milliAmperes
MACE	major adverse cardiac events
MBF	myocardial blood flow
MCQ	multiple-choice question
MI	myocardial infarction
MIP	maximum intensity reconstruction
ML	machine learning
MPI	myocardial perfusion imaging
MPR	multiplanar reconstruction
MR	mitral regurgitation
mSv	millisievert
MRI	magnetic resonance imaging
MV	mitral valve
NICE	National Institute for Health and Care Excellence
NSTE-ACS	non-ST elevation acute coronary syndrome
PA	pulmonary artery
PAU	penetrating atherosclerotic ulcer
PCI	percutaneous coronary intervention
PDA	posterior descending artery
PTP	pretest probability
PV	pulmonary vein
PVE	prosthetic valve endocarditis
RCA	right coronary artery
RCT	randomized clinical/controlled trial
RV	right ventricle
RVEF	right ventricle ejection fraction
RVOT	right ventricular outflow tract
SAVR	surgical aortic valve replacement
SCCT	Society of Cardiovascular Computed Tomography
SPECT	single photon emission CT
SVC	superior vena cava
TAVI	transcatheter aortic valve implantation
TEVAR	thoracic endovascular aortic repair
TMVR	transcatheter mitral valve replacement

TOE	transoesophageal echocardiography
TSH	thyroid stimulating hormone
2D	two-dimensional
ViMAC	valve-in-mitral annular calcification
ViR	valve-in-ring
VSD	ventricular septal defect

Chapter 1.1

Key hardware components of a cardiac-enabled CT scanner

Sebastian Vandermolen, Marcel van Straten,
and Francesca Pugliese

Teaching points

- Contemporary CT scanners comprise a rotating gantry onto which the X-ray tube(s) and the detector array(s) are housed.
- Collimators determine the shape of the emitted X-ray beam to maximize image quality and minimize radiation exposure to patients.
- Detectors receive and transform the signal necessary to reconstruct CT images.
- The term 'multidetector' or 'multislice' CT refers to the ability to image multiple sections of the patient's anatomy along the z-axis during one gantry rotation.
- 'Dual-source' CT contains two X-ray sources coupled with two detector arrays mounted at an (approximately) 90-degree angle. Dual-source CT allows doubling of the temporal resolution compared to a single-source system with the same gantry rotation time.
- A motorized scanner table, the electrocardiogram (ECG) synchronization system, and power injection are further key requirements to deliver cardiac CT in clinical practice.

Gantry

The gantry is the ring-shaped structure that houses the X-ray tube and the detector array.

- In contemporary scanners, the gantry can rotate continuously thanks to (contactless) slip-ring technology. Slip-ring technology allows fast transfer of power and data to and from the gantry without the need of power cables. Power cables would require unwinding every few turns, which would prevent continuous rotation and require reversal of gantry rotation. Cables can be replaced by brush technology that is in permanent electrical contact with the gantry and allows continuous rotation.
- The switch-mode power supply allows construction of a small and light but efficient power supply that can be housed in the gantry while generating very

high voltages with limited heat production. In general, this works by converting alternating current (AC) to direct current (DC) using a switch circuit. The DC current is reconverted to AC at a higher frequency.

- The gantry rotation time is a key determinant of temporal resolution, a paramount scanner requirement for cardiac CT (discussed in Chapter 1.2). In a single-source (one X-ray tube) scanner, approximately half a revolution is needed for the acquisition of data required to reconstruct one image (half-scan algorithm). A single-source CT scanner with a rotation time of 300 ms can sample data for one image in 150 ms, which is the temporal resolution of this scanner.

X-ray tube

The X-ray tube is the component where X-ray generation occurs (Figure 1.1.1).

- A tungsten filament is heated by current and emits electrons (thermionic emission).

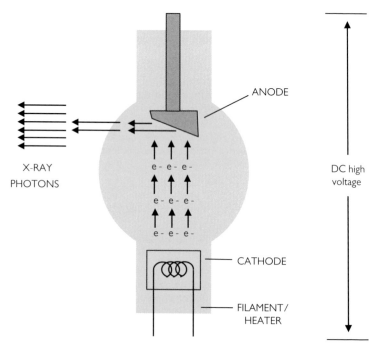

Figure 1.1.1 Simplified structure of an X-ray tube.

- By applying a potential difference (kilovoltage, kV) between the cathode and the anode, the electrons are accelerated towards a positively charged anode.
- The resulting flow of electrons represents the tube current, measured in milliAmperes (mA).
- The electrons gain energy proportional to the voltage applied (kV).
- The electron beam hits the focal spot of the anode. About 4% of the energy of the beam leads to the generation of X-ray photons; the rest is dissipated as heat.
- The emitted X-ray beam displays a range of different energies (polychromatic X-ray spectrum), from a few kiloelectron volts (keV) to the nominal value of the applied tube voltage (discussed further in Chapter 1.3, Figure 1.3.1).
- If the applied voltage is 100 kV, the average energy of the X-ray beam is 50–60 keV.
- Lower-energy X-rays are removed from the X-ray beam by the tube housing and by filtration: this is because energies at the lower end of the spectrum would otherwise be absorbed by tissue before reaching the detector and would contribute to patient dose but not to image formation.
- The X-ray tube voltage determines the average energy of the X-ray beam; the X-ray tube current determines how many X-ray photons the X-ray beam is comprised of, without affecting their energy.
- The intensity of the X-ray beam decreases with the inverse of the distance from the source squared.
- When traversing tissue, the intensity of the X-ray beam decreases as X-ray photons interact with atoms (Chapter 1.3). The transmitted intensity depends on the initial intensity, the thickness of the tissue/material traversed, and their linear attenuation coefficient. The latter depends not only on the atomic number of the tissue/material, but also on photon energy and is generally higher at lower energy.

Collimators

The term 'collimation' refers to the process of restricting or confining a beam of particles.

- Beam collimators are used to shape the X-ray beam emitted, reduce unnecessary radiation, and maximize image quality.
- Pre-patient collimators determine the width of the beam (fixed and adjustable collimators).
- Post-patient collimators reduce scatter radiation.
- The heart is centrally located in the patient's axial cross section; image quality can be reduced in peripheral regions that are of limited interest. Additional shaped filters in cardiac CT may reduce radiation exposure for peripheral organs and tissues.

Detectors

The detection of X-rays constitutes the key 'signal' to form projection images needed to reconstruct CT images.

• Current CT detector technology is based on solid-state rare earth ceramics.

• Incident X-rays are absorbed with release of light photons.

• Light photons are detected by photodiodes and converted into an electrical signal.

Detector terminology and configuration

The term 'multidetector' or 'multislice' CT refers to the ability to image multiple sections of the patient's anatomy along the z-axis during one gantry rotation (see also Chapter 1.2 and Figure 1.2.2).

• Detector element size is the width of the detector row in the x–y plane and is related to in-plane spatial resolution.

• Detector row width is the width of the detector row in the z-axis, determining the minimum slice thickness and the through-plane (longitudinal) spatial resolution (fixed hardware characteristics of the detector array).

• In the past, detector configurations varied across manufacturers and scanner models. Modern cardiac CT systems feature isotropic detector configuration, meaning that detector rows have constant width.

• Detector rows can be combined to increase slice thickness to a multiple of the detector width. The decision to do so can be made at the time of scanning to increase signal and reduce dose, at the expense of though-plane spatial resolution. This approach is not typically used in cardiac CT, where the highest spatial resolution is mandatory.

• It is possible to increase slice thickness post-scanning, by reconstructing thicker slices to reduce image noise (e.g. very large patients).

Dual-source CT

While single-source CT systems contain one X-ray tube and one detector array, 'dual-source' CT contains two X-ray sources coupled with two detector arrays mounted at an (approximately) 90-degree angle (Figure 1.1.2).

• Dual-source CT is a scanner design solution that allows the doubling of temporal resolution without decreasing gantry rotation time.

• The two-tube detector systems simultaneously generate X-rays and acquire data so that a 90-degree gantry revolution (instead of 180-degree) is sufficient to acquire data for the reconstruction of one image.

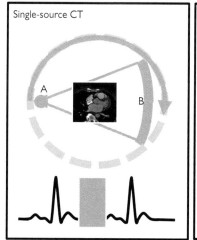 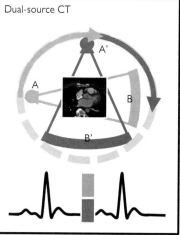

Figure 1.1.2 The simplified geometries of single- and dual-source CT.
A, A': X-ray tube(s); B, B': detector array(s).

Dual-energy CT

- Dual-source CT allows dual-energy applications. In dual-source dual-energy CT, different X-ray tube voltages are applied to each of the X-ray tubes. This is done to exploit the differential ability of tissues (with different atomic numbers) to attenuate X-rays of variable energy, with the goal of differentiating tissues on the images.
- Different approaches to dual-energy (or multiple-energy) CT do not require dual-source CT. Dual-layer detectors comprise two layers made of different scintillating materials that selectively detect X-rays of different energy. Ultrafast kV switching involves rapid changes in X-ray tube potential with generation of X-ray beams of different energy.
- Dual-energy CT is not widely applied in cardiac imaging. Potential applications include subtraction of coronary artery calcium (Chapter 2.1), plaque imaging (Chapter 2.6), and characterization of myocardial enhancement such as in perfusion and scar imaging (Chapter 2.5).

Other hardware components

- The scanner table is the motorized platform to move the patient in and out of the gantry. The longitudinal coverage of the scanner is often smaller than the region of interest. Multiple acquisitions can be made at different table positions (sequential scanning). The table can move continuously through the gantry during scanning (helical or spiral scanning).

- Electrocardiogram (ECG) recording capability allow for the synchronization of image acquisition and reconstruction with specific phases of cardiac cycle. Four ECG electrodes are usually required
- A power injector is required to allow rapid injection of contrast agent to depict cardiac chambers and coronary tree. A power injector consists of (i) injector 'head'—allows insertion of syringes of contrast; (ii) piston plungers—push the contrast from syringe into patient; and (iii) pressure tubing—connects the syringe to the patient's intravenous access.

Further reading

Goldman LW. Principles of CT and CT technology. *J Nucl Med Technol* 2007; 35: 115–28.

Mamourian AC. *CT Imaging. Practical Physics, Artifacts and Pitfalls*. Oxford: OUP, 2013.

Stirrup J, Bull R, Williams M, Nicol E (eds). *Cardiovascular Computed Tomography*, 2nd edn. New York: Oxford Medical Publications, 2020.

Chapter 1.2

Technical requirements for cardiac CT scanning

Ulrike Haberland and Thomas Allmendinger

Teaching points

- High-quality cardiac CT imaging depends on motion-free images. In half-scan mode, temporal resolution can be defined as the time required to acquire data to reconstruct one CT image. Therefore, temporal resolution depends not only on the scanner's rotation time, but also on the number of X-ray sources and the availability of multisegment reconstruction.

- Some manufacturers have introduced coronary motion correction algorithms to reduce image motion blur.

- The scanner's detector coverage influences the number of cardiac cycles needed to complete the scan range and depends on physical collimation, number of slices, and detector element size (slice width). The scan pitch also influences through-plane (z-axis) coverage in the spiral scanning mode. Wide area detectors aim to cover the heart in a single cardiac cycle without table movement.

- The typical size of coronary artery lesions is in the sub-millimetre range. Spatial resolution is the ability to discern two objects as separate from one another. In-plane and through-plane (isotropic) spatial resolution depends on focal spot size, individual detector element size, number of detector channels, number of projections/views, system geometry, and reconstruction filter/kernel.

- Coronary artery CT angiography is based on high iodine contrast imaging, which can be optimized by adjusting the X-ray tube kilovoltage (kV) to influence iodine enhancement and the tube current (mAs) to mitigate noise.

Resting phases

Given that the heart moves continuously, the primary aim of a cardiac CT scan is to 'image during the resting phase(s)'.

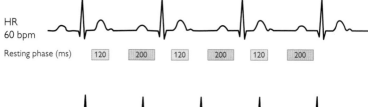

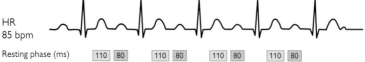

Figure 1.2.1 The resting phases in patients with a heart rate (HR) of 60 beats/min (bpm; upper panel) and 85 bpm (lower panel). Of note, there is significant shortening of the diastolic resting phase (blue) with increasing HR, while the systolic resting phase (green) remains fairly stable.

- Diastole has a typical resting phase duration of approximately 200 ms at a heart rate (HR) of 60 bpm, which rapidly decreases towards higher HRs.
- Systole also has a resting phase at its end but is significantly shorter at about 120 ms; however, to some extent, it is relatively constant over a wider HR range (Figure 1.2.1).
- These physiological findings build the basis for the established strategies of coronary CT angiography (CCTA) imaging: end-diastolic imaging for low-to-intermediate HRs; and end-systolic imaging for high HRs (see also Chapters 1.5 and 1.9, and Figure 1.5.1). The ill-defined range in between often requires images from both diastolic and systolic phases in order to achieve diagnostic image quality.

Temporal resolution

Owing to the short duration of cardiac 'rest phases', optimizing CT acquisition and reconstruction towards speed to 'freeze motion' is essential. Temporal resolution is the time required to acquire data to reconstruct one CT image. CT images consist of individual X-ray data projections recorded during the rotation of the CT system. The minimum amount of parallel projection data required for a single CT image in a half-scan, filtered back projection-based image reconstruction is 180 degrees (see also Chapter 1.1). In single-source CT, data corresponding to a time span of half gantry rotation contribute to a single cardiac image; hence, the temporal resolution is defined as ½ times the rotation time. Any movement during this time leads to blurred images.

Optimization of the temporal resolution can be achieved by:

- Faster gantry rotation times, which are limited by increasing G-force experienced by the rotating components, data transmission rate increase, and tube power.

- Using CT systems with two tubes (dual-source technology). The required 180 degrees of data consist of two separate, simultaneously recorded data fragments of approximately 90 degrees (see Chapter 1.1). The in-plane temporal resolution is decreased to around $1/4$ of the rotation time.

- Multisegment reconstruction. This approach involves acquisition of data over several cardiac cycles at the same table position, with combination of the data in the reconstruction process. Typical numbers of segments are 2, 3, 4, and 5 (vendor-specific; Figure 1.2.2). Ideally, this results in a temporal resolution of $1/4$ (two-segment), $1/6$ (three-segment), $1/8$ (four-segment), or $1/10$ (five-segment) of the rotation time. This can only be achieved for specific HRs, which makes the effectiveness of this approach difficult to predict. Segmented reconstructions require stable HRs and can suffer from blurring due to beat-to-beat variability. The amount of recorded data must be increased, which usually leads to a higher radiation dose.

- Intelligent coronary wall motion correction algorithms track the vessel path and velocity to compensate adaptively for residual image motion (blur) on a per-vessel and segment basis.

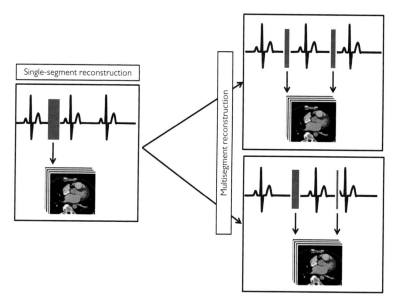

Figure 1.2.2 The principle of single-segment (left) and multisegment reconstruction (right; two segments in this case). Image data at the same table position are acquired over several cardiac cycles and combined in the reconstruction process. Segmented reconstructions require stable heart rates (upper right panel) and can suffer from heart rate variability (lower right panel).

- In wide-area detector scanners, if the entire cardiac scan range can be covered in one gantry rotation, the scanner table remains stationary. All images in the scan range will be simultaneously acquired during one cardiac cycle.

Detector coverage

The typical scan length of CCTA or calcium scoring examinations is around 14 cm. Notable exceptions are CCTA bypass examinations with longer scan ranges of around 16–22 cm.

- Ideally, the required scan length is covered in a single scan of a single cardiac cycle.
- In all other cases, the acquisition is spread over multiple cardiac cycles, which results in a block-wise combination of the reconstructed images based on data from multiple cardiac cycles, covering the entire examination range.
- A basic assumption is the equality of heart motion state and anatomical position in all contributing cardiac cycles. This explains the need for good patient breath-hold, a regular sinus rhythm, and constant HR. Wider detectors are beneficial in terms of the required number of blocks and scan time, with fewer requirements related to the patient being in sinus rhythm and complying with a relatively long breath-hold time.

A CT detector is typically banana shaped, consisting of many thousand individual elements focused onto the focal spot of the X-ray source (Figure 1.2.3).

- The layout of the CT detector can be described along the fan direction by the number of detector channels in each individual detector row. This geometry is replicated over multiple slices along the (longitudinal) z-axis, resulting in a multislice detector. A modern CT system suitable for cardiac imaging should provide at least 64 detector rows.
- The width of each individual detector row or element is typically in the range of 0.5–0.8 mm at the iso-centre.
- The total detector coverage in z-axis direction (detector collimation/physical collimation) is the product of the number of slices times the width of the detector element (slice width). A 64-row system with 0.625 mm slice width has a detector collimation of 40 mm at the iso-centre.
- The physical collimation is the primary factor determining the number of cardiac cycles required in a single cardiac scan range when different CT systems are compared. The comparison needs to be done using the same acquisition technique (e.g. prospective step-and-shoot and retrospective ECG-gated spiral) as there are large systematic differences between them.
- CT systems with a periodic motion of the tube focal spot in the z-direction (z-flying focal spot) create an oversampling of the slices in z-direction and 'double' their slices in the reconstruction process. These CT systems are often referenced by their effective doubled slice count instead of their physical detector slice count.

The key parameters of current selected cardiac CT scanners are described in Table 1.2.1.

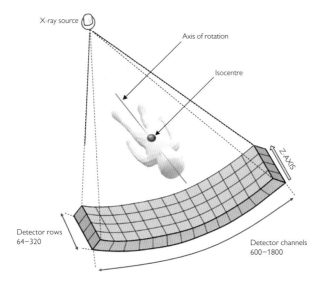

X-ray source

Axis of rotation

Isocentre

Z-AXIS

Detector rows
64–320

Detector channels
600–1800

Figure 1.2.3 Illustration of a detector array.
Adapted from Malajikian, K. and Finelli, D. *Basics of Computed Tomography, Multimodality Imaging Guidance in Interventional Pain Management*. Oxford University Press.

Spatial resolution

Spatial resolution is the ability to discern two objects as separate from one another.

- Spatial resolution plays an important role in the assessment of the severity of coronary stenosis and the overall interpretability of CCTA images. The term 'isotropic' indicates similar spatial resolution achieved in the in-plane (x- and y-axes) and through-plane (z-axis) directions.

- Sufficient spatial resolution is required for a detailed analysis of coronary plaque components.

- Insufficient spatial resolution leads to partial volume effects that may result in blooming artefacts from high-attenuating objects (calcified plaque, coronary stents), which can lead to overestimation of object size and the severity of stenosis

The spatial or high-contrast resolution of a CT system can be determined experimentally from phantom measurements of high-contrast objects with a very large 'signal-to-noise' ratio. The test measures the system's ability to resolve objects of decreasing sizes by scanning, for example, a wire phantom or an aluminium bar pattern phantom. A CT system's maximum spatial resolution, which can be achieved given a suitable reconstruction filter/kernel, is typically provided in units of 'line-pairs per cm' (lp/cm). This 'maximum' resolution is closely:

Table 1.2.1 Key parameters of current selected cardiac CT scanners

Vendor	Model	Physical element (slice width; mm)*	No. of slices (physical detector row count)	Physical collimation (mm)†	Gantry rotation time (ms)	Temporal resolution (ms)‡
Canon	Aquilion ONE/GENESIS Edition	0.5	320	160	275	137.5
Canon	Aquilion ONE/GENESIS 320	0.5	160	80	350	175
Canon	Aquilion PRIME	0.5	80	40	350	175
GE Healthcare	CardioGraphe	0.5	280	140	240	120
GE Healthcare	Revolution Frontier	0.625	64	40	350	175
GE Healthcare	Revolution HD	0.625	64	40	350	175
GE Healthcare	Revolution CT/Apex	0.625	256	160	280	140
Philips	iCT Elite	0.625	128	80	270	135
Philips	IQon Elite Spectral CT	0.625	64	40	270	135
Siemens Healthineers	SOMATOM Definition Edge	0.6	64	38.4	285	142
Siemens Healthineers	SOMATOM Force (dual source)	0.6	(2x) 96	(2x) 57.6	250	66
Siemens Healthineers	SOMATOM X.cite	0.6	64	38.4	300	150

*Although unusual in cardiac mode, slice width could be larger than detector element depending on acquisition modes and reconstruction methodology.
†Also referred to as z-axis coverage.
‡In-plane physical temporal resolution based on half-scan time; multisegment reconstruction or software applications not reflected.

- tied to the in-plane detector resolution limits given by the number of detector elements and their size;
- influenced by the size of the tube focal spot and the number of projections acquired per rotation;
- influenced by system geometry and reconstruction filter/kernel.

Clinical routine CCTA imaging does typically not achieve maximum spatial resolution of the system, as the necessary 'signal-to-noise' ratio is not accessible for the following reasons:

- on the signal side, the contrast between iodine-enhanced blood, soft tissue, low attenuation, and calcified plaque is considerably smaller compared with a 'true' high-contrast object;
- on the noise side, the strong focus on temporal resolution limits the accumulation of X-rays into the image over time;
- together with radiation dose considerations, this yields higher noise levels than 'true' high-contrast examinations (e.g. inner ear).

The routine working point of CCTA imaging is in the intermediate resolution range, mostly determined by the user-selected reconstruction kernel/filter. Advances in terms of realized detector resolution over the last decade pushed the accessible range of reconstruction kernels/filter into the intermediate-to-sharp region.

X-ray tube kilovoltage and current

Low kilovoltage (kV) scanning has been widely applied in CT angiography (CTA) imaging as it increases X-ray photon absorption and substantially increases the relative vascular attenuation, which results in a desired contrast increase in the CT image. High contrast allows loosening of the image noise requirements as contrast image quality is primarily driven by the realized contrast-to-noise ratio. With restrictions imposed by patient size, this typically results in considerable radiation dose reduction compared to a 'standard' 120 kV acquisition.

- There is an approximate squared relation between radiation dose and tube voltage ($dose \propto V^2$).
- Radiation dose is linear to the tube current output ($dose \propto mAs$).
- Image noise in standard filtered back projection reconstruction is inversely proportional to the square root of the tube current output ($noise \propto 1/\sqrt{mAs}$).
- Increased tube current reduces noise but does not affect relative vascular attenuation.

Based on these relationships, the application of low kV CT angiography scanning requires adjustments towards higher tube current output (mAs) to maintain the desired contrast-to-noise ratio at a low kV.

The impact of image reconstruction approaches on contrast and noise is discussed in Chapter 1.6.

Further reading

Abbara S, Blanke P, Maroules CD, Cheezum M, Choi AD, Han BK, et al. SCCT guidelines for the performance and acquisition of coronary computed tomographic angiography: a report of the society of Cardiovascular Computed Tomography Guidelines Committee: Endorsed by the North American Society for Cardiovascular Imaging (NASCI). *J Cardiovasc Comput Tomogr* 2016; 10: 435–49.

Achenbach S, Ropers D, Holle J, Muschiol G, Daniel WG, Moshage W. In-plane coronary arterial motion velocity: measurement with electron-beam CT. *Radiology* 2000; 216: 457–63.

Hausleiter J. Estimated radiation dose associated with cardiac CT angiography. *JAMA* 2009; 301: 500–7.

Lu H, Zhuo W, Xu B, Wang M. Organ and effective dose evaluation in coronary angiography by using a 320 MDCT based on in-phantom dose measurements with TLDs. *J Radiol Prot* 2015; 35: 597–609.

Meyer M, Haubenreisser H, Schoepf J, Vliegenthart R, Leidecker C, Allmendinger T, et al. Closing in on the K edge: coronary CT angiography at 100, 80, and 70 kV—initial comparison of a second- versus a third-generation dual-source CT system. *Radiology* 2014; 273: 373–82.

Chapter 1.3

Physical background: X-ray generation, interaction with matter, and radiation dosimetry concepts

Martina Chantal de Knegt, Jens Dahlgaard Hove, and Alexia Rossi

Teaching points
• X-rays interact with matter, affecting image quality and patient radiation dose.
• Effective radiation dose is the parameter currently used to express radiation risk.
• Tissue damage due to radiation is classified as either deterministic or stochastic.

X-ray generation

In an X-ray tube, a heated coil filament (cathode) emits electrons by thermionic emission. These electrons are accelerated from the negatively charged cathode toward a positively charged target (anode; also see Figure 1.1.1). The energy of the electrons that strike the anode is determined by the tube voltage (kilovolt, kV). When the electrons hit the anode, they interact with its atoms. This interaction generates X-ray photons through the formation of bremsstrahlung and characteristic radiation. The resultant X-ray beam consists of a continuum of photon energies (polychromatic X-ray beam) known as the X-ray emission spectrum (Figure 1.3.1). The X-ray energy is measured in kiloelectron volts (keV).

When X-rays pass through tissue, they are attenuated. Attenuation provides the basis for all CT image creation and is the process by which photons are removed from an X-ray beam as it passes through the body. The major mechanisms leading to attenuation are photoelectric absorption and Compton scattering. The probability of occurrence of one mechanism rather than the other depends mainly on tissue characteristics and the energy of the incident X-ray photons.

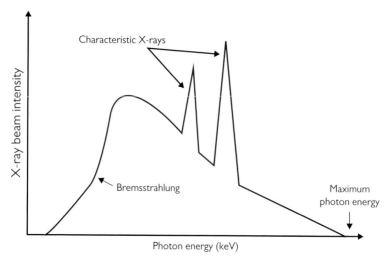

Figure 1.3.1 X-ray emission spectrum.

The lowest photon energies produced are usually 15–20 kiloelectron volts (keV), whereas the highest energy equals the maximum tube potential applied. Most photons have much lower energies than the maximum keV, resulting in a mean energy of the X-ray beam usually around one-third to one-half of the maximum energy. Characteristic line spectra of the tungsten or characteristic X-rays are emitted when a fast-moving electron collides with a K-shell electron. The electron in the K-shell is ejected leaving a hole behind. An outer-shell electron fills this hole from the L-shell with an emission of a single X-ray photon with an energy level equivalent to the energy level difference between the outer- and inner-shell electron involved in the transition.

Photoelectric absorption

Photoelectric absorption occurs when an incident photon interacts with a tightly bound inner shell (K-shell) electron. During this process, the energy of the photon is completely absorbed, and the electron is ejected as a photoelectron from its shell, causing ionization of the atom. Consequently, an electron from an outer shell drops down to fill the vacancy in the inner shell, resulting in the production of a characteristic X-ray (see Figure 1.3.2).

Photoelectric absorption is related to the effective atomic number (Z), tissue density (ρ), and energy level of the X-ray beam (E) by the formula $Z^3\rho/E^3$.

- The likelihood of photoelectric absorption decreases dramatically with increasing incident photon energy. Conversely, its probability of occurrence increases when the energy of the incident photon is close to the binding energy of the electron in the K-shell.

- The higher the effective atomic number, the higher the X-ray absorption. If Z doubles, photoelectric absorption is increased by a factor of 8.

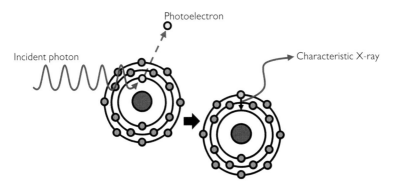

Figure 1.3.2 Photoelectric absorption.

As K-shells are typically low-energy shells, photoelectric absorption is the predominant interaction between low-energy photons and high Z materials, such as iodinated contrast material. Lowering X-ray energy therefore improves vessel contrast in CT angiography (CTA). Specifically, photoelectric absorption is the major contributor to X-ray attenuation up to energy levels of approximately 30 keV.

Compton scattering

Compton scattering occurs when an incident photon interacts with a loosely bound outer shell electron. During this process, the energy of the photon is partially absorbed by the electron. This results in the ejection of the electron (Compton electron) and the scattering of the resultant lower-energy Compton photon in a different direction (Figure 1.3.3).

Compton scattering leads to:

• increased patient radiation dose due to the absorption of scattered photons;

• reduced image quality due to increased image noise caused by the scattered photons.

Compton scattering is directly proportional to tissue density but, unlike photoelectric absorption, it is independent of the material's effective atomic number. Compton scattering is the predominant interaction of X-ray photons with soft tissue in the energy range 30 keV to 30 meV.

Principles of dual-energy CT

Materials or tissues with different elemental composition (atomic numbers and tissue density) can have identical or very similar ability to absorb X-rays, leading to similar Hounsfield units (HU) being assigned to them in the process of CT image formation. This makes tissue differentiation a challenge on CT.

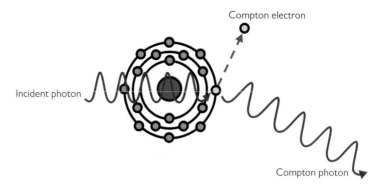

Figure 1.3.3 Compton scattering.

- Calcium/bone and iodine differ in their atomic numbers. However, depending on calcium/bone mass density and on the iodine concentration in the blood, calcified atheroma and iodinated blood may display the same brightness on CT images.
- Another problem is that the presence of multiple tissue types in a voxel hinders the accuracy in measuring material concentration. When measuring the amount of iodine enhancement in the myocardium (e.g. perfusion imaging), the measured mean HU reflects not only the enhancement due to iodine, but also the HU of the underlying tissue.

The reason underlying these challenges is that the measured HU in a CT voxel is related to its linear attenuation coefficient $\mu(E)$, which is not unique for any given material, but is a function of material composition, mass density, and photon energies interacting with the material.

- Dual-energy CT uses attenuation measurements acquired with different energy spectra along with known changes in attenuation between the two spectra, to differentiate and quantify material composition (Figure 1.3.4).
- Technical approaches to dual-energy CT are described in Chapter 1.2.

Current and emerging clinical applications of dual-energy CT include:

- Virtual monoenergetic imaging, automated bone removal in CTA, perfused blood-volume imaging, virtual non-contrast-enhanced imaging, plaque removal, virtual non-calcium imaging, urinary stone characterization, imaging of crystalline arthropathies, and the detection of silicone from breast implants.
- Applications of dual-energy CT in cardiac imaging are not in widespread use at the time of publication. The most promising applications include subtraction of coronary artery calcium (Chapter 2.1), plaque imaging (Chapter 2.6), and characterization of myocardial enhancement such as in perfusion and scar imaging (Chapter 2.5).

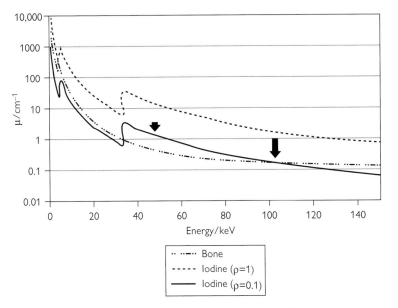

Figure 1.3.4 Dual-energy CT. Linear attenuation coefficients as a function of X-ray energy.

Linear attenuation coefficients for bone (assuming ρ = 1 g/cm³), iodine (assuming ρ = 1 g/cm³), and iodine with lower density (assuming ρ = 0.1 g/cm³) as a function of X-ray energy (in kiloelectron volts (keV)). Assuming monoenergetic X-rays were used, at 100 keV the same linear attenuation coefficients can be measured for bone and iodine (arrow). Measuring attenuation at a second energy, 50 keV, enables the differentiation of the two materials (arrowhead). Although X-ray tubes for diagnostic use generate a polyenergetic spectra, the general principle remains true.

Source: Reproduced from McCollough CH, Leng S, Yu L, Fletcher JG. (2015) Dual- and Multi-Energy CT: Principles, Technical Approaches, and Clinical Application. *Radiology*, 276(3):637–53. doi: 10.1148/radiol.2015142631 with permission from RSNA.

Radiation dose in cardiac CT

Several variables are commonly used to describe radiation dose in CT (Table 1.3.1). In particular, the effective dose is an index of radiation risk and describes the biological effects of ionizing radiation according to the different organ radiation sensitivities (radiosensitivity). The effective dose is expressed in millisievert (mSv).

$$\text{Effective dose (mSv)} = 0.028 \times \text{scan DLP (mGy*cm)}$$

To account for differences in tissue radiosensitivity, a tissue-weighting factor (K-factor) is used to calculate the effective dose from the dose length product. Although a factor of 0.014 mSv·mGray (mGy)⁻¹·cm⁻¹ has been traditionally used

Table 1.3.1 Radiation dose parameters

Term	SI unit	Definition
Absorbed dose	Gy	The amount of energy deposited in radiated tissue per mass
CT dose index (CTDI)	mGy	The average dose in the z-plane from a single rotation
Weighted CTDI (CTDI$_w$)	mGy	The weighted average of the CTDI at the periphery and centre of a standardized phantom
Volume CTDI (CTDI$_{vol}$)	mGy	CTDI$_w$ divided by the pitch. CTDI$_{vol}$ allows for comparison of radiation output dose between CT scanners
Dose length product (DLP)	mGy*cm	The total amount of incident radiation on the patient. DLP is obtained by the formula: CTDI$_{vol}$ × scan range. DLP allows for comparison of radiation dose between patients
Equivalent dose	mSv	A measure of the absorbed dose weighted for the effectiveness of the radiation type by applying specific radiation-weighting factors
Effective dose	mSv	A measure of the equivalent dose weighted for the radiosensitivity of the exposed organs and tissues by applying specific tissue-weighting factors. In CT, effective dose is derived using the formula: DLP × tissue-weighting factor

Gy, Gray; Sv, Sievert.

(ICRP, 1991) for cardiac CT, recent studies have derived higher values, particularly a K-factor of 0.028. With the accumulation of newer data, the K-factor is likely to be periodically updated. Examples of tissues with higher and lower radiosensitivities are breast (weighting factor 0.12) and skin tissue (weighting factor 0.01), respectively.

As with all radiological procedures, the ALARA ('as low as reasonably achievable') principle should always be employed (see Chapter 1.7). Thanks to technological advancements and new scan protocols, the radiation dose has decreased considerably in the last decades, while preserving image quality.

The biological effects of radiation

Ionizing radiation damage to DNA may result in base destruction and strand breaks. Damage may be direct or indirect. Indirect damage is caused by the ionization of water and the resultant formation of radical components. Affected cells attempt to repair any DNA damage, which may result in successful repair, incomplete repair and cell mutation, or unsuccessful repair and cell death or degeneration.

The biological effects of radiation depend on a variety of exposure factors and include type (whole-body/local, internal/external, etc.), radiation dose (high-dose/

low-dose), and time (acute/chronic). Tissues with actively dividing cells that are less differentiated, such as haemopoietic cells, tend to be more radiosensitive than tissues with cells that no longer undergo cell division.

The biological effects of radiation can be divided into two groups:

1. Deterministic effects

   Deterministic effects are caused by cell death or degeneration. These effects have a threshold dose, below which they do not occur (see Figure 1.3.5). The severity of deterministic effects increases with dose. Examples include:

   • acute disorders such as acute radiation syndromes, hair loss, skin injury, and sterility;

   • late-onset disorders such as radiation-induced cataract formation;

   • fetal disorders.

2. Stochastic effects

   Stochastic effects are caused by cell mutation and occur by chance. According to the linear no-threshold (LNT) theory, the probability of stochastic effects is proportional to the radiation dose but, unlike deterministic effects, they do not have a threshold dose (Figure 1.3.5). Examples include:

   • late-onset disorders such as cancer and leukaemia;

   • hereditary effects (i.e. damage to DNA in reproductive cells that allows for transmission to future generations).

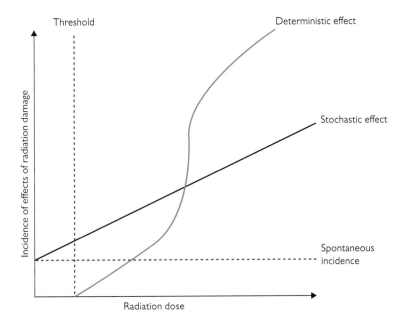

Figure 1.3.5 Deterministic and stochastic effects of radiation.

Reference

ICRP. 1990 Recommendations of the International Commission on Radiological Protection. Available at: https://www.icrp.org/publication.asp?id=icrp%20publication%2060 (1991, accessed 8 June 2022).

Further reading

Bushberg JT. The AAPM/RSNA physics tutorial for residents—X-ray interaction. *Radiographics* 1998; 18: 457–68.

Halliburton SS, Abbara S, Chen MY, Gentry R, Mahesh M, Raff GL, et al. SCCT guidelines on radiation dose and dose-optimization strategies in cardiovascular CT. *J Cardiovasc Comput Tomogr* 2011; 5: 198–224.

McCollough C, Leng S, Yu L, Fletcher JG. Dual- and multi-energy CT: principles, technical approaches, and clinical applications. *Radiology* 2015; 276: 637–53.

Trattner S, Halliburton S, Thompson CM, Xu Y, Chelliah A, Jambawalikar SR, et al. Cardiac-specific conversion factors to estimate radiation effective dose from dose-length product in computed tomography. *JACC Cardiovasc Imaging* 2018; 11: 64–74.

Chapter 1.4

Patient selection and preparation

Ronak Rajani and Mihály Károlyi

Teaching points

- Appropriate patient selection and preparation is vital to ensure patient safety, minimize ionizing radiation, and improve diagnostic accuracy by avoiding artefacts.
- Patient selection should be considered in accordance with appropriate local and international guidelines.
- Preparation for cardiac CT should be individualized according to the clinical question, the patient's characteristics, and possible contraindications.
- A focused anamnesis and safety checklist before the examination is helpful in avoiding undesired events and optimizing diagnostic ability.

Patient selection

- Indications for cardiac CT should be vetted for appropriateness against standard cardiac CT appropriate-use criteria.
  - Patients' pretest probability should be considered when choosing coronary CT angiography (CCTA) to assess coronary artery disease (CAD), and generally considered for patients with a low-to-intermediate clinical likelihood of obstructive CAD.
  - For non-coronary cardiac CT, knowing the previous and planned cardiac procedures is important.
- General contraindications for CT and specific contraindications for cardiac CT on the planned protocol must be evaluated.
  - Non-compliance and inability to follow breathing instructions: anaesthesia might be helpful (especially in paediatric patients) or consider the use of a high-pitch acquisition mode where available.
  - Unstable clinical condition: postpone CT and consider an alternative test.
  - Known history of severe and/or anaphylactic contrast reaction: obtain a full medical history, and consider other type of contrast agent and/or premedication (see Chapter 1.10).

- Renal insufficiency and risk of contrast-induced nephropathy: all requests for examinations involving iodinated contrast administration should be accompanied by a recent estimated glomerular filtration rate (GFR) blood result, ideally within 3 months. In at-risk patients (with known impaired renal function) determine GFR on the day of CT; if the GFR is >30 ml/min/ 1.73 m^2 perform the CT, otherwise critically measure the risk/benefit (see Chapter 1.11).

- Hyperthyroidism: if the patient is at risk of thyrotoxicosis measure their thyroid stimulating hormone (TSH) level; when hyperthyroidism is treated and TSH level is normal, perform the CT. Otherwise, postpone and consult an endocrinologist.

- Pregnancy: generally considered as an absolute contraindication. Strictly evaluate the benefit of the test for patient and risks for the fetus.

- Breastfeeding: no restrictions; breastfeeding can be continued uninterrupted.

- Contraindications to heart rate (HR) control medications: use a cardio-selective, short-acting beta-blocker, consider alternative drugs, and consult the referring physician (see Table 1.4.3).

- Contraindications to nitroglycerin: use of phosphodiesterase inhibitors (e.g. sildenafil (Viagra™)); stop them 24–48 h before CT and consult the referring physician.

- Ongoing metformin therapy:
  - before CT examination no restrictions, continue metformin until CT;
  - after CT examination no restrictions for patients with a GFR >30 ml/min/ 1.73 m^2, continue metformin;
  - after CT examination suspend metformin for 48 h in patients with a GFR <30 ml/min/1.73 m^2 and avoid nephrotoxic agents (including non-steroidal anti-inflammatory drugs).

- Patient characteristics that potentially restrict cardiac CT or degrade image quality have to be considered.
  - Obesity: most CT tables accommodate patients weighing >200 kg; increase tube voltage, adjust tube potential, and use iterative reconstruction during CT for the best image quality.
  - High HR or arrhythmia: measure HR before CT and in between HR control medication administration (in inspiration). Consider increased padding in prospective triggering and retrospective triggering >70–80 beats per minute (bpm; scanner dependent), and electrocardiogram (ECG) editing (note: high HR variability degrades image quality more than tachycardia; in heart transplant patients coronary CT can be performed with good image quality even with rapid HRs, owing to low HR variability; see Chapter 2.10).
  - Difficulties understanding and following breathing instructions, or lying in a supine position with both arms raised and maintaining the position: change the wording/language of the instructions, review the breathing instructions, and consider alternative positioning.

Patient preparation

- Patient information: adequate information about the procedure should be provided, along with advice for appropriate preparation. This should include the specific advice provided in Box 1.4.1.
- History: all patients should complete a CT safety checklist (Table 1.4.1) upon arrival. This should accompany the request form, and should clearly state the indications and prior relevant cardiac and medical history for the cardiac CT. In patients at risk for contrast-induced nephropathy where an estimated GFR is unavailable, the scan should be deferred unless point-of-care testing exists at the host institute.

Contrast-induced nephropathy risk assessment

The risk of contrast-induced nephropathy (CIN) in patients with normal renal function is <2% (see also Chapter 1.10). This is increased with:

- pre-existing renal impairment;
- diabetes mellitus in combination with chronic kidney disease;
- heart failure;
- volume depletion;
- sepsis;
- hypotension;
- age ≥75 years;
- renal transplant;
- high total dose of contrast media;
- intra-arterial administration of contrast;
- all patients with acute kidney injury.

A CIN checklist should be completed for each patient (Figure 1.4.1).

Box 1.4.1 Information about the procedure

1. Ongoing cardiac medication can potentially conflict with the exam:
   (a) Avoid phosphodiesterase inhibitors for 24 h.
   (b) Continue all other medications, especially beta-blockers.
2. Clear fluids (water) may be consumed up until the scan appointment.
3. No food for 4 h prior to the appointment.

Note: Special considerations for myocardial stress perfusion: beta-blockers might conflict with the exam protocol and caffeinated products should be avoided for a minimum of 12 h prior to the appointment.

Table 1.4.1 CT safety checklist		
Medical history	Prior cardiac surgery	(Y/N)
	Prior coronary stenting	(Y/N)
	Pacemaker implantation	(Y/N)
	Hypertension	(Y/N)
	Asthma	(Y/N)
	Diabetes	(Y/N)
	Kidney disease	(Y/N)
	Liver disease	(Y/N)
	Haematological disease	(Y/N)
	Thyroid disease	(Y/N)
Medications	Beta-blockers	(Y/N)
	Verapamil	(Y/N)
	Metformin	(Y/N)
	Respiratory inhalers	(Y/N)
	Phosphodiesterase inhibitors	(Y/N)
	Other:	
Allergies	Medication allergies and specify	(Y/N)
	Prior severe allergic reaction:	(Y/N)
	Prior allergic reaction to X-ray dye in the past	(Y/N)
Female patients	Breastfeeding	(Y/N)
	Possibility of pregnancy	(Y/N)

Low risk (eGFR ≥ 60)
- Diuretics, NSAIDs gentamicin, amikacin, and vancomycin witheld for 24 hours pre-scan where possible
- Oral fluids advised post-procedure
- Continue taking metformin normally

Moderate (eGFR 30–59)
- As per low risk and
- ACE inhibitors and angiotensin II receptor blockers witheld 24 hours pre-procedure
- eGFR to be checked 48–72 hours post-procedure
- Continue taking metformin normally

High (eGFR <30)
- Diuretics, NSAIDs gentamicin, amikacin, and vancomycin witheld for 24 hours pre-procedure where possible
- Patient's volume status assessed with IV fluids prescribed pre- and post-procedure in cases of hypovolaemia
- Metformin witheld on day of scan and for 48 hours post-procedure
- ACE inhibitors and angiotensin II receptor blockers witheld
- 24 hours pre-procedure
- eGFR to be checked within 48–72 hours
  Restart metformin if renal function has not changed significantly

Figure 1.4.1 Contrast-induced nephropathy checklist.

eGFR: estimated glomerular filtration rate; NSAIDs: non-steroidal anti-inflammatory drugs; ACE: angiotensin-converting enzyme; IV: intravenous.

Courtesy of Guy's and St Thomas' NHS Foundation Trust and King's College London, United Kingdom.

Examination

Once a safety checklist has been completed, a set of baseline observations should be performed and documented prior to the patient entering the CT room. The minimum data set should include:

- heart rate—alert thresholds (HR <50 bpm and > 100 bpm);
- blood pressure—alert thresholds (<100 mmHg and >170 mmHg systolic);
- oxygen saturations—alert threshold on room air (<96%);
- height—no threshold;
- weight (alert threshold is dependent on scanner specifications).

All deviations from these thresholds should be communicated to the supervising clinician and radiographer, as additional tests may be necessary, the scan protocol may need to be adapted, or the examination cancelled.

Actions

'Prescan actions' (Table 1.4.2) are designed to modify patient-related factors that can influence scan quality, irrespective of CT vendor or technology. These are broadly categorized into reduction of respiratory and cardiac/coronary motion artefact, and ensuring that good volumes of contrast reach the vessel lumen.

Table 1.4.2 Prescan actions		
Action	Aim	Specific
Intravenous cannulation (out of scan room)	Adequate iodine delivery rate within the coronary lumen	18–20 G cannula in good-sized vein. Ability: minimum 5–7 ml/s
Discussion with patient: use ambient lighting and background music, where available (in and out of scan room)	Reduce anxiety and heart rate	Provide information as to what to expect during the scan and the feeling to expect during contrast injection
Practice breath holds (in and out scan room)	Freeze respiratory motion during cardiac CT acquisition to reduce artefact	Practice breath holds with patient until satisfied the patient can adhere to instructions for required duration. Ask patient to hold breath for 10 s
ECG (in scan room)	Good ECG signal to enable ECG gating and review of arrhythmias	Move electrode positions until satisfactory trace achieved
Pharmacotherapy (in scan room after ECG check)	Coronary vasodilation and heart rate control <65 bpm with reduction in R-R variability	See Table 1.4.3
ECG: electrocardiogram; bpm: beats/min.		

Pharmacotherapy

Ideally, CCTA should be performed at a HR of <65 bpm and with coronary vaso-dilation. Preloading with oral beta-blockers or prescan intravenous (IV) metoprolol are standard approaches. A recommended HR control scheme is summarized in Figure 1.4.2. Results with alternative rate-controlling medication such as diltiazem and verapamil IV have been disappointing and should only be used in special circumstances with appropriate expertise. To achieve coronary vasodilation, sublingual nitroglycerin spray or tablets are administered (Table 1.4.3).

Heart rate control scheme for cardiac CT

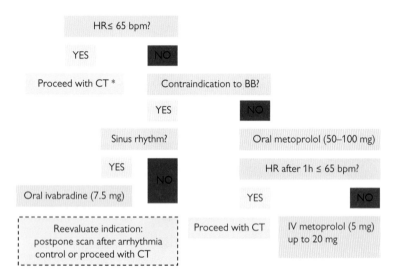

Note: Measure HR and HR variability in breath hold and determine blood pressure at arrival, before scan and if IV BB used.

* Consider low dose BB to reduce HR variability.

Figure 1.4.2 Possible algorithm for heart rate (HR) control.
BB: beta blocker; bpm: beats/min; IV: intravenous.

Table 1.4.3 Examples of premedication

Medication	Indications/dosing	Contraindications
Metoprolol tartrate PO (DOA: 5–8 h; TTO: 1 h; PHL: 3–7 h)	Resting HR >65 bpm/dosing: 50–100 mg 1 h prescan; 100 mg if HR >80 bpm; 50 mg if HR 65–80 bpm	• HR <60 bpm • SBP <100 mmHg • Decompensated heart failure • Allergy to beta-blocker • Asthma or COPD, regular B2 agonist with prior hospitalization, unstable symptoms, or nebuliser at home • Acute bronchospasm • Second- or third-degree AV block • Sinoatrial disease (i.e. sick sinus syndrome) • Severe peripheral vascular disease • Severe aortic stenosis
Metoprolol IV (DOA: 5–8 h; TTO: 5–10 min; PHL: 3–7 h)	Resting HR >65 bpm/dosing 2.5–5 mg IV each 5 mins, maximum dose 20 mg	As per metoprolol PO
Bisoprolol PO (DOA: 24 h; TTO: 1–4 h; PHL: 7–15 h)	Resting HR >65 bpm/dose: 2.5–5 mg 2 days before scan and on morning of scan	As per PO metoprolol
Ivabradine PO (DOA: 6 h; TTO: 1–3 h; PHL: 2 h)	Resting HR >65 bpm • Beta-blockers contraindicated • HTX patients Dose: 7.5–15 mg 1–3 h prescan	• HR < 60 bpm • Decompensated heart failure • SBP < 100 mmHg • Second- or third-degree AV block • Sinoatrial disease (i.e. sick sinus syndrome) • Recent stroke
Nitroglycerin SL spray or tablets (TTO: 3–5 min; PHL 1–3 min)	Coronary vasodilation 1 or 2 sprays (dose: 400–800 μg)	• SBP <100 mmHg • Constrictive pericarditis • Severe aortic or mitral stenosis • Hypotension • Cerebral haemorrhage and brain trauma • Angina caused by HOCM • Cardiogenic shock • G6PD deficiency • Concomitant use with phosphodiesterase inhibitors. • Hypersensitivity to ethanol or peppermint oil
GTN SL tablets	Coronary vasodilation/ dose: 500 μg–1 mg	As per SL GTN excluding hypersensitivity to ethanol or peppermint oil

PO: per os; DOA: duration of action; TTO: time to onset; PHL: plasma half-life; HR: heart rate; bpm: beats/min; SBP: systolic blood pressure; COPD: chronic obstructive pulmonary disease; AV: atrioventricular; IV: intravenous; HTX: heart transplant; SL: sublingual; HOCM: hypertrophic obstructive cardiomyopathy; G6PD: glucose-6-phosphate dehydrogenase; GTN: glyceryl trinitrate.

Safety and logistics

- All cardiac CT scans should be conducted with at least one certified clinician or radiographer trained in advanced life support.
- Blood pressure, HR, ECG trace, scan indications, and checklists should be reviewed prior to the administration of any pharmacotherapy.
- It is preferable that the IV beta-blocker and nitroglycerin are given early and as soon as the ECG electrode and safety checks have been performed, to allow peak plasma concentrations to be achieved before commencing calcium scanning. This also minimizes disruption once the scan protocol has begun.
- If any of the prescan 'actions' cannot be completed satisfactorily, consider the suitability of scanning the patient.
- Once the scan is complete, if the patient has been administered sublingual nitroglycerin alone or is on an oral metoprolol regime, the patient can usually leave the department as soon as no adverse reaction to the contrast has been established.
- Patients receiving IV metoprolol should normally be observed in the department for 30 minutes.

Pharmacotherapy bailout

- For significant bradycardia, atropine 500 µg IV may be administered and repeated up to a maximum of 3 mg. Transcutaneous pacing may be employed for refractory bradyarrhythmias.
- For acute bronchospasm, inhaled salbutamol 100–200 µg (1–2 puffs) may be administered. For severe cases, administer nebulized salbutamol 2.5–5 mg.
- In cases of severe hypotension—a rapid bolus of 250–500 ml IV fluid should be administered, with the patient's legs raised to increase preload.
- For severe life-threatening anaphylaxis, adrenaline 1:1000 (500 µg intramuscularly) with a repeat dose at 5 minutes if no change, along with an IV fluid challenge; hydrocortisone 200 mg slow IV and chlorphenamine 10 mg slow IV, as appropriate.

Further reading

Abbara S, Blanke P, Maroules CD, Cheezum M, Choi AD, Han BK, et al. SCCT guidelines for the performance and acquisition of coronary computed tomographic angiography. *J Cardiovasc Comput Tomogr* 2016; 10: 435e449.

European Society of Urogenital Radiology (ESUR). ESUR guidelines on contrast agents. Available at: http://www.esur.org/esur-guidelines/ (accessed 9 June 2022).

Knuuti J, Wijns W, Saraste A, Capodanno D, Barbato E, Funck-Brentano C, et al. 2019 ESC Guidelines for the diagnosis and management of chronic coronary syndromes. *Eur Heart J* 2020; 41:407–77.

Schoepf UJ (ed.). *CT of the Heart*. 2nd edn. Totowa, NJ: Humana Press.

Chapter 1.5

Scanner setup, cardiac protocols, and contrast injection

Ulrike Haberland, Thomas Allmendinger, and Francesca Pugliese

Teaching points

- A typical examination of the heart includes sequential steps. The scout view (topogram) and the monitoring scan are acquired first for planning purposes.

- The calcium score scan is a plain (non-contrast-enhanced) acquisition for the quantitative measure of coronary artery calcification (Agatston calcium score). This scan uses standardized tube voltage (120 kV) and reconstruction slice thickness (3 mm).

- Coronary CT angiography (CCTA) aims to achieve motion-free images of the coronary arteries during optimal intravascular contrast enhancement. In modern scanners, scan parameters (kV, mAs) are automatically adjusted based on patient size (optimal image quality, minimal radiation exposure).

- CCTA uses two primary acquisition techniques: the prospective electrocardiogram (ECG)-triggered sequential mode (step-and-shoot or axial scanning) and the retrospectively ECG-gated spiral (or helical) mode.

- For all scan modes and protocols, motion-free imaging depends on the patient's heart rate and the scanner's temporal resolution, which in turn will affect the 'phase(s)' of the cardiac cycle selected for image acquisition and reconstruction.

- Optimal contrast delivery in CCTA is achieved by employing power injector systems. The desirable intracoronary attenuation of 250 HU or higher can be accomplished with an iodine delivery rate of 1.6–2 g iodine per second.

Scanner setup

Prior to scan acquisition, a few key aspects of equipment and patient setup need to be addressed.

Equipment setup

- Complete scanner safety checks (automated warm-up, X-ray tube checks).
- Connect electrocardiogram (ECG) leads to the scanner.
- Switch on the power injector, and load with contrast medium and saline.
- Prepare a tray with saline flush and prescan medication, where required.

Patient setup

- Position the patient head first or feet first on the scanner table, depending on manufacturer and/or scan protocol.
- Apply ECG electrodes on the patient's chest and connect the leads.
- Recap the key procedural aspects and breathing instructions, to ensure the patient's compliance.
- Centre the patient in the gantry so that the scout view (topogram) starts at the level of the lung apices.
- Connect the patient to the contrast injector line.
- During the exam, ensure communication with the patient via the microphone/speaker.

Preparing for image acquisition

A coronary CT angiography (CCTA) exam typically includes subsequent scans, starting with planning scans.

- Scout view or topogram: an anteroposterior view of the chest ranging from lung apices to base of the heart. Used to set the scan range in subsequent acquisitions.
- Calcium scan (optional): plain scan for quantification of the coronary calcium.
- Control scan (optional): single image positioned at the tracheal bifurcation to estimate the level of the ascending aorta for contrast agent arrival monitoring (for bolus tracking); the control scan is not necessary when a calcium score data set is available.
- Test bolus scan: this can be used to monitor the arrival of contrast agent in the ascending aorta to time the main angiographic scan accurately; an alternative approach is the bolus tracking algorithm, which allows 'live' monitoring of attenuation in the ascending aorta leading to automatic or manual triggering of the main angiographic scan.
- CCTA: scan range planned based on calcium scan (if performed); scan protocol chosen based on clinical indication and patient's heart rhythm (see Scan protocols).

Scan protocols

Coronary calcium scoring

Coronary calcium imaging is a non-contrast examination that aims to detect and quantify coronary artery calcification using a standardized acquisition approach.

- Fixed tube voltage of 120 kV or 130 kV (vendor dependent). The application of low kV techniques for dose savings would result in a systematic shift of the Agatston score and require adjustment of the Agatston thresholds or other dedicated technical solutions.
- The tube current can be adjusted based on the patient's body mass index (BMI).
- Protocol on single-source systems: prospectively triggered sequential acquisition restricted to a single cardiac phase in mid-/late diastole. In the presence of arrhythmia or fast heart rate (HR; e.g. above 80 beats per minute (bpm)) a single-phase acquisition in end-systole based on an absolute millisecond delay is preferable (e.g. 350 ms, vendor dependent).
- Protocol on dual-source systems: high-pitch mode acquisition in late diastole is typically chosen independent of the patient's HR.
- Standardized image reconstruction for the Agatston score: reconstructed image slice width of 2.5–3 mm (depending on manufacturer) with an image increment of 1.5 mm. The reconstruction kernel/filter is medium–soft and the reconstruction technique is filtered back projection.
- Caution is advised regarding iterative reconstruction, owing to the quantitative nature of the image evaluation. Increasingly, vendor-specific solutions are receiving clearance from a regulatory perspective and may become available.

Coronary CT angiography

CCTA is based on iodine contrast-enhanced imaging of the coronary arteries. The approach to planning CCTA can be broken down to two primary questions:

- Which parts of the cardiac cycle need to be acquired to ensure enough data for a complete volume of motion-free images (e.g. narrow or wide padding window, mid-/late diastole or end systole, or both)?
- What acquisition technique is the most appropriate based on the clinical question (e.g. prospective axial scanning, retrospective spiral scanning, high-pitch, or volume scanning)?

Most modern CT scanners feature functionalities enabling the automatic adjustment of technical parameters based on measured patient characteristics.

- Tube voltage and tube current automatically controlled by patient size/body diameter (automatic exposure control).
- The 'standard' tube potential for CCTA was previously 120 kV. This has shifted towards lower kV values.
- Automatic exposure is preferred over manual threshold-based selection methods (e.g. patient BMI/weight) as these are usually overly simplistic and often not reflective of the actual limitations of the X-ray tube. If a manual tube voltage choice is necessary, generally a suitable selection is 100 kV for patients weighing <100 kg and BMI <30 kg/m^2, and 120 kV otherwise. A lower kilovoltage (70–90 kV) can be used in lighter patients (50–70 kg).
- The cardiac phase for data acquisition is determined by the patient's HR and rhythm prior to acquisition, in combination with a dedicated breath-hold command.

- Iodine delivery rates of around 2 g/s are generally recommended to achieve an intracoronary attenuation of around 250 Hounsfield units (HU) or (ideally) higher. In adult patients, this can be reached using contrast agents with high iodine concentrations (270–400 mg/ml) and injection rates between 5 and 7 ml/s (see also Chapter 1.10).

Choice of appropriate cardiac phase(s)

The Wiggers diagram (Figure 1.5.1) shows the events of the cardiac cycle with electrographic trace lines. From a CCTA point of view, the primary time points of interest are the 'diastasis' in mid-/late diastole and the slot directly after the end of systole, when diastole starts with its 'isovolumic relaxation' phase. Ideally, one of these two cardiac phases provides motion-free images. Occasionally, a single cardiac CT image volume does not provide motion-free images in all segments of the coronary arteries. In this case, multiple reconstructions at different time points of the cardiac cycle maybe necessary.

The most common target cardiac phase is mid-/late diastole (just before atrial contraction), typically realized at around 75% of the RR interval (see Chapters 1.9 and 1.11). Prerequisites are:

- A sufficiently slow HR: maximum HR of 63–65 bpm for single-source systems with a temporal resolution <160 ms, or maximum HR closer to 68–70 bpm for dual-source systems with temporal resolution <80 ms.
- Regular sinus rhythm: this is needed to predict adequately the next upcoming R-peak and target phase. Increasing the reach of the system can be achieved by adding a padding window around the target phase of ±5% to ±10% (e.g. 70%–80% or 65%–85%).

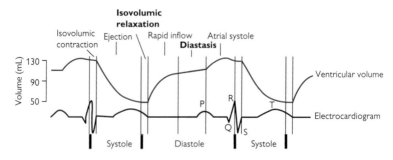

Figure 1.5.1 Wiggers diagram.

Marked in blue are the most likely coronary artery resting periods used for end systolic and mid-/late diastolic acquisition.

In patients with higher HRs:

- In single-source CT systems, with increasing HRs above 70 bpm up to 85 bpm, it is advisable to include the systolic solution in the acquisition window, shifting the start of the acquisition to ~35%–45%, while the stop point remains at ~85%.

- In HRs above 85 bpm, the diastolic target phases can be omitted as the systole target provides consistently better results. Changes to the acquisition mode might be necessary to increase the temporal resolution of single-source systems to values below 100 ms by means of multisegment acquisition and reconstruction techniques

- In dual-source CT systems, a direct transition from the diastolic target phase to the systolic target phase at a HR of around 75 bpm can be realized with a ±5 to ±10% padding window for either solution.

Arrhythmic patients with atrial fibrillation, bigeminy, or otherwise irregular R-R interval lengths (see also Chapter 1.11):

- In these patients the 'unpredictability' of the next R peak invalidates approaches based on a relative percentage-based cardiac phase definition. Instead of the latter, one aims at the end systole target cardiac phase by means of an absolute delay-based window definition starting at around 300 ms up to 450–500 ms, based on the assumption that the duration of the systolic contraction phase stays rather constant across all HRs.

Acquisition modes and scan protocols

Cardiac CT uses two primary acquisition techniques: the prospective ECG-triggered sequential mode (also known as step-and-shoot or axial scanning) and the retrospective ECG-gated spiral (or helical) mode. The term 'mode' refers to the sequential or spiral/helical approaches for CT data acquisition (Figure 1.5.2). In cardiac CT, the term 'protocol' is commonly used to indicate the scan mode associated with the specific algorithm for data synchronization (i.e. prospectively ECG-trigged or retrospectively ECG-gated acquisition; Figure 1.5.3). The principles described above linking the patient's HR and the appropriate cardiac phase(s) for data acquisition apply to both primary cardiac acquisition modes and protocols.

In the prospective ECG-triggered axial sequential mode, the user-defined cardiac phase window is applied to the X-ray tube to generate photons.

- In sequential acquisition, data are acquired in a step-by-step approach over multiple separate cardiac cycles with a fixed table feed between the sequence steps. The table feed is independent of the patient's HR and rhythm.

- The axial sequential mode should be considered as the default scan mode of choice for CCTA with at least 64-slice cardiac CT systems, over a wide range of HRs.

- The main advantage of a prospective sequential acquisition over a retrospective spiral acquisition is lower radiation dose.

- The availability of padding windows can increase robustness in patients with a fast HR but will increase dose.

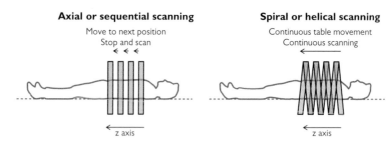

Axial or sequential scanning

Move to next position
Stop and scan

z axis

Spiral or helical scanning

Continuous table movement
Continuous scanning

z axis

Figure 1.5.2 Axial (sequential) and spiral (helical) scan modes.

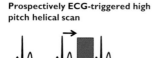

Retrospectively ECG-gated helical scan (tube current modulation 4–20%)

Prospectively ECG-triggered axial (or sequential) scan

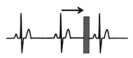

Prospectively ECG-triggered high pitch helical scan

Prospectively ECG-triggered volume scan

Figure 1.5.3 Scan protocols for cardiac CT.

In the retrospective electrocardiogram (ECG)-gated helical scan, the X-ray tube is on throughout the cardiac cycle. The phase for image reconstruction can be arbitrarily chosen. In order to reduce radiation exposure to patients, the X-ray tube current is generally reduced during phases of the RR interval, where the highest image quality is not necessary. In the prospective ECG-triggered axial scan, the X-ray tube emits X-ray photons at prespecified phase(s) of the cardiac cycle, (typically) over 2–4 cardiac cycles to cover the heart range, while the table is stationary. In the prospectively ECG-triggered high-pitch helical scan, fast table movement allows coverage of the scan range starting at a prespecified cardiac phase, during one RR interval. In the prospectively ECG-triggered volume scan, the entire scan range is acquired in one RR interval during a prespecified phase without movement of the scanner table.

- This is also the default scan mode for wide-detector CT systems, which provide coverage of the entire heart in a single cardiac cycle without movement of the scanner table.

In the retrospective ECG-gated spiral mode, data are acquired continuously over the entire scan time over multiple cardiac cycles, typically with a fixed, low-pitch value (automatically set based on the patient HR).

- The pitch is defined as the distance travelled by the scanner table during one rotation divided by the X-ray beam width (Figure 1.5.4).

- The continuous data stream enables multiphase reconstructions over the full cardiac cycle followed by a functional evaluation of the images (e.g. ventricular ejection fraction).

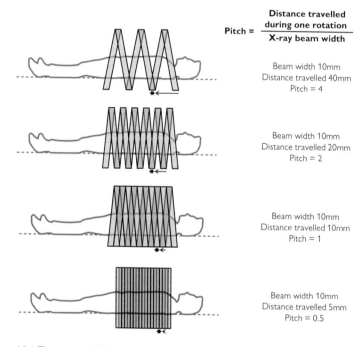

$$\text{Pitch} = \frac{\text{Distance travelled during one rotation}}{\text{X-ray beam width}}$$

Beam width 10mm
Distance travelled 40mm
Pitch = 4

Beam width 10mm
Distance travelled 20mm
Pitch = 2

Beam width 10mm
Distance travelled 10mm
Pitch = 1

Beam width 10mm
Distance travelled 5mm
Pitch = 0.5

Figure 1.5.4 The concept of CT pitch.

With pitch >1, the distance travelled by the scanner table is larger than the beam width (data gaps). With pitch <1, the distance travelled is smaller than the beam width (overlap).

- Retrospectively ECG-gated protocols are generally used with ECG tube current modulation. A phase window can be set, resulting in strong modulation of the applied tube current towards very low levels outside the user-defined window (see Figure 1.5.3).
- Any unexpected significant drop in HR during acquisition can lead to gaps in the data, which can result in interpolation artefacts (see Chapter 1.8). The pitch of a retrospective ECG-gated spiral cardiac CT scan is typically very conservative and quite low relative to the measured HR just prior to the scan.
- Low pitch, in combination with continuous data acquisition over the entire examination, results in a significantly increased average radiation dose compared with a prospectively ECG-triggered axial sequence, even if wider padding is applied to the latter.
- Towards higher HRs, the adjustment of the pitch to the actual HR yields significant shortening of the scan acquisition time compared with a sequential acquisition, which can be beneficial in terms of patient breath-hold and contrast injection timing. This also aligns with the fact that multisegment acquisition and reconstruction options, which may be necessary in single-source systems for high HRs, often exist only as ECG-gated spiral acquisition mode.

The high-pitch spiral acquisition (flash) is only available on dual-source systems.

- Prospectively triggered dual-source spiral scan with a pitch of up to 3.4 enables the acquisition of CCTA in a single cardiac cycle.
- Prospectively triggered start phase set to 60–65% (system dependent).
- The cardiac phase of each reconstructed image is slightly shifted.
- No redundant data are acquired: very dose-efficient acquisition.
- Prerequisite is a low and regular HR to 'hit' the start phase prospectively with precision. The upper HR limits for the application of this mode are 63 and 68 bpm (second- and third-generation dual-source CT, respectively).

Contrast injection for coronary CT angiography

Adjacent tissues with high natural contrast, such as bone and lung tissue, are easily distinguished on CT. Blood vessels and surrounding soft tissues, or the vessel wall and the blood contained in the vessel lumen, have similar densities and will display similar X-ray attenuation (low contrast). To achieve ideal contrast between these structures, iodinated contrast agents are used (for the properties of contrast agents, see Chapter 1.10).

The concentration of iodinated contrast agents is expressed in mg of iodine per ml of contrast volume.

- Typical contrast agent concentrations used for CCTA are 300, 320, 350, 370, and 400 mg/ml
- Typical contrast injection rates are 4–7 ml/s.
- The contrast concentration (mg/ml) multiplied by the injection rate (ml/s) defines the iodine delivery rate (mg/s or g/s). The desired intracoronary

attenuation of 250 Hounsfield units (HU) or (ideally) higher can be achieved with iodine delivery rates of 1.6–2 g/s.

- The contrast volume used for a standard CCTA exam is often fixed (e.g. 50 ml, concentration 400 mg/ml, injection rate 5 ml/s).

- The contrast volume can be individualized based on the patient's weight (either with a fixed dose (e.g. 300 mg/kg body weight) or with variable dose (e.g. 270 mg/kg) in patients weighing <50 kg, 300 mg/kg in patients weighing 51–85 kg, and 400 mg/kg in patients weighing >85 kg).

- Lighter patients will be imaged with lower kV settings and may be injected with a smaller dose of contrast agent (see also Chapter 1.2).

- To enable the typical injection rates of CCTA, a 20 G intravenous cannula is the minimum requirement. Ideally, this should be positioned in the right antecubital vein. Injection through smaller cannulas may increase the risk of contrast extravasation.

- Programmable double-headed power injectors, with a contrast and a saline syringe, are routinely used for precise and consistent contrast volume delivery, flow rate, and timing of the injection. As a safety feature to prevent extravasation, power injectors automatically stop the injection if pressure in the delivery system rises above a set threshold.

- The saline flush (chaser) is useful to achieve a compact contrast bolus (optimize enhancement) and facilitate its advancement from the injection site to the coronary circulation, minimizing the total contrast volume and reducing streak artefacts from concentrated contrast in the superior vena cava and/or brachiocephalic vein.

- Contrast agent injection through central venous catheters, tunnelled central venous catheters, or dialysis catheters is not recommended.

Further reading

Achenbach S, Marwan M, Schepis T, Pflederer T, Bruder H, Allmendinger T, et al. High-pitch spiral acquisition: a new scan mode for coronary CT angiography. *J Cardiovasc Comput Tomogr* 2009; 3: 117–21.

Agatston AS, Janowitz WR, Hildner FJ, Zusmer NR, Viamonte Jr M, Detrano R. Quantification of coronary artery calcium using ultrafast computed tomography. *J Am Coll Cardiol* 1990; 15: 827–32.

Deseive S, Pugliese F, Meave A, Alexanderson E, Martinoff S, Hadamitzky M, et al. Image quality and radiation dose of a prospectively electrocardiography-triggered high-pitch data acquisition strategy for coronary CT angiography: The multicenter, randomized PROTECTION IV study. *J Cardiovasc Comput Tomogr* 2015; 9: 278–85.

Ghekiere O, Salgado R, Buls N, Leiner T, Mancini I, Vanhoenacker P, et al. Image quality in coronary CT angiography: challenges and technical solutions. *Br J Radiol* 2017; 90: 20160567.

Heartflow. CCTA resources. CCTA Acquisition Protocols: Acquisition and Reconstruction Techniques for Coronary CT Angiography. Available at: https://www.heartflow.com/education/ccta-resources (accessed May 2020).

Saini S, Rubin GD, Kalra MK. (eds) *MSCT: A Practical Approach*. Milan: Springer Verlag, 2006.

Chapter 1.6

Image reconstruction, postprocessing, and fundamentals of image analysis

Jamal Khan, Sarah Moharem-Elgamal, and
Francesca Pugliese

Teaching points

- Image reconstruction is the process that produces diagnostic images from raw CT data and uses two main algorithms: filtered back projection and iterative reconstruction.
- A CT image consists of a defined matrix of pixels, typically a square matrix of 512 × 512 pixels.
- Pixels are assigned a CT number (Hounsfield units (HUs)) that reflects the mean attenuation of the tissues included in the corresponding voxel; HUs are affected by the energy of the X-ray beam and are normalized by the attenuation coefficient of water.
- The CT number scale in the image is mapped to a visual grey scale; window settings (level/width) allow adjustment of the way CT numbers are mapped to the grey scale, and determine image brightness and contrast.
- It is recommended that scans are checked for image quality/completeness before the patient leaves the scanner.
- Although coronary CT angiography raw data are first reconstructed in a series of axial images, image data are isotropic and coronary artery stenosis analysis is based on multiplanar reconstructions (MPRs) and curved MPRs constructed along the vessel of interest.
- Maximum intensity projection and volume-rendered views display anatomical relationships between structures and are not primarily intended for fine coronary stenosis assessment

---

Image reconstruction

Image reconstruction is the process that allows the generation of diagnostic images from raw CT raw. Image reconstruction requirements must meet the clinical need to diagnose disease in small, submillimetre vessel anatomy in an arbitrary orientation.

The primary image reconstruction result of a coronary CT angiography (CCTA) examination is therefore a medium, sharp, thin-slice image volume, which provides isotropic resolution at an acceptable image noise level (see Chapter 1.2).

The scanner detector elements record the incident X-ray photon intensity as the beam exits the patient' body. The detected intensity is inversely related to the attenuation of the tissues traversed (see Chapter 1.3). As the gantry rotates around the patient's body, the beam partially traverses the same tissues and organs with different angles, leading to multiple projections or measurements. A rotation of 180 degrees plus fan beam width provides sufficient views to allow the reconstruction of one image. The higher the number of projections per gantry rotation, the better the spatial resolution of the images. With modern technology, the projections acquired are in the region of 1000–2000 per rotation. These measurements are processed and 'purged' from errors to form the raw CT data. Image reconstruction is the process that produces diagnostic images from raw CT data and uses two main approaches: filtered back projection (FBP) and iterative reconstruction.

Filtered back projection

- A ray path is the trajectory line between beam focus and any detector element in the scanner detector array.
- The number of detector elements determines the number of X-ray paths in the X-ray beam.
- In back projection, ray paths are used to trace the attenuation coefficient of the tissues/organs that the X-ray beam has traversed.
- A picture of the tissue or organ of interest is formed by combining ray paths obtained from data generated at different angular positions of the gantry.
- The tracing of tissue mean attenuation following the trajectory of ray paths causes smearing effect and 'star artefacts'.
- Convolution kernels or filters are mathematical functions (sets of coefficients) applied during the reconstruction process and mitigate these issues: this process is called 'filtered back projection'.
- Convolution kernels also control whether an image appears with 'soft' edges and lower image noise, or if it results in 'sharp' edges at the expense of higher image noise. These are among the selectable reconstruction parameters.
- In most cases a medium-sharp kernel is selected for coronary artery evaluation as sharper images are often too noisy given the available signal contrast. Sharper reconstructions can be added optionally in the case of very high coronary calcium burden or presence of coronary stents.
- In FBP, there is typically a relationship between selected image sharpness and reconstructed noise level. This relationship can be removed with advanced, typically iterative, reconstruction methods (see next subsection).

Iterative reconstruction
- FBP is a fast reconstruction technique. The main limitation of FBP is that raw CT data contain noise from various sources: X-ray scattering; photon flux statistical

variation; and electronic noise at the detector level. Smooth convolution kernels can only partly compensate for this.

- Iterative reconstruction algorithms aim to reduce or correct image noise. These algorithms can be used in addition to (mixed or hybrid reconstruction techniques) or in place of FBP.

- Early iterative reconstruction techniques were based on selective noise reduction algorithms (iterative noise-reduction techniques). These techniques reduce local variation in pixel values within uniform areas, without affecting the edges and spatial resolution. These algorithms operate either on FBP-reconstructed images (image space or image domain) or on raw data (raw data domain) before FBP reconstruction.

- A different approach involves the generation of synthetic raw data based on an image data set reconstructed by simulating the acquisition process. The synthetic and real raw data are compared and corrections made to the initial reconstructed image (iterative forward projection and comparison techniques). The process can be repeated either until the synthetic raw data accurately model the actual raw data, or at completion of a preset number of iterations.

- Techniques where the forward projection phase of synthetic raw data generation is modelled as closely as possible on the real acquisition process, including noise from all sources, system acquisition geometry, X-ray source, and detector features (model-based iterative reconstruction techniques), harness a high potential for noise reduction and spatial resolution improvement. These techniques are computationally intensive and time consuming.

- Pragmatically, it is useful to mix limited iterative reconstruction (without a full model-based algorithm) with FBP to optimize noise reduction, kernel smoothing, or sharpening, as well as reconstruction speed.

- Iterative reconstruction is sometimes considered to be a dose-reduction technique because lower image noise implies that it may be possible to lower patient radiation exposure without observing a net increase in image noise. As a caveat, very aggressive noise reduction may affect image spatial resolution and edge detail. Most commercial iterative reconstruction techniques are developed as proprietary algorithms; quantitative image analysis (calcium scoring, attenuation measurement, coronary plaque evaluation) could be affected (see Chapter 1.5).

Reconstruction parameters

Image quality, edge enhancement, noise, and artefacts are influenced by a wide variety of parameters, which are often subject to vendor-specific terminology and vocabulary. In most cases, an initial set of suitable reconstruction parameters is provided with the CT system, recommended as a starting point. Owing to the difficulty of generalizing between the different vendors and CT systems, this section focuses on selected generic reconstruction parameters.

- The reconstruction field of view (FoV) refers to the portion of the scan field that ends up in the reconstructed image, with individually selected in-plane dimensions. The image matrix size refers to the number of pixels along each axis of the reconstructed images. Typical reconstructions for coronary artery evaluation are built on a FoV of 200–250 mm using a 512 × 512 matrix size. Larger matrix sizes are usually only needed in combination with large FoVs and sharp reconstruction settings (e.g. full thorax lung imaging).

- The reconstruction kernel or filter affects spatial resolution and image noise. Typically in FBP one is traded against the other (see 'Filtered back projection'). The filter selectively enhances the spatial frequency content of the data to smooth or sharpen the images according to the user's needs. Convolution kernels are generally named based on their main effect of smoothing or sharpening an image (e.g. smooth, sharp, medium-smooth, or medium-sharp); however, terminology varies with scanner manufacturers.

- The reconstructed slice thickness should enable isotropic resolution in all three spatial dimensions in the case of coronary artery evaluation. Therefore, the selected slice thickness needs to match the in-plane kernel resolution. For coronary artery reconstructions the slice thickness is typically between 0.5 mm and 0.8 mm, and quite often equal to the smallest possible slice width on the CT system.

- The reconstruction increment (distance between the reconstructed slices) should be 50% of the slice thickness.

- Immediate review the images after reconstruction, either by a trained radiographer or physician, is recommended while the patient is still on the CT table, in order to confirm sufficient quality of data acquisition (Table 1.6.1).

Table 1.6.1 Example of reconstruction parameters suitable for coronary artery evaluation

Siemens	Axial reconstruction. Slice thickness: 0.6 mm; increment: 0.3 mm; medium-sharp convolution kernel Bv40 (older systems B26). If available, iterative reconstruction SAFIRE/ADMIRE, strength 3. In case of a high calcium burden or in case of stents use an additional sharper convolution kernel: Bv49 (older systems B46)
Philips	Reconstructions: standard, iDose level: 3–5; filter: XCB and XCC; FoV limited to the heart; slice thickness 0.8 mm, increment 0.4 mm
GE	Slice thickness: 0.625 mm; recon type: standard; iterative reconstruction: ASiR-V™: 50%
Canon	FoV limited to the heart (200–220 mm); slice thickness 0.5 mm, increment 0.25 mm. CTA settings: kernel FC03, OSR cardiac, iterative reconstruction AIDR 3D, filter OFF. In the case of stents: kernel FC05

SAFIRE: sinogram affirmed iterative reconstruction; ADMIRE: advanced model iterative reconstruction; XCB: medium smooth kernel, Philips platform; XCC: standard-sharp reconstruction kernel, Philips platform; ASiR: adaptive statistical iterative reconstruction; FoV: field of view; CTA: CT angiography; 3D: three-dimensional.

Key concepts of image postprocessing

A CT image consists of a defined matrix of pixels, typically a square matrix of 512 × 512 pixels.

- Pixel stands for 'picture element', the smallest part of an image that can be displayed in the x,y plane. Pixel size depends on the size of the FoV and the image matrix.
- Z-axis directional information confers volumetric dimension to a 'volume element' or voxel. The z-dimension of a voxel is determined by the slice width on the CT system.
- The use of small pixel size when reconstructing an image is limited by the spatial resolution of the scanner.
- Image noise is inversely related to pixel size.

After FBP reconstruction, voxels are assigned an attenuation value that reflects the mean attenuation of the tissues included in the voxel. However, these values are affected by the X-ray beam energy (see Chapter 1.2). Values in tissues are normalized to the attenuation coefficient of water. Normalization yields CT numbers measured in Hounsfield units (HUs), reflecting the relative attenuation of tissue compared to water (Table 1.6.2):

$$CT \text{ number } [HU] = [LAC\,(tissue) - LAC\,(water)]\,/\,LAC\,(water) * 1000,$$
$$where\,LAC = linear\ attenuation\ coefficient$$

Image windowing is an important aspect of image visualization.

- The CT number scale is mapped to a visual grey scale, the range of which is generally exceeded by the dynamic range of the CT numbers.
- 'Windowing' allows adjustment of the way CT numbers are mapped to the grey scale.

Table 1.6.2 Normalization yields CT numbers measured in Hounsfield units (HU), reflecting the relative attenuation of tissue compared to water	
Tissue	CT number (HU)
Water	0 (by definition)
Adipose tissue	−30 to −190
Air	−1000 HU
Bone	+400 to +1000
Blood	+40 to +60
Metal devices	>1000

- The range of CT numbers of interest defines the display window.
- Display window settings are defined by window level (or centre; i.e. the CT number around which the window is centred) and window width (i.e. the range of CT numbers displayed by the window, defined as difference between the upper and lower limits of the window). CT numbers above the upper limit of the window width will be displayed in white; CT numbers below the lower limit of the window width will be displayed in black.
- The window width defines the contrast displayed in an image. A narrow window displays a small range of CT numbers over a large grey scale.
- Typically used CT window settings (level/width) vary depending on the tissues under evaluation: mediastinum (25/350 HU); lungs (−500/1500 HU); bone (300/1500 HU).

Fundamentals of image analysis

To evaluate image quality and scan completeness, review of the acquired data immediately after reconstruction, while the patient is still on the scanner table, is advised.

- Assess the electrocardiogram (ECG) trace: heart rate (HR) will determine which cardiac phase is likely to display the best CTCA image quality; HR variability may help explain artefacts; ectopic beats may cause stairstep artefacts, although algorithms for arrhythmia rejection during prospectively ECG-triggered scanning are available on most modern scanners (Figure 1.6.1); location of ECG abnormality (first, second, or third cardiac cycle) suggests the position of the expected artefact in the image data set, as stacks are scanned sequentially (typically in the craniocaudal direction); in retrospectively ECG-gated scans, ectopic beats can be removed with ECG editing (see Chapter 1.11 and Figure 1.11.1).
- Calcium score scan: ensure standard parameters are applied for image reconstruction (slice thickness, increment) to allow calcium quantification (see Chapter 1.5).

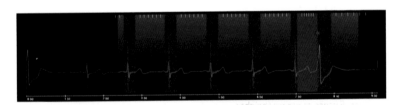

Figure 1.6.1 From a prospectively electrocardiogram (ECG)-triggered protocol, the ECG trace shows a regular sinus rhythm with one ventricular ectopic beat (asterisk) during the fifth cardiac cycle. The scanner detected the anomalous beat and rejected data acquisition (purple box) during this cardiac cycle to avoid motion artefact.

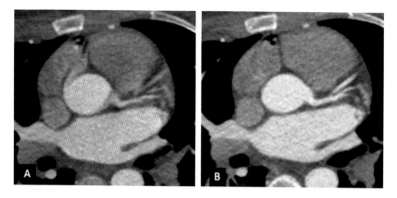

Figure 1.6.2 Selection of the optimal cardiac phase in patient with a well-controlled heart rate of 57 beats/min during the scan.

(A) Systolic phase, 40% of RR interval, shows motion artefact and blurring of the left coronary system (asterisk). (B) Diastolic phase, 70% of RR interval, shows improved image quality.

- Wide FoV data sets: ensure that appropriately sized FoV and reconstruction kernels (lung, mediastinum) are applied for review of extracardiac pathology (see Chapter 3.15). This data set can inform on the presence of respiratory motion artefacts (see Chapter 1.8).
- CTCA raw data are reconstructed in a series of axial images (typically 200–300). Review the primary axial data set to ascertain diagnostic quality and determine which phase (if multiple acquired) has the least amount of residual motion and should be the primary data set for coronary analysis (Figure 1.6.2). Reconstruction thickness (typically 0.5–0.75 mm) can be increased (1 mm) if contrast-to-noise ratio is particularly poor, such as, for instance, in very large patients.

Image formats and viewing settings:

- The axial data set is the primary source for all post-processing methods.
- The axial data set is further postprocessed in different image formats, such as multiplanar reconstruction (MPR) and curved MPRs (cMPR), maximum intensity projection (MIP) images, and volume-rendered technique views.
- A combination of these image formats is typically used on dedicated workstations, with MPR and cMPR representing the workhorse of cardiac CT analysis.
- Appropriate window settings optimize the displayed image brightness and contrast. Excess contrast/brightness can increase the 'blooming effect' (i.e. a hyperdense halo around X-ray dense structures (e.g., calcification and metal; see Chapter 1.8)). Insufficient image contrast can lead to underestimation of stenosis severity (Figure 1.6.3).

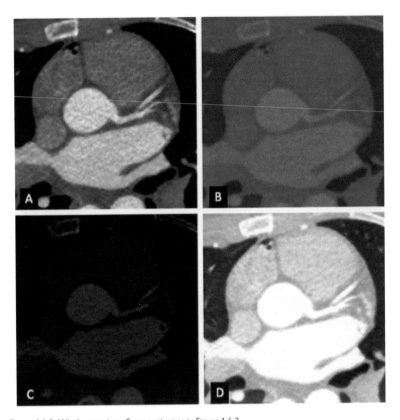

Figure 1.6.3 Window settings. Same patient as in Figure 1.6.2.

(A) Optimized window level/width. (B) Insufficient contrast (width too high). (C) Insufficient brightness (level too high). (D) Excessive brightness (level too low).

- Heavily calcified coronary arteries and vessels with implanted stents may be better visualized on images reconstructed with a sharp convolution kernel. The latter typically decreases the 'blooming effect' at the expense of increased image noise. It is advisable to review this data set in addition to the data set with a standard reconstruction kernel (Figure 1.6.4).

Multiplanar reconstruction (MPR) and curved MPR

- The spatial resolution of the axial data set is isotropic (see Chapter 1.2), which implies that the data volume can be cut and displayed in any arbitrary plane.

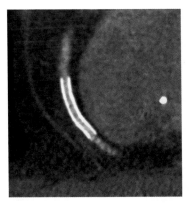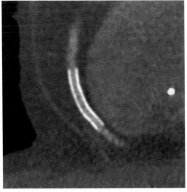

Figure 1.6.4 Patient with stent implanted in the mid-right coronary artery.

Multiplanar reconstructed images reconstructed with conventional medium-soft (left) and sharp (right) reconstruction kernels. The sharp reconstruction kernel improves in-stent lumen visualization (larger area of the in-stent lumen is visualized without superimposed brightness from stent struts), which is useful in excluding in-stent restenosis. Wider window width is also useful to improve in-stent lumen visualization.

- An MPR is a two-dimensional (2D) view of the data volume. MPRs can follow standard radiological planes such as axial, coronal, and sagittal (Figure 1.6.5), or assume any oblique orientation.

- The orientation plane of a specific MPR can cause false appearances of artefactual stenoses ('pseudostenoses') or lead to underestimation of lesion severity. Interactive manipulation of the CT data set is mandatory. Review of static reformatted MPRs is generally not sufficient for accurate CTCA interpretation.

- By default, the thickness of an MPR view is the same as the data set slice thickness. A 'thick MPR' results from summing adjacent slices in parallel planes. Thick MPR provides views with improved contrast-to-noise ratio; however, the spatial resolution is decreased

- Curved MPR is a type of MPR where the image plane orientation is curved, automatically or manually sampled along the curved centreline of a coronary vessel, which can then be visualized in its entirety on a single, flattened 2D plane (Figure 1.6.6).

- It is generally possible to rotate curved MPRs around the centreline providing 360-degree radial views of the coronary artery; views perpendicular to the centreline provide cross-sectional images of the coronary vessel.

- Accuracy of the vessel centreline is crucial to generate good quality curved MPRs. It is good practice to ensure that the centreline (automated or manually drawn) accurately tracks the vessel long axis to avoid postprocessing artefacts ('pseudostenoses'; data replication/mirroring).

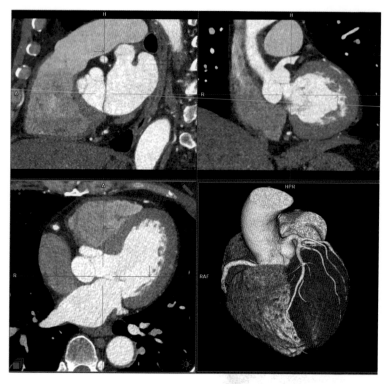

Figure 1.6.5 Clockwise, from top-left: multiplanar reconstructions of the heart according to standard radiological planes: sagittal view (y,z), coronal view (x,z), and axial view (x,y). Lower right: volume-rendered image of the heart. These are common starting views provided as default by various coronary CT angiography analysis software tools.

Maximum intensity projection

- A MIP image is a stack of images orientated according to an arbitrary plane, like a thick MPR; however, the MIP selectively displays the brightest voxels contained within the stack (Figure 1.6.7).
- Contrast in the MIP will be primarily determined by structures with high attenuation (calcium, bone, metal, dense contrast agent, etc.) at the expense of lower attenuation structures and tissues.
- The brightest voxels may be contained in different slices within the stack. MIP may give the impression of flattening or overlapping structures in a plane
- MIP thickness can be selected by the operator; 3 mm or 5 mm are typically used and often default options. However, MIPs can be made thicker.

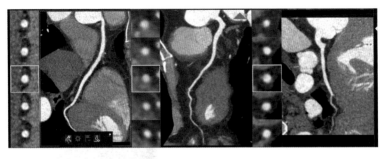

Figure 1.6.6 Curved multiplanar reconstructions (cMPRs).

From left to right: curved MPRs demonstrate the right coronary artery, the left anterior descending artery, and the left circumflex artery, all of which have an unobstructed appearance. Vessel cross sections are also displayed.

- In cardiac CT, MIPs are useful because they allow rapid visualization of the vessel course (e.g. anomalous vessel, long course of coronary artery bypass grafts, pulmonary vein configuration, identification of motion artefacts, etc.). Complete assessment should always be followed by evaluation with MPR.
- MIPs discard spatial resolution; they are not intended for fine obstruction assessment and should not be used for this purpose.

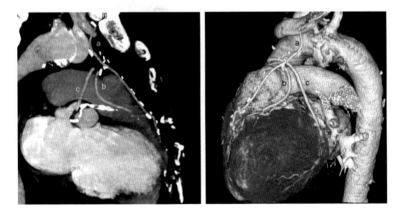

Figure 1.6.7 In a patient with (a) a left internal mammary artery graft to the left anterior descending artery and venous grafts to a (b) diagonal branch and an (c) obtuse marginal branch, a maximum intensity projection image (on the left) and volume-rendered image (on the right) provide quick visualization of the grafts' courses and anatomical relationship to the surrounding structures.

Volume rendering or volume-rendering technique

- This type of three-dimensional view is constructed based on a view line that goes from the viewer's eye through the image volume. The contribution of each voxel along this line is weighed in the final image. Different tissues are assigned variable colour, transparency, and shadow settings (Figure 1.6.7). These settings are modifiable by the user.

- Volume rendering allows realistic visualization of spatial relationships between anatomical structures, making it a useful tool to display complex anatomy, congenital pathology, aortic and pulmonary vein configuration, course of anomalous coronary vessels, and coronary artery bypass grafts.

- Volume rendering can be an effective tool to demonstrate cardiac anatomy to clinicians less familiar with standard techniques for CT image interpretation.

- Volume rendering is not intended for fine stenosis assessment and should not be used for this purpose.

Further reading

Abbara S, Blanke P, Maroules CD, Cheezum M, Choi AD, Han BK, et al. SCCT guidelines for the performance and acquisition of coronary computed tomographic angiography. *J Cardiovasc Comput Tomogr* 2016; 10: 435e449.

Budoff M, Shinbane J. *Cardiac CT Imaging*. New York: Springer, 2010.

Heartflow. CCTA resources. CCTA Acquisition Protocols: Acquisition and Reconstruction Techniques for Coronary CT Angiography. Available at: https://www.heartflow.com/education/ccta-resources (accessed May 2020).

Leipsic J, Abbara S, Achenbach S, Cury R, Earls J.P, Mancini GJ, et al. SCCT guidelines for the interpretation and reporting of coronary CT angiography: a report of the Society of Cardiovascular Computed Tomography Guidelines Committee. *J Cardiovasc Comput Tomogr* 2014; 8: 342–58.

Concepts of radioprotection

Anna Beattie and Francesca Pugliese

Teaching points

- Justification and optimization (the ALARA principle ('as low as reasonably achievable') of radiation exposure associated with imaging procedures are the pillars of radioprotection.
- Increases in scan range, X-ray tube voltage and current, use of retrospectively electrocardiogram (ECG)-gated protocols are typically associated with increased radiation exposure.
- Automated exposure control based on patient's size, use prospectively ECG-triggered CT and routine application of X-ray tube current modulation in retrospectively ECG-gated CT, good patient heart rate control, and staff training are typically associated with decreased radiation exposure.

The ALARA principle

The International Commission on Radiological Protection (ICRP) is a non-governmental organization that provides guidance and recommendations concerning radioprotection and the use of ionizing radiation for medical and diagnostic purposes. To ensure good practice, the ICRP has framed the matter of radioprotection using three principles.

- Justification: patient exposure can be justified when the benefit derived to the patient (e.g. from the diagnostic information obtained) exceeds the risk from radiation exposure. All available diagnostic alternatives should be evaluated when deciding to perform a test with radiation. Patient, as well as staff, exposures should be justified.

- Optimization: radiation exposure to patients and staff members must be 'as low as reasonably achievable' (the ALARA principle). Patient exposure can be optimized by controlling the radiation dose so that it is appropriate for a given diagnostic procedure. As benchmark for good clinical practice, national diagnostic reference levels, and/or the scientific literature are used. Radiation exposure to staff can be optimized by controlling patient exposure and applying further measures, for instance appropriate shielding of staff working in the CT control room; for interventional procedures, this also includes the use of lead apron, minimizing exposure time, and maximizing distance from the X-ray source and patient.

- Limitation: the ICRP recommends dose limits for members of staff and the public that should not be exceeded.

Relationship between scan parameters and dose

- The relationship between scan range and radiation dose is linearly proportional. The larger the scan range, the larger the dose.
- The relationship between X-ray tube voltage and radiation dose is exponential. Dose increases proportionally to the square of the tube kV.
- The relationship between the X-ray tube current and radiation dose is linear. Radiation dose increases in linear proportion with the tube current (mAs or mAs/rotation).
- In scanners that express X-ray current in mAs or mAs/rotation, radiation dose varies inversely with pitch; in scanners than express X-ray current in effective mAs or mAs/rotation, radiation dose is independent of pitch.

- As a general rule, with the level of image noise kept constant, the relationship between slice thickness and radiation dose is inversely proportional (the thicker the slice thickness, the higher the intensity of the signal detected). A small increase in mAs is usually sufficient as improved spatial resolution compensates for image noise.
- For certain manufacturers, larger in-plane FoV may require slower table feed between prospectively electrocardiogram (ECG)-triggered stacks, leading to increased exposure.

See also Chapter 1.5.

Scanner features and scan protocols that affect dose

- Scanners with faster gantry rotation times have improved temporal resolution than scanners with slower rotation times. If X-ray tube voltage, current, and scan time remain the same, faster gantry rotation does not have implications on a patient's exposure. However, if the scan time is shorter, exposure time (and hence overall exposure) will be decreased. The same consideration is valid for dual-source CT. Dual-source CT geometry does not *per se* have implications on a patient's radiation exposure.
- Prospectively ECG-triggered axial protocols are dose efficient, in that most of the projection data contribute to the formation of diagnostic images (see also Chapter 1.2). Exposure is affected by the scan parameters (kV, mAs) and the width of temporal padding. Whether the approach is a volume stationary scan,

sequential step-and-shoot axial scan, or high-pitch spiral, this does not greatly affect exposure.

• Retrospectively ECG-gated protocols acquire redundant data (X-rays emitted throughout the scan duration) and are generally less dose efficient than prospectively ECG-triggered approaches. Exposure is affected by scan parameters (kV, mAs), the length within the RR interval where X-ray tube current modulation is applied, and its intensity (4% or 20% of maximum tube output).

Radiation dose optimization

Some key steps can be systematically followed to ensure radiation exposure to patients is minimized (Table 1.7.1).

Table 1.7.1 How to minimize patient radiation exposure	
Patient preparation	Apply optimal heart rate control (see Chapter 1.4) as this is more likely to lead to the selection of a highly dose-efficient scan protocol (e.g. prospectively ECG-triggered or high-pitch spiral scan)
Planning	• Tailor the scan range to each patient and clinical question (larger unnecessary scan range, larger dose) • Tailor the FoV to each patient and clinical question (FoV may cause dose penalty)
Scan parameters	Apply automated exposure control based on patient's specific anatomy (see also Chapter 1.5). If a manual tube voltage choice is necessary, generally a suitable selection is 100 kV for patients weighing <100 kg and a BMI <30 kg/m², and 120 kV otherwise. In patients with lower body weights, lower kV settings (70–90 kV) may also be viable options (see also Chapter 1.5)
Scan protocol	If appropriate to answer the clinical question, prefer prospective ECG-triggering over retrospective ECG-gating
Dose-saving algorithms	Routinely apply X-ray tube current modulation in retrospective ECG-gated scans, with width and intensity appropriate to meet the clinical question
Contrast delivery	Optimize contrast agent delivery for maximum contrast-to-noise ratio
Image reconstruction	Review the default reconstruction approach or blending of approaches; optimize slice reconstruction thickness and convolution kernels to improve contrast-to-noise ratio
Team building	• Ensure all members of staff receive appropriate application training • Liaise with the local medical physics expert for advice where necessary
ECG: electrocardiogram; FoV: field of view; BMI: body mass index.	

Further reading

Gimelli A, Achenbach S, Buechel RR, Edvardsen T, Francone M, Gaemperli O, et al. Strategies for radiation dose reduction in nuclear cardiology and cardiac computed tomography imaging: a report from the European Association of Cardiovascular Imaging (EACVI), the Cardiovascular Committee of European Association of Nuclear Medicine (EANM), and the European Society of Cardiovascular Radiology (ESCR). *Eur Heart J* 2018; 39: 286–94.

Gosling O, Loader R, Venables P, Rowles N, Morgan-Hughes G, Roobottom C. Cardiac CT: are we underestimating the dose? A radiation dose study utilizing the 2007 ICRP tissue weighting factors and a cardiac specific scan volume. *Clin Radiol* 2010; 65: 1013–17.

Stirrup J, Bull R, Williams M, Nicol E (eds). *Cardiovascular Computed Tomography.* 2nd edn. New York: Oxford Medical Publications, 2020.

Trattner S, Halliburton S, Thompson CM, Xu Y, Chelliah A, Jambawalikar SR, et al. Cardiac-specific conversion factors to estimate radiation effective dose from dose–length product in computed tomography. *JACC Cardiovasc Imaging* 2018; 11: 64–74.

Chapter 1.8

Common CT imaging artefacts

Oliver Gaemperli

Teaching points

- Cardiac CT image artefacts can be patient- or scan-related.
- Failure to recognize artefacts may result in either under- or overdiagnosis of disease.
- Anticipate artefacts! Artefacts can be avoided or mitigated by appropriate patient selection, optimal patient preparation, and specific adjustments in protocols/reconstruction algorithms.
- The most common cardiac CT artefact is motion (mostly cardiac); hence, the most effective measure to improve image quality is to decrease the heart rate and heart rate variability (see Chapter 1.4).

Over the years, technological improvements such as faster gantry rotation, increased number of detectors, and larger z-axis coverage have resulted in improved image quality in coronary CT angiography (see Chapters 1.1 and 1.2). However, images may still be affected by a number of artefacts from patient- and scan-related issues. Recognizing common CT artefacts is crucial to avoid inappropriate diagnoses. Table 1.8.1 provides an overview of the most common CT artefacts relevant to cardiac CT.

Some practical tips are provided in Box 1.8.1.

Table 1.8.1 Overview of the most common cardiac CT artefacts: C, causes; A, appearance; M, measures to prevent/avoid

Cardiac motion (Figure **1.8.1**)	
C	Motion (cardiac, respiratory, gross patient) is the most common CT artefact. *Cardiac* motion artefacts occur when the system is unable to adequately temporally resolve heartbeat motion (see Chapter 1.2 and 1.5). Most often this is the case when the cardiac resting period is too narrow for the system's temporal resolution (fast HR), or in the case of failure to trigger during the best resting period (irregular HR, premature beats)
A	• Blurring, ghosting, streaking (in-plane and through-plane) • Dense objects: dark shadows
M	• Decrease HR and variability (beta blockers; see Chapter 1.4) • Fast scanner gantry rotation • Dual-source CT technology • Multisegment reconstruction (see Chapters 1.5 and 1.9) • Multiple reconstruction phases (limited with prospective ECG triggering) • Intracycle motion compensation (vendor-dependent) • Edge enhancement/correction (vendor-dependent)

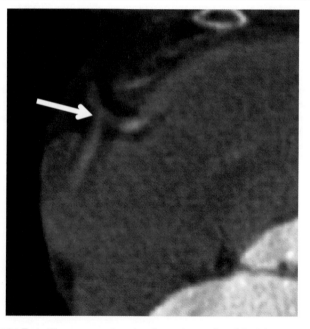

Figure 1.8.1 Typical Y- or crescent-shaped cardiac motion artefact of the right coronary artery (arrow).

Table 1.8.1 Continued

Discontinuity artefacts (Figure 1.8.2)

C	Discontinuity (or stair-step or displacement) artefacts are also caused by cardiac motion. They occur from misalignment between the reconstructions of sequential heartbeats. The cause is an irregular HR (e.g. atrial fibrillation or premature beats) with the heart not being in an identical position during consecutive beats
A	• Through-plane: discontinuity, stair-stepping, linear bands • Cave: in oblique coronary artery reconstructions, this artefact may mimic a lesion/stenosis
M	• Decrease HR and variability (beta blockers) (see Chapter 1.4) • Wide detector technology • High-pitch helical protocol on dual-source systems (decreases displacement artefacts but may increase cardiac motion blurring) • ECG editing (only with retrospective ECG-gated helical scanning; vendor-dependent)

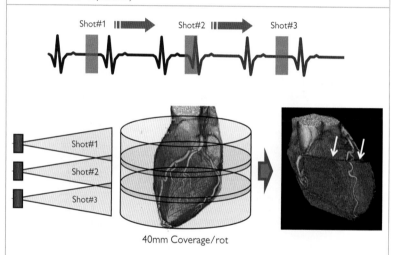

40mm Coverage/rot

Figure 1.8.2 Discontinuity artefacts (stairstep artefacts) occur when image slabs from different heartbeats are combined.

In the presence of an irregular heart rate, image acquisition may occur during different phases of the RR cycle, causing misalignment between image slabs (arrows). This artefact is intrinsic to scanners with limited z-axis coverage (scanners with wide detectors and single-beat acquisitions are exempt from this artefact).

(continued)

Table 1.8.1	Continued
Respiratory or gross patient motion (Figure 1.8.3)	
C	Increased respiratory rate or continued breathing, voluntary patient motion
A	• Through-plane: discontinuity • Cross-sectional: stair-stepping, blurring, ghosting, streaking • Sternal and rib motion
M	• Review breathing instructions with the patient (see Chapter 1.4) • Hyperventilate patient before the scan • Oxygen supplementation • Prefer scanners with low gantry rotation time • Wide z-axis coverage • High-pitch helical scanning • Shorten scan range • Swift acquisition

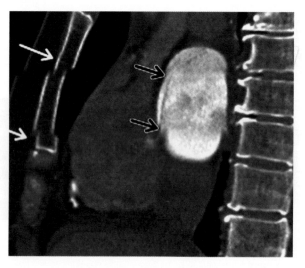

Figure 1.8.3 Discontinuity of the sternum and left atrial wall due to respiratory motion (arrows).

Table 1.8.1 Continued

Partial volume averaging/blooming (Figure 1.8.4)

C	Partial volume averaging occurs when objects smaller than the spatial resolution of the system are scanned: the attenuation of a given voxel becomes the weighted average of each of the tissue densities contained in that voxel (Figure 1.8.4A). The effect is especially pronounced at interfaces with substantially differing densities (e.g. coronary artery lumen and calcified plaque or stent)
A	Blooming/blurring and size overestimation
M	• Decrease collimated detector width • Increase reconstruction filter or kernel sharpness • Increase tube potential (up to 140 kVp; see Chapters 1.5 and 1.9) • Decrease reconstructed slice thickness • Virtual monoenergetic images at high energies (only if dual-energy available) • Iterative reconstruction • Increase display window width

(A)

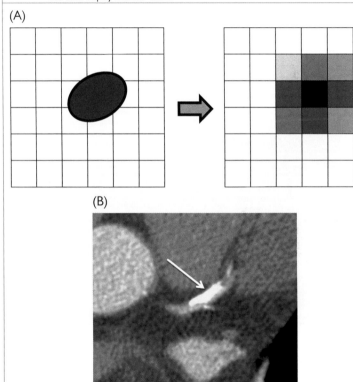

(B)

Figure 1.8.4 (A) Partial volume averaging occurs for small objects in the range of the spatial resolution of the scanner: when pixels are only partially filled by the dense object, the signal is averaged over the entire pixel resulting in blooming (objects appears larger) and blurring. (B) Calcium blooming in the left main and anterior descending artery (arrow).

(continued)

Table 1.8.1 Continued

Beam hardening (Figure 1.8.5)

C	X-ray beams produced from a CT source are composed of a spectrum of energies (polyenergetic or polychromatic; see Chapter 1.3). As they pass through a dense object (metal, calcium, bone), preferentially low-energy photons are absorbed and the mean beam energy is increased (i.e. the X-ray beam becomes 'harder'). The high-energy photons better penetrate surrounding tissues and the recorded signal hitting the detector becomes higher. Beam hardening typically results in two distinct types of artefacts: streaking and cupping
A	• Dark and bright streaks around high-attenuating objects (streaking is the result of the polychromatic X-ray being 'hardened' at different rates according to the rotational position of the tube/detector) • Cupping (the centre of a dense structure appears to have lower calculated attenuation than the periphery)
M	• Increase tube potential (up to 140 kVp; see Chapter 1.5 and 1.9) • X-ray beam filtration (flat or bowtie filter) • Detector calibration • Contrast agent protocol modification • Iterative reconstruction • Virtual monoenergetic images at high energies (only if dual-energy available)

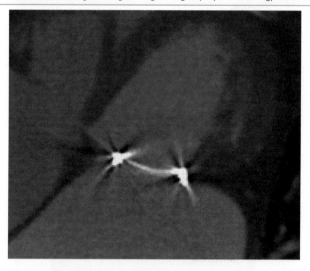

Figure 1.8.5 Streaking artefacts from beam hardening around metallic mitral annuloplasty ring.

Table 1.8.1 Continued

High image noise (Figure 1.8.6)

C	Image noise is not so much an artefact than a basic image characteristic. However, excessive noise should prompt steps to reduce it. Image noise occurs secondary to a low photon count reaching the detector. The main cause for excessive image noise is a large body size. Another common cause for localized high image noise may be *photon starvation*: behind high attenuation areas, typically metal implants, the X-ray beam is strongly attenuated and insufficient photons reach the detector, resulting in amplified noise
A	Grainy image Characteristic streaks of high image noise behind metal implants
M	• Increase tube current • Increase tube potential • Increase reconstructed slice thickness • Decrease reconstruction filter or kernel sharpness • Higher volume of contrast agent • Iterative reconstruction

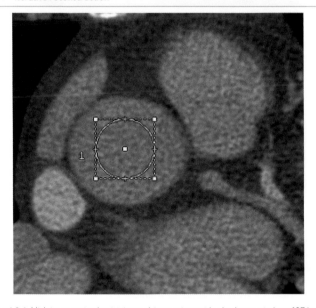

Figure 1.8.6 High image noise (grainy images) in a patient with a body mass index of 37 kg/m².

Common CT imaging artefacts

65

(continued)

Table 1.8.1	Continued

Slab or banding artefacts (Figure 1.8.7)

C	Slab or banding artefacts occur when image acquisition is performed during different phases of contrast enhancement. They reflect slightly varying levels of contrast enhancement over the course of a scan
A	Thick bands of differing contrast enhancement
M	• Increase z-axis coverage per cardiac cycle • Decrease number of imaged cardiac cycles • Maintain homogenous level of contrast enhancement

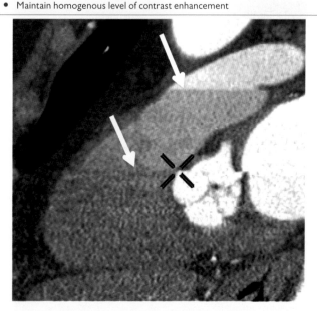

Figure 1.8.7 Slab or banding artefacts (arrows).

Insufficient contrast enhancement (Figure 1.8.8)

C	Low contrast enhancement may result from inappropriately low contrast volume/density/flow rate, extravasation of contrast agent, improper bolus tracking, or poor circulation (i.e. low cardiac output with contrast pooling in the venous system)
A	Decreased attenuation of vascular structures
M	• Increase volume/density/flow rate of contrast • Proper bolus tracking and timing • Use timing bolus • Decrease tube potential • Virtual low monoenergetic images (only if dual-energy available)

Table 1.8.1 Continued

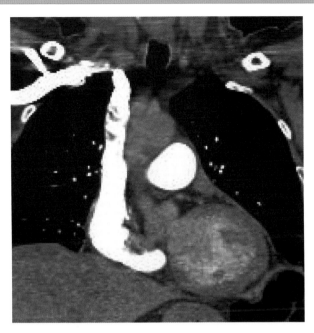

Figure 1.8.8 Low contrast in the left ventricle due to inappropriate bolus timing.

Data gaps/missing data/interpolation artefacts	
C	Inappropriate pitch (occurs only with helical CT acquisition; i.e. too high for a given HR)
A	One or more heavily blurred slices between relatively normal slices
M	• Use conservative pitch (as low as needed to ensure complete coverage) • Practice breath-hold manoeuvres before scan (and observe HR decrease)

HR: heart rate.

Common CT imaging artefacts

67

Box 1.8.1 Anticipate artefacts! Practical tips

- **Rapid heart rate:**
  - aggressive beta blockade (oral and/or intravenously);
  - prefer scanners with rapid gantry rotation or with a dual source;
  - retrospective electrocardiogram (ECG)-gated helical scan or prospective scan with padding/high energy during 30%–50% of RR cycle;
  - consider multisegment reconstruction;
  - use vendor-specific algorithms (e.g. ECG editing and intracycle motion compensation).
- **Atrial fibrillation:**
  - all of the above (except multisegment reconstruction).
- **Stents, pacemakers, and metallic implants:**
  - high tube voltage (140 kVp);
  - avoid motion artefacts;
  - use sharp kernel or filter;
  - iterative reconstruction;
  - reconstruct with thin slice thickness (e.g. 0.5–0.6 mm);
  - consider dual energy (if available).
- **Obesity:**
  - high tube current and tube voltage;
  - high contrast volume/density/flow rate;
  - iterative reconstruction;
  - reconstruct thicker slices (e.g. 1.0–1.5 mm);
  - if no calcium/metal, use soft kernel/filter.

  See also Chapters 1.8 and 1.9.

Further reading

Abbara S, Blanke P, Maroules CD, Cheezum M, Choi AD, Han BK, et al. SCCT guidelines for the performance and acquisition of coronary computed tomographic angiography. *J Cardiovasc Comput Tomogr* 2016; 10: 435e449.

Kalisz K, Buethe J, Saboo SS, Abbara S, Halliburton S, Rajiah P. Artifacts at cardiac CT: physics and solutions. *Radiographics* 2016; 36: 2064–83.

Schoepf UJ (ed.). *CT of the Heart*. 2nd edn. Totowa, NJ: Humana Press.

Chapter 1.9

Tips and tricks to improve image quality

Mohamed Marwan and Mihály Károlyi

> **Teaching points**
>
> - Adequate patient preparation is key to achieving diagnostic image quality with reasonably low radiation dose.
> - Scan protocols should be adapted to the clinical question and patient characteristics.
> - Advanced reconstruction techniques and postprocessing tools can help to remove or diminish the effects of image artefacts and improve image quality.

Tips and tricks for coronary CT angiography acquisition

Prior to image acquisition

Patient selection

- Patients with marked obesity, severe rhythm disturbances or patients who cannot adhere to breathing commands are not ideal candidates for coronary CT angiography (see Chapter 1.4).

Heart rate control

- Even with high-end scanners with wide detectors and high temporal resolution, lowering the heart rate (HR) to 60 beats per minute (bpm) is crucial for obtaining artefact-free images (see Chapter 1.4).
- Note: HR control is especially important in patients with stents and heavily calcified coronary arteries (consider a target HR of ≤60 bpm).

Patient positioning and scout scan

- To avoid scatter artefacts remove necklaces and other high-density materials from the chest surface, and scout for high-attenuation objects.
- Place the electrocardiogram (ECG) electrodes outside of the heart contours.
- Centre the patient with their arms raised above their head.

- It is important to achieve a comfortable position (consider supporting the legs and/or arms).
- Note: an uncomfortable patient position may result in an increased HR.

Explain the procedure and the breath-hold commands
- Non-compliance with breath-hold commands is a major source of artefacts.
- To ensure perfect breath-hold compliance for a cardiac examination, a slow and long sequence of breath-hold instructions is recommended ('breathe in—breathe out—breathe in—hold your breath' over about 15 seconds), as well as practising that command prior to data acquisition, to ensure that the patient can comfortably follow the command and hold their breath for the required time interval.

Electrocardiogram
- Acquire a clear ECG signal with a high R peak amplitude.
- Never start the scan without a well-defined QRS complex.

Secure a good intravenous access
- Cardiac CT requires a high contrast flow rate. For this reason, a stable intravenous access—preferably 18 G in the right antecubital region—should be placed and tested prior the procedure (see also Chapter 1.10).

Nitrates
- To achieve coronary dilatation and hence improve image quality and ease reporting of the coronaries, nitrates should be given around 5 minutes prior to acquisition of the angiography data set either as a sublingual spray or tablets (see also Chapter 1.4).

Image acquisition

Acquisition parameters

- Check the native scan prior to the CT angiography (CTA) as it provides information about the degree of coronary calcification, helps to determine the CTA scan length, and allows patient cooperation to be checked (i.e. proper breath-hold technique).
- In patients with no or mild coronary calcification, low-dose acquisition parameters could be used for the contrast-enhanced acquisition.
- Furthermore, using a higher tube voltage and tube current is important in obese patients, in order to avoid excessive image noise, and in patients with heavily calcified coronaries or with coronary stents, in order to reduce blooming artefacts. See Box 1.9.1.

Acquisition protocol
- The choice of protocol for image acquisition depends on the required information (e.g. functional assessment), HR and heart rhythm, as well as the available scanner technology (see Table 1.9.1).

Table 1.9.1 Acquisition protocol recommendations based on heart rate (HR) and regularity	
Stable sinus rhythm with a HR around or below 60 bpm	• Prospectively triggered axial acquisition or high-pitch spiral acquisition (depending on the available scanner technology; see Table 1.9.2) with a trigger typically around 70% of the peak R-wave to R-wave (note: depends on the vendor (some vendors use the centre of scan duration, whereas others use the start of scan window as the reference)
Mildly unstable rhythm or HR between 60 and 70 bpm (despite beta blockers)	• Prospectively triggered acquisition protocols (Table 1.9.2) may be used with modern scanners. However, it is recommended that the acquisition window is widened (typically from 40% to 70% of the peak R-wave to R-wave) to allow for flexible timing of the reconstruction if needed • It is of note that for dual-source scanners providing high-pitch spiral acquisition protocols, the stability of the HR is crucial in achieving high image quality and in patients with even the slightest irregularities in HR, a prospectively triggered axial acquisition would be preferred
High HR (>70 bpm) or irregular rhythm (extrasystoles or non-sinus rhythm)	• For modern scanner platforms, using a prospective axial acquisition in systolic phase is recommended (commonly, an absolute delay and trigger somewhere between 250 and 350 ms after the peak R-wave (corresponding to the peak of the T-wave) will provide adequate image quality (see Figure 1.9.1) • For patients with rhythm irregularities or high HRs despite beta blockers a spiral acquisition with ECG modulation (maximum output between 40% and 70% of the cardiac cycle with reduction of tube output outside this window; Table 1.9.2) and retrospectively ECG-gated image reconstruction (Table 1.9.2) is preferable (note: for certain vendors, the estimated HR during the acquisition of spiral scans should be provided to adjust the table pitch and hence avoid artefacts (e.g. interpolation artefacts; see Chapter 1.8 and Figure 1.9.2)

HR: heart rate; bpm: beats per minute; ECG: electrocardiogram.

Practical tips for acquisition

71

• Note: HR should be assessed in deep inspiration, as deep inspiration usually causes the HR to decrease substantially.

Contrast injection
• For adequate opacification of the coronary arteries, a minimum flow rate of 5 ml/s is recommended to be increased up to 7 ml/s for obese patients or, for example, patients with stents if the intravenous access allows.
• Furthermore, dual-head injectors capable of providing a chaser with some degree of contrast (commonly 20% contrast, 80% saline) allow for better contrast enhancement of right heart structures and hence better image quality (see Chapter 1.10).

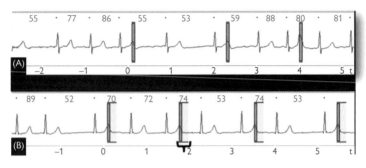

Figure 1.9.1 Electrocardiogram traces from two patients with atrial fibrillation examined with prospective axial acquisition.

(A) Trigger at 300 ms after the R-wave. (B) Prospective axial acquisition with widened window between 300 and 400 ms, as marked by the braces.

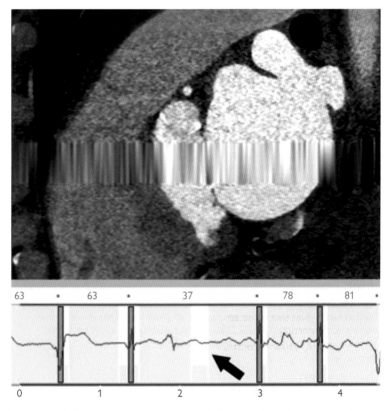

Figure 1.9.2 Typical interpolation artefact caused by missing information at the marked area (arrow).

Box 1.9.1 General tips for achieving high image quality

- Be present during the scan to optimize protocol and review images.
- Know the patient, the clinical context, and adopt a protocol tailored to the patient's HR, rhythm, and indication.
  - Heavily calcified coronaries and stents: achieving a HR of <60 bpm is important, use a higher tube voltage, irrespective of the patient's body weight.
  - Obese patients (weighing >100 kg or with a BMI >30 kg/m^2): increase the tube voltage and current, increase the contrast volume and flow rate, consider 360-degree (full-scan rotation) reconstruction, create 'averaged' resp. 'thick' multiplanar reconstructions at postprocessing, and use iterative reconstruction algorithms.
  - Rapid HR (>65 bpm), arrhythmia: prospective ECG-triggering to systolic phase, wider acquisition window, or use retrospective ECG gating (Table 1.9.2).
  - With an indication to clarify coronary anomaly or pulmonary vein angiography, do not necessarily aim for excellent images of the coronaries at the cost of a higher radiation dose.
- Know the capabilities (and limitations) of your scanner.

After image acquisition

Prospectively ECG-triggered axial acquisitions

- Several vendors provide image interpolation of structural displacement between acquisitions (slabs).
- These reconstructions could potentially mimic coronary artery stenoses at areas with step artefacts (see Chapter 1.8).
- If this is suspected, it is also important to reconstruct original images without interpolation to allow for differentiation between areas of step artefacts and 'false' or 'mimicked' stenosis.

Retrospective acquisition

- After acquiring a retrospectively gated spiral CT data set, it is important to make use of the available information.
- In the case of HR irregularities, some vendors provide the ability to edit the ECG (i.e. deactivate or move trigger points) to change the timing of the reconstructed window in order to obtain artefact-free images.

Tips for ECG editing
- Avoid the P-waves that cause atrial contraction and artefacts, especially of the right coronary artery.
- Try to maintain regular reconstruction time points (at the same phase of the cardiac cycle).
- Reconstruct away from ventricular extrasystoles and fill information gaps to avoid interpolation (e.g. see Figure 1.9.3).

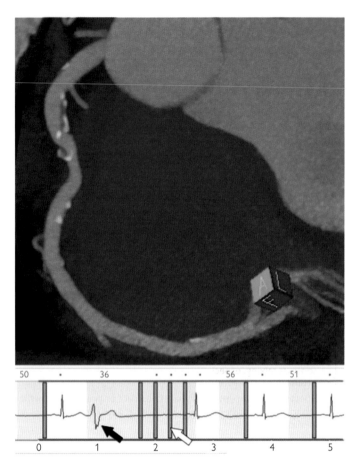

Figure 1.9.3 Multiplanar reconstruction of the right coronary artery after electrocardiogram (ECG) editing with very good image quality.

The ECG trace shows regular sinus rhythm with a single ventricular ectopic beat (black arrow). Additional reconstruction time points added beyond the extrasystole (white arrows) to fill in the missing information.

Tips and tricks for non-coronary cardiac CT acquisition

• For non-coronary CT acquisition in the context of structural heart disease or planning of structural interventions, spiral acquisition with retrospective ECG-gated image reconstruction is usually needed to allow for multiphase assessment through the entire cardiac cycle (functional CT assessment), for example in analysis of the aortic valve annulus prior to transcatheter valve replacement (see Chapters 3.3–3.6).

Table 1.9.2 Comparison of electrocardiogram-gating techniques		
	Prospective triggering	Retrospective gating
Position of the acquisition time window	Predicted, fixed in advance	At arbitrary phase of RR, freely selectable offline
Scan mode	Axial (sequential)	Helical (spiral)
Main applications	Calcium scoring, CCTA in low HR, dynamic perfusion	CCTA in high HR, functional/dynamic imaging
Advantages	Low radiation dose	4D data sets, flexibility
Limitations	Limited number of phases, susceptible to HR variations, obese patients (weighing >120 kg)	High radiation dose
CCTA: coronary CT angiography; HR: heart rate; 4D: four-dimensional.		

- In addition, adjustment of the contrast protocol or the acquisition protocol depends on the clinical question or the structure to be evaluated.
- For example, for assessment of right-sided structures, a triphasic contrast protocol (contrast followed initially by saline/contrast mix and then pure saline) to allow for adequate opacification of the right side with no contrast streak artefacts in the right atrium is recommended (see Chapters 3.9–3.12).
- Similarly, amending the acquisition protocol, for example in cases of left atrial appendage assessment with a delayed phase scan, may be necessary to allow for adequate contrast mixing, especially in patients with atrial fibrillation (Figure 1.9.1; see Chapter 3.7).
- Note: within the context of structural heart disease assessment, the application of nitrates is not necessary and lowering the HR is usually not needed.

Chapter 1.10

CT contrast agents and injection protocols

Casper Mihl and Bibi Martens

> **Teaching points**
>
> - Diagnostic image quality in coronary CT angiography is influenced by scan and contrast media (CM) parameters, as well as patient-related factors.
> - CT CM are iodinated agents with variable osmolarity, ionicity, and iodine concentrations.
> - Contrast injection protocols need to be individually tailored to obtain optimal opacification of the cardiac structures of interest.
> - Adverse reactions to CT contrast agents may range from mild to (very rarely) severe. Appropriate precautions, rapid identification. and practical knowledge on their treatment are fundamental for all physicians and technical staff involved in cardiac CT imaging.

Iodinated contrast media agents

- Osmolarity: (high/low/iso), ionicity (ionic/non-ionic), benzene rings (monomer/dimer).
- Non-ionic low or iso-osmolar contrast media (CM) predominantly used in coronary CT angiography (see Table 1.10.1).

Parameters influencing image quality in coronary CT angiography

Contrast media parameters

- Temperature:
  - higher temperature decreases viscosity.
- Concentration:
  - 240–400 mg/ml;
  - higher concentration equals higher viscosity.

Table 1.10.1 Concentrations of different iodinated contrast media agents

Osmolarity	Generic name	Ionicity	Available concentrations (mgI/ml)
Low	Iopadimol	Non-ionic (monomer)	150, 200, 250, 300, 370
	Iohexol	Non-ionic (monomer)	180, 200, 240, 300, 350
	Iopromide	Non-ionic (monomer)	150, 180, 200, 240, 300, 350, 370, 400
	Ioversol	Non-ionic (monomer)	160, 240, 300, 320, 350
	Ioxaglate	Ionic (dimer)	160, 200, 320, 350
	Iomeprol	Non-ionic (monomer)	150, 200, 250, 300, 350, 400
	Iobitridol	Non-ionic (monomer)	250, 300, 350
Iso	Iodixanol	Non-ionic (dimer)	150, 270, 320

Trade names and indications may vary in different countries. Contact the representative of the firm for availability and indications.

- Flow rate:
  - recommended range of 4.0–7.0 ml/s;
  - high flow rates are possible with proper intravenous cannulas;
  - lower flow rates may be appropriate in lower tube voltages.
- Iodine delivery rate (IDR), in g/s:
  - concentration (mgI/ml) × flow rate (ml/s);
  - recommended range of 1.5–2.0 g/s iodine;
  - should ideally be adapted to body weight and tube voltage.
- Volume:
  - depending on the image acquisition protocol and CM concentration;
  - range of 50–120 ml;
  - shorter scan acquisition time can reduce CM volume;
  - should be adapted to body weight and tube voltage.
- Total iodine load:
  - CM concentration (mg/ml) × CM volume (ml).
- Saline chaser:
  - pushes residual CM out of central venous system and right heart;
  - reduces artefacts caused by CM in the subclavian or brachiocephalic vein (streaking);
  - same flow rate as CM bolus.

CM injection protocols

Timing

- Test bolus technique:
    - Test bolus injection (e.g. 10–20 ml CM) followed by a saline chaser, both injected at the anticipated injection rate.
- Bolus tracking:
    - automated scan triggering by monitoring the arrival of CM bolus with repetitive single-slice scans at a prespecified anatomical level (region of interest);
    - the scan is triggered when the attenuation reaches predefined threshold.

For further details, please see Chapter 1.5.

Two-phase contrast media injection protocol

- CM bolus followed by saline chaser (40–50 ml).
- Right heart cavities ideally washed out (reduction of streak artefacts).

Three-phase contrast media injection protocol

- Right heart opacification (e.g. left ventricle geometry and right ventricle abnormalities).
- CM bolus injection followed by a second bolus injection at a lower injection rate (e.g. CM at lower flow rate or mix of CM with saline at a standard flow rate, saline chaser (Figure 1.10.1)).

Four-phase contrast media injection protocol

- To decrease the risk of vein injury.
- Starts with a pacer saline bolus at a lower injection rate to open up the vein for the large CM load, then continues as per a three-phasic protocol (Figure 1.10.1).

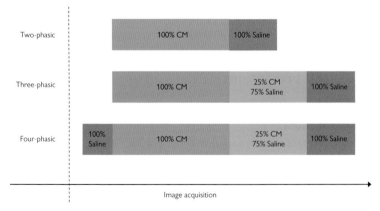

Figure 1.10.1 Overview of contrast media injection protocols. Individual volumes and flow rates for each injection phase may vary based on patient characteristics and scan parameters.

Delayed contrast media injection protocol
- To rule out atrial thrombus, a second CM injection separated by 30–60 seconds after the first (main) injection.

Patient-related parameters

- (Lean) body weight/body mass index/body surface area:
  - impact on attenuation and time to peak.
- Injection site:
  - preferred—antecubital/large forearm vein;
  - preferred—large cannula (e.g. 18 G cannula);
  - smaller cannula results in a lower maximum flow rate.
- 24 G: 0.5–1.5 ml/s, maximum 50–100 psi.
- 22 G: 2–3.5 ml/s, maximum 100–300 psi.
- 20 G: 3–5 ml/s, maximum 300 psi.
- 18 G: 4–6.5 ml/s, maximum 300 psi.

Scanner-related parameters

- Tube voltage:
  - preferable usage of automated tube voltage selection techniques (for more details see Chapters 1.2 and 1.5).
  - remember—the higher the tube voltage, the lower the iodine opacification is (lower Hounsfield units). Thus, higher tube voltage translates into a lower image contrast-to-noise ratio for a given IDR.
- Tube current:
  - preferable use of automated tube current modulation techniques.

10 to 10 rule
- A reduction in tube voltage of 10 kV should be followed by a 10 % reduction in IDR and vice versa.

Safety and precautions

For contrast-induced nephropathy, see Chapter 1.4.

Allergic reactions

Please also see the European Society of Urogenital Radiology guidelines for further details on the management and dosing of various reactions.
- Estimated incidence of recurrent reaction: 8–60%.
- Increased risk of a hypersensitivity reaction with:
  - a history of asthma/bronchospasm;
  - multiple allergies.

See Table 1.10.2.

Table 1.10.2 Grading of general adverse reactions and treatment

Grading	Characteristics	Treatment
Minor	<ul><li>Mild urticaria/itching</li><li>Erythema</li><li>Warmth/chills</li><li>Nausea/vomiting</li><li>Vasovagal reaction</li></ul>	<ul><li>Sustain IV access</li><li>Usually self-limiting</li><li>Observation</li></ul>
Moderate	<ul><li>Marked urticaria</li><li>Mild bronchospasm</li><li>Severe vomiting</li><li>Facial/laryngeal oedema</li><li>Vasovagal reaction</li></ul>	<ul><li>Antihistamine</li><li>Adrenaline</li><li>Oxygen by mask (6–10 l/min)</li><li>Check blood pressure/heart rate</li><li>IV fluids</li><li>Elevate legs</li></ul>
Severe	<ul><li>Hypotensive shock</li><li>Respiratory arrest</li><li>Cardiac arrest</li><li>Arrhythmia</li><li>Convulsion</li></ul>	<ul><li>Call resuscitation team</li><li>Suction airway if needed</li><li>Elevate patient's legs</li><li>Oxygen by mask (6–10 l/min)</li><li>Adrenaline (IM): adults: 0.5 ml (0.5 mg); 6–12 years: 0.3 ml (0.3 mg); <6 years: 0.15 ml (0.15 mg)</li><li>IV fluids</li><li>Antihistamine</li></ul>
Delayed reaction (60 min–1 week after CM administration)	Skin reactions	<ul><li>Consider antihistamines, topical steroids and emollients</li><li>Drug prophylaxis not recommended</li></ul>
Extra precautions	Increased risk of hypersensitivity reaction	<ul><li>History of asthma/bronchospasm</li><li>Multiple allergies</li><li>Previous severe reaction</li></ul>
	History of thyrotoxicosis and hyperthyroidism	Monitoring by endocrinologist

IV: intravenous; IM: intramuscular; CM: contrast media.

CM extravasation
Incidence may increase with:

- smaller cannula;
- more peripheral injection sites;
- use of an already existing venous access

Serious complications:

- Compartment syndrome:
  - ulceration;
  - tissue necrosis.

Treatment may vary according to protocol and may include:
- elevation;
- warm or cold compresses;
- surgical consultation.

Symptoms indicating possible surgical consultation:
- progressive pain or swelling;
- decreased capillary refill;
- paraesthesia, skin ulceration, or blistering.

Further reading

Abbara S, Blanke P, Maroules CD, Cheezum M, Choi AD, Han BK, et al. SCCT guidelines for the performance and acquisition of coronary computed tomographic angiography: a report of the Society of Cardiovascular Computed Tomography Guidelines Committee Endorsed by the North American Society for Cardiovascular Imaging (NASCI). *J Cardiovasc Comput Tomogr* 2016; 10: 435–449.

Bae KT. Intravenous contrast medium administration and scan timing at CT: considerations and approaches. *Radiology* 2010; 256: 32–61.

European Society of Urogenital Radiology (ESUR). ESUR guidelines on contrast agents. Available at: http://www.esur.org/esur-guidelines/ (accessed 9 June 2022).

Chapter 1.11

How to deal with challenging scenarios

Ricardo P.J. Budde, Sarah Moharem-Elgamal,
and Francesca Pugliese

> **Teaching points**
>
> - Awareness of potential difficulties prior to scanning is important so that measures can be taken to prevent and/or reduce their influence on image quality.
> - After image acquisition, changing the image reconstruction parameters can mitigate some factors that negatively influence image quality

General principles

Multiple factors, circumstances, and patient characteristics may negatively influence CT image acquisition and quality. It is important to be aware of these and of the measures that can be taken to reduce their influence. An overview is provided of the most common difficulties encountered before, during, or after the CT scan acquisition, how they affect the procedure, and which measures can be taken to prevent, avoid, or reduce their negative effect on image quality and diagnostic yield.

- Review the CT scan request beforehand (ideally days before) so there is time to prepare the scan optimally.
- Always evaluate the reason for performing the scan and determine whether other imaging modalities may be better options in patients with expected difficulties.

Impaired renal function

Impaired renal function poses the risk that the patient may develop contrast-induced nephropathy as a consequence of iodinated contrast agent injection (see Chapter 1.10).

- Obtain a recent estimated glomerular filtration rate.
- Consider non-contrast-enhanced CT acquisition or an alternative imaging technique (e.g. cardiac magnetic resonance (CMR) or echocardiogram).

- If contrast CT imaging cannot be replaced by another modality, prehydrate the patient prior to the scan according to the institutional protocol (see Chapter 1.4).
- Use low-kilovoltage (kV) scanning where possible to increase contrast attenuation, so that reduced contrast volume can be injected at a slower injection rate (see Chapter 1.5).
- Increasing the reconstruction slice thickness (1 mm instead of 0.6–0.75 mm) and the application of iterative reconstruction (higher strength than normal, in mixed reconstruction) may compensate for a loss of signal induced by a low contrast volume injection (see Chapter 1.6).

Known allergy to iodinated contrast agent

This scenario requires risk assessment for severe contrast reaction (see Chapter 1.10).

- Collect from patient accurate contrast allergy history.
- Ascertain whether allergy occurred in association with older, ionic iodinated contrast agents (no longer in use), or whether this occurred with non-ionic contrast agents that are more recent and still in use today.
- If the history is consistent with severe allergy to non-ionic contrast, consider non-contrast-enhanced CT acquisition or an alternative imaging technique (e.g. CMR and echocardiogram).
- Antiallergy medication (as per institutional protocol) are used in clinical practice, when the occurrence of severe allergy appears extremely unlikely and there are no viable diagnostic alternative in the specific clinical scenario (see Chapter 1.10).
- Antiallergy medication does not provide 100% protection against the occurrence of allergic reactions and should not be considered as totally safe.

Poor intravenous access

Situations where the patient has poor intravenous access with the availability of only small or distant access (typically in the hand) pose the risk of suboptimal contrast enhancement. Small peripheral veins may not be suitable for injection rates of 4–5 ml/s. Slower injection rates will cause a reduction in the iodine delivery rate (see Chapter 1.5).

- Place a cannula commensurate to the size of the peripheral vein and reduce the injection rate accordingly (2–3.5 ml/s) to avoid contrast extravasation.
- Time the main scan based on the new injection rate; with a reduced injection rate, it will take longer to inject the same contrast volume.
- Slower injection may allow more contrast dilution with poorer contrast/ noise images.
- Use low-kV scanning where possible.

- Apply iterative reconstruction (or higher iterative reconstruction strength in mixed reconstruction) to compensate for image noise.
- As an extreme solution, plan a second emergency scan in the examination planning platform—delayed imaging may yield slight contrast enhancement, but only start one if the first scan is non-diagnostic.
- The use of central venous catheters for contrast injection is generally not recommended.

Contraindications to beta blockers and nitroglycerin

This scenario may lead to a fast heart rate (HR) during the scan, which in turn leads to motion artefacts and reduced coronary dilatation.

- Practice breath holds and assess their effect on HR (HR usually drops during breath hold).
- Reassure the patient, try to reduce anxiety.
- Adapt the acquisition protocol for fast HRs (see Chapter 1.5).
- Consider alternative medication (see Chapter 1.4).

Obesity, morbid obesity, and large-body habitus

This situation may lead to increased X-ray scatter and poor contrast/noise images. This affects the delineation of small vessels and atherosclerotic plaques, particularly if non-calcified.

- Take extra care with patient positioning (e.g. for cardiac imaging in females, try to move the breasts outside the scan range, where possible).
- Optimize kV and mAs settings (automated exposure control) for an acceptable level of image noise (see Chapter 1.5).
- Consider modifying the contrast injection protocol towards an increased iodine delivery rate (increased iodine concentration or increased contrast injection rate if allowed by the available venous access).
- Increase reconstruction slice thickness (typically 1 mm instead of 0.6–0.75 mm; see Chapter 1.6).
- Increase the strength of iterative reconstruction in a mixed filtered back projection/iterative reconstruction approach.
- Apply dedicated scan protocols and/or reconstruction approaches (e.g. retrospectively electrocardiogram (ECG)-gated protocol with best diastolic/systolic phases reconstructed from 'longer' reconstruction windows of 105, 125, or 165 ms. This approach trades in temporal resolution to increase image contrast and therefore requires good HR control).

Metallic implants

Metallic devices (e.g. stents and pacemaker leads) in the scan range may cause high-density artefacts and limit the interpretability of the study.

- Application of a higher kV may be necessary. This will help reduce metal-related high-density artefacts in the images (see Chapter 1.5).
- Apply dedicated high-frequency reconstruction kernels (see Chapter 1.6).
- Use of dual-energy scanning and reconstruction of high monochromatic energy data sets may also reduce high-density artefacts.

Fast heart rate, ectopic beats, and atrial fibrillation

High-quality cardiac CT images ideally require regular, stable, and slow HRs. Prospectively ECG-triggered scans are particularly sensitive to cardiac arrhythmias leading to misregistration and artefacts. Retrospectively ECG-gated protocols offer more flexibility as data are acquired continuously during the cardiac cycle and images can be reconstructed in various parts of the RR interval.

In general:

- Consider an alternative test or defer imaging until the arrhythmia is controlled, if possible.
- Apply arrhythmia rejection protocols if available (see example in Figure 1.6.1).
- Recommended scan protocols include prospectively ECG-triggered scan with generous padding, prospectively ECG-triggered scan during systole, and retrospectively ECG-gated scan.
- Consider reconstructing images with an absolute time delay (milliseconds) instead of % phases.
- Store raw data on scanner until the time of image analysis and reporting, to allow for additional image reconstruction, if necessary.
- Patients with premature beats are best suited for retrospectively ECG-gated scanning followed by ECG editing (manufacturer dependent). In ECG editing, data acquired during the premature beat are removed with the additional reconstruction window placed in the compensatory pause of the following cardiac cycle (see the examples in Figure 1.6.2 and Figure 1.11.1). Premature atrial contraction may be more challenging to compensate for. The lower the underlying sinus rhythm, the higher the chance of successful ECG editing.
- In patients with sinus tachycardia or atrial tachycardia, the normal motion of the coronary vessel is exacerbated. Imaging in the systolic phase may be the best option in these scenarios.
- In patients with atrial fibrillation (5% of patients over the age of 70 years), cardiac cycles can vary in duration, which represents a challenging scenario for ECG synchronization, especially with a prospective approach. The high temporal resolution of dual-source CT and single heartbeat wide-detector scanning are generally sufficient to overcome this limitation and provide dose-efficient, diagnostic image quality in most patients with atrial fibrillation. With

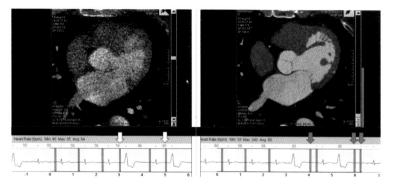

Figure 1.11.1 Example of electrocardiogram (ECG) editing in a patient with recurring ectopic beats.

Reconstructed CT images and ECG traces in a patient with ectopic beats during the scan. The blue vertical bars on the ECG traces represent the reconstruction windows (i.e. the portions of the RR interval whose data were used for image reconstruction). In the ECG trace on the left, there are two premature beats occurring during the scan. Reconstruction windows were automatically positioned during these ectopic beats (white arrows). The resulting image on the left is affected by motion artefacts and noise. In the ECG trace on the right, with ECG editing reconstruction bars were removed from the ectopic beats and new bars were added during the following compensatory diastole (orange arrows). As a result, the image on the right is of improved quality and motion free.

single-source 64-slice CT systems, it is important to achieve good control of the ventricular response. With retrospectively ECG-gated scanning, multiple-phase data sets will be obtained, increasing the chances of fully diagnostic image quality

Non-collaborative patients/non-compliance with breathing instructions

- Practice breath holds before scanning.
- Use multilanguage voice commands on scanner, when needed.
- Use fast scan acquisition protocols (e.g. high pitch) to allow for shorter breath hold.
- Use a test bolus injection for contrast timing instead of region of interest contrast tracking, to reduce scan time and impose shorter breath holds.

Patients with dyspnoea

- Plan and prepare the scan as best and fast as possible to ensure the patient is kept in a prone position for as short a time as possible.
- Reduce the volume of contrast agent and consider adjusting the injection rate.
- Use fast scan acquisition protocols (e.g. high pitch).
- Consider oxygen administration.

Chapter 2.1

Coronary artery calcium imaging

Martin J. Willemink

Teaching points

- The presence or absence of coronary artery calcium in asymptomatic individuals is a robust measure of subclinical atherosclerosis, allowing for risk reclassification for the primary prevention of atherosclerotic cardiovascular events.
- The optimal calcium scoring acquisition protocol is a prospectively electrocardiogram-triggered non-contrast-enhanced CT scan.
- The Agatston score is the most validated coronary artery calcium quantification method.
- The Coronary Artery Calcium Data and Reporting System (CAC-DRS) is a standardized method to communicate coronary artery calcium findings on non-contrast CT scans.
- Coronary artery calcium scoring is recommended in asymptomatic adults at intermediate cardiovascular risk. In select cases of adults with low-to-intermediate risk coronary artery calcium may be used to further evaluate risk.

Coronary artery calcium has shown to be a strong predictor of the long-term risk for atherosclerotic cardiovascular disease in asymptomatic individuals. Coronary artery calcium can be quantified with a non-contrast CT scan. Coronary artery calcium can be used to reclassify asymptomatic individuals at intermediate cardiovascular risk. The absence of coronary artery calcium on a CT scan is a strong marker for identification of individuals at very low 10-year risk. Elevated coronary artery calcium scores indicate that the individual is likely to benefit from treatment.

Acquisition protocol

Patient preparation

- There is no need for beta-blockers, nitroglycerin, or other medications. Calcium CT scans are performed without iodinated contrast agents.
- Patients do not need to fast before the exam.
- Patients should be able to lie still and hold their breath for 3–5 seconds.

Image acquisition

- Prospectively electrocardiogram (ECG)-triggered non-contrast CT is the most optimal protocol due to the relatively low radiation exposure.
- Recommended tube potential is 120 kVp, while tube current can be adjusted based on patient size.
- Reducing the tube potential to 100 kVp results in a substantial radiation dose reduction. However, low-voltage acquisition is not routinely performed because it changes the calcium scores. This can be partially corrected by adjustment of the Hounsfield unit (HU) threshold.
- The effective radiation dose should be approximately 1 mSv, or lower.
- Reconstructed slice thickness should be 2.5 or 3.0 mm, depending on the CT manufacturer.
- Iterative reconstruction algorithms are currently not recommended for calcium imaging because this method results in lower calcium scores.
- In general, convolution kernels with medium sharpness are used for calcium scoring, to compromise between noise and blooming of calcifications. The selection of convolutional kernel depends on the vendor.
- Besides dedicated ECG-triggered CT scans, the calcium burden can be semi-quantified on non-gated chest CT exams. Visual interpretation (as discussed later) may be used to quantify coronary calcium on these exams, but Agatston scores cannot be calculated on non-gated chest CT.

See also Chapter 1.5.

Calcium quantification

Agatston score

- The Agatston score is the most validated quantification method for coronary calcium.
- A calcification within the coronary arteries is defined as a ≥ 1 mm^2 area with a CT density of ≥ 130 HU.
- The Agatston score per calcification is calculated by multiplying the area of each calcification by a density weighting factor related to the maximum attenuation within the calcification:
  - 130–199 HU: factor 1;
  - 200–299 HU: factor 2;
  - 300–399 HU: factor 3;
  - ≥ 400 HU: factor 4.
- The total Agatston score is calculated by taking the weighted sum of each calcification.
- A basic interpretation of the absolute Agatston score with regard to coronary plaque burden:
  - Agatston score = 0, no identifiable disease;
  - Agatston score = 1–99, mild disease;

- Agatston score = 100–399, moderate disease;
- Agatston score ≥400, severe disease.

Volume and mass scores

- Besides the Agatston score, coronary calcium can be quantified as volume and mass (Table 2.1.1).
- The calcium volume (mm^3) is calculated by multiplying the number of voxels within calcified plaques with an attenuation of >130 HU by the volume of each voxel.
- Calcium mass (mg) is calculated by multiplying the mean attenuation of each calcified plaque by the plaque volume. A correction factor based on the attenuation of water is used to calculate the mass.
- Volume and mass have better reproducibility than the Agatston score; however, they are less validated for cardiovascular outcomes. Volume and mass are thus rarely used in the clinical setting.

Reporting

Coronary Artery Calcium Data and Reporting System

- The Coronary Artery Calcium Data and Reporting System (CAC-DRS) is a standardized method to communicate coronary calcium findings on non-contrast CT scans.
- CAC-DRS can be determined based on dedicated calcium scans and non-contrast chest CT, irrespective of the indication.
- CAC-DRS classification is applied on a per-patient basis and represents the total calcium score and the number of involved arteries.
- Modifiers:
  - scoring system, can be either A = Agatston or V = visual estimation;
  - number of vessels with coronary artery calcium ($n = 1–4$) is not used to change risk categories, but may be reported.
- Example CAC-DRS score for an Agatston score of 75 with calcium in the left main, left anterior descending, and circumflex arteries would be CAC-DRS A1/N3.

Table 2.1.1 Comparison of coronary artery calcium quantification methods

	Agatston score	Calcium volume	Calcium mass
Unit of measure	None	mm^3	mg
Benefit	Well validated	Good reproducibility	Good reproducibility

Table 2.1.2 CAC-DRS scoring methods and treatment recommendations according to Agatston score on dedicated calcium scoring CT and visual score on chest CT

Agatston score	Coronary artery calcium score	Risk	Treatment recommendation
CAC-DRS A0	0	Very low	Statin generally not recommended*
CAC-DRS A1	1–99	Mildly increased	Moderate intensity statin
CAC-DRS A2	100–299	Moderately increased	Moderate- to-high-intensity statin + ASA 81 mg
CAC-DRS A3	>300	Moderately to severely increased	High-intensity statin + ASA 81 mg
Visual score			
CAC-DRS V0	0	Very low	Statin generally not recommended*
CAC-DRS V1	1	Mildly increased	Moderate intensity statin
CAC-DRS V2	2	Moderately increased	Moderate-to-high intensity statin + ASA 81 mg
CAC-DRS V3	3	Moderately to severely increased	High-intensity statin + ASA 81 mg

*Excluding familial hypercholesterolaemia. ASA: acetylsalicylic acid.

- CAC-DRS classification and treatment recommendations are listed in Table 2.1.2 and displayed in Figure 2.1.1.

Coronary calcium risk prediction nomogram

- For each risk factor, draw a vertical line from the corresponding axis to the 'points' line in Figure 2.1.2. The 'total points' can be calculated by summing the total points for all risk factors.
- Draw a vertical line down from the 'total points' axis to estimate 5-, 10-, and 15-year survival probabilities.
- For dichotomous numbers, no is 0 and yes is 1. Coronary artery calcium score categories: none is 0, 1–100 is 1, 101–400 is 2, 401–1000 is 3, and >1000 is 4.

Pitfalls

- Proper identification of calcium located within the coronary artery walls is essential. A common pitfall is to include calcifications from other anatomical structures such as the aortic valve or mitral annulus.

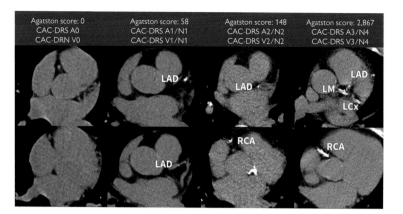

Figure 2.1.1 Four example cases with different Coronary Artery Calcium Data and Reporting System (CAC-DRS) scores.
LAD: left anterior descending artery; RCA: right coronary artery; LM: left main artery; LCx: left circumflex artery.

- Different causes of motion artefacts may be present. Breathing during the exam causes breathing artefacts, and heart rate irregularities that occur during scanning (e.g. premature heartbeat) may cause cardiac motion artefacts.
- The relatively thick image slices of calcium CT (3.0 mm or 2.5 mm) may result in missing small and low-density calcifications due to the partial volume effect.

Clinical application

Asymptomatic individuals

European Society of Cardiology guidelines state that calcium scoring may be considered as a risk modifier to reclassify asymptomatic individuals into low- or high-risk groups. Moreover, it is emphasized that the calcium score is not recommended to identify individuals with obstructive coronary artery disease.

American College of Cardiology/American Heart Association guidelines include the following recommendations.

- Intermediate-risk individuals:
- calcium scoring is recommended in adults at intermediate cardiovascular risk (7.5% to <20% 10-year atherosclerotic cardiovascular disease risk).
- Low-to-intermediate-risk individuals:
  - in select cases of adults with borderline increased risk (5% to <7.5% 10-year atherosclerotic cardiovascular risk), a calcium score may be used to further evaluate risk.
- Low- or high-risk individuals:
  - calcium imaging is not recommended in adults at low (<5% 10-year risk) or high risk (≥20% 10-year risk).
- Calcium scoring may be considered in adults aged between 40 and 75 years.

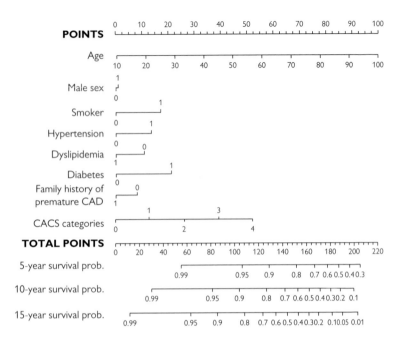

Figure 2.1.2 Coronary calcium risk prediction nomogram.

CAD: coronary artery disease; CACS: coronary artery calcium score.

Source: Reproduced from Ó Hartaigh B, Gransar H, Callister T, et al. (2018) Development and validation of a simple-to-use nomogram for predicting 5-, 10-, and 15-year survival in asymptomatic adults undergoing coronary artery calcium scoring. *JACC Cardiovasc Imaging*, 11(3):450–458 with permission from Elsevier (Creative Commons 4.0 – https://creativecommons.org/licenses/by-nc-nd/4.0/)

Elderly individuals

- Calcium scoring may be used for risk reclassification in asymptomatic, elderly individuals as it has proven to be an independent predictor for long-term coronary heart disease.

Women

- Compared to men of similar age and cardiovascular risk category, women have less coronary calcium. However, the prognostic value of the calcium score in women is equal to men. Generally, 10-year cardiovascular risk is assessed to be lower in women than in men.

Ethnicity

- While the likelihood of having detectable coronary calcium differs between ethnic groups, the predictive value is similar within various ethnicities.
- Both in men and women, coronary calcium is more prevalent in white people than in Chinese, Hispanic, and African American people.

Symptomatic patients

- Although a zero-calcium score reduces the probability of having significant coronary artery stenosis in symptomatic patients, a calcium scan is not recommended in this population.
- Calcium imaging is not recommended in symptomatic patients as its specificity for coronary artery disease is low.

Progression

- In individuals who have coronary calcium (score >0) monitoring of calcium progression is not recommended, as management is rarely adjusted. This is especially the case with higher calcium scores (>100).
- In asymptomatic individuals without coronary calcium (score 0) a follow-up calcium scan may be considered after 5 years if the individual is still at low-to-intermediate or intermediate risk.
- Efficacy of cholesterol reduction therapy should not be assessed with serial calcium imaging.

Decision-making

The treatment decision-making process is listed in Table 2.1.3.

Table 2.1.3 Decision-making table				
Patient's 10-year atherosclerotic cardiovascular disease (ASCVD) risk estimate:	<5%	5–7.5%	>7.5–20%	>20%
Consulting ASCVD risk estimate alone	Statin not recommended	Consider for statin	Recommend statin	Recommend statin
Consulting ASCVD risk estimate + CAC If CAC score = 0 If CAC score >0	Statin not recommended Statin not recommended	Statin not recommended Consider for statin	Statin not recommended Recommend statin	Recommend statin Recommend statin
Does CAC score modify treatment plan?	× CAC not effective in this population	✓ CAC can reclassify risk up or down	✓ CACcan reclassify risk up or down	× CAC not effective in this population

CAC: coronary artery calcium.

Source: Reproduced from Greenland P, Blaha MJ, Budoff MJ, Erbel R, Watson KE. Coronary calcium score and cardiovascular risk. *J Am Coll Cardiol* 2018 Jul 24;72(4):434-477. doi: 10.1016/j.jacc.2018.05.027 with permission from Elsevier.

Further reading

Cury RC, Abbara S, Achenbach S, Agatston A, Berman DS, Budoff MJ, et al. CAD-RADS(TM) Coronary Artery Disease–Reporting and Data System. An expert consensus document of the Society of Cardiovascular Computed Tomography (SCCT), the American College of Radiology (ACR) and the North American Society for Cardiovascular Imaging (NASCI). Endorsed by the American College of Cardiology. *J Cardiovasc Comput Tomogr* 2016; 10: 269–81. Greenland P, Blaha MJ, Budoff MJ, Erbel R, Watson KE. Coronary calcium score and cardiovascular risk. *J Am Coll Cardiol* 2018; 72: 434–47.

Hecht HS, Blaha MJ, Kazerooni EA, Cury RC, Budoff M, Leipsic J, Shaw L. CAC-DRS: Coronary Artery Calcium Data and Reporting System. An expert consensus document of the Society of Cardiovascular Computed Tomography (SCCT). *J Cardiovasc Comput Tomogr* 2018; 12: 185–91.

Mach F, Baigent C, Catapano AL, Koskinas KC, Casula M, Badimon L, et al. 2019 ESC/EAS Guidelines for the management of dyslipidaemias: lipid modification to reduce cardiovascular risk. *Eur Heart J* 2020; 41: 111–88.

Chapter 2.2

Coronary CT angiography interpretation and reporting

Bálint Szilveszter, Csilla Celeng, Richard Takx
and Pál Maurovich-Horvat

Introduction

CT imaging of the heart plays a central role in modern cardiovascular care by providing not only diagnostic information on ischaemic heart disease, but also in refining risk and guiding patient management. Coronary CT angiography (CCTA) allows for the robust assessment of coronary plaque burden, degree of luminal stenosis, and plaque morphology (see Chapter 2.6). A detailed knowledge of cross-sectional cardiac and coronary anatomy is crucial for the accurate interpretation of CCTA images. For details on patient preparation, image acquisition, and postprocessing please see Chapters 1.4–1.6, and for tips to improve image quality see Chapter 1.9.

Anatomy of the coronary arteries

The left ventricular myocardium is supplied by the left (LCA) and right coronary arteries (RCA). This anatomical pattern is quite predictable in humans, while the branching pattern of the coronary arteries may be more variable. Both coronary arteries originate from the aortic sinus (sinus of Valsalva) at the level or slightly below the sinotubular junction; the left and right coronary sinuses are those facing the right ventricular outflow tract anteriorly. Anomalies of coronary origin are discussed separately in Chapter 2.8. The aortic sinus lies embedded between the following structures: right ventricular outflow tract (leftwards anterior), right atrium (to the right), and left atrium (posterior; see Figure 2.2.1).

Left coronary artery

- The LCA runs usually approximately 1–2 cm behind the pulmonary trunk before it bifurcates into the left anterior descending (LAD) and left circumflex artery (LCX). This segment is called left main artery (LMA). Occasionally, it may be very short (Figure 2.2.1A) or missing altogether (separate ostia of LAD and LCX, see Chapter 2.8).

- The LAD is generally the largest coronary artery and runs in the anterior interventricular groove (see Figures 2.2.1B–D and 2.2.2B). The LAD is divided into three segments: the proximal, the mid, and the distal portion (Figure 2.2.2B).

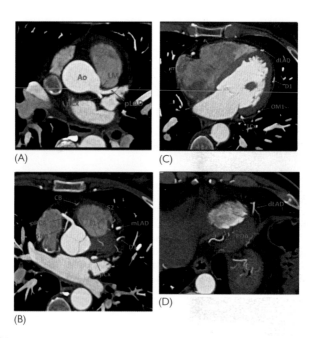

(A) (C)

(B) (D)

Figure 2.2.1 Axial coronary anatomy at (A) the level of left main (LM) artery origin, (B) the level of right coronary artery (RCA) origin, and (C) mid-ventricular and (D) axial level.

Ao: aorta; pCX: proximal circumflex artery; pLAD: proximal left anterior descending artery; CB: conus branch; pRCA: proximal RCA; SNB: sinoatrial nodal artery; S1: first septal branch; S2: second septal branch; D1: first diagonal; mLAD: mid-left anterior descending artery; OM1: first obtuse marginal; AM: acute marginal; dLAD: distal left anterior descending artery; PDA: posterior descending artery.

- The LAD gives two types of branches: the diagonal branches supply the anterolateral myocardium, and the septal branches supply most of the interventricular septum. Branches are ordered numerically from proximal to distal (Figures 2.2.1B, C and 2.2.2B).

- Occasionally, the LMA trifurcates into a third additional branch called the ramus intermedius supplying the basal anterolateral myocardium.

- The LCX runs posteriorly in the atrioventricular groove. Its branches are called obtuse marginal or posterolateral branches, and supply the anterolateral or posterolateral portions of the myocardium, respectively (Figures 2.2.1B, C and 2.2.2B).

Right coronary artery

- The RCA travels first anteriorly and then downwards in the right atrioventricular groove to reach the posterior surface of the heart (Figures 2.2.1A–C and 2.2.2A). It is divided into a proximal, mid, and distal portion.

- Until reaching the crux cordis (the point where the atrioventricular groove and the inferior interventricular groove meet), the RCA gives only small branches (sinus node artery, conus branch; Figure 2.2.2B). Rarely, these branches have their separate origin from the right coronary sinus. The small

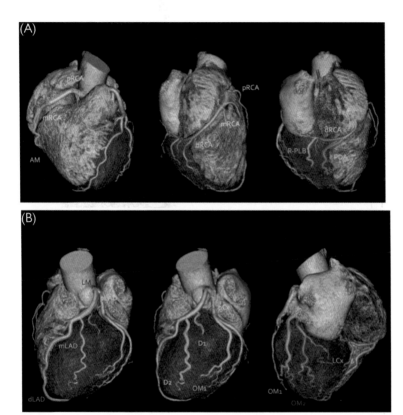

Figure 2.2.2 Three-dimensional coronary anatomy based on volumetric reconstruction coronary CT angiography.

Coronary segments are marked with different colours. (A) The right coronary artery (RCA) originates from the right sinus of Valsalva and runs in the right atrioventricular groove, curving posteriorly at the acute margin of the right ventricle and bifurcating into the posterior descending artery (PDA) and posterolateral branches (PLB) at the crux of the heart. (B) The left main (LM) artery arises from the left sinus of Valsalva and divides into its two main branches, the left anterior descending artery (LAD) and left circumflex artery (LCx).

pRCA: proximal RCA; mRCA: mid-RCA; dRC: distal RCA; R-PLB: right PLB; pLAD: proximal LAD; mLAD: mid-LAD; dLAD: distal LAD; pCX: proximal circumflex artery; D1: first diagonal artery; D2: second diagonal artery; OM1: first obtuse marginal; LCx: left circumflex artery; OM2: second obtuse marginal.

branches supplying the free wall of the right ventricular myocardium are called marginal branches.

- In a right-dominant system, the RCA bifurcates into a posterior descending artery (PDA) and one or more right posterolateral branches when reaching the crux cordis (Figure 2.2.2A). The PDA runs in the inferior interventricular groove and may reach the apex. It supplies small septal perforators the supplying the inferior septal myocardium.

Coronary dominance

The dominance of the coronary circulation is determined by the circulation that gives rise to the PDA and the posterolateral branches. Representative cases of coronary dominance are provided in Figure 2.2.3.

Coronary venous anatomy

- Knowledge of coronary vein anatomy may be important for certain interventional procedures such as cardiac resynchronization therapy, coronary sinus reducer implantation, and indirect mitral annuloplasty procedures.

- The coronary sinus (CS) runs posteriorly in the atrioventricular groove and drains into the right atrium, It collects blood from the great cardiac vein (GCV), the middle cardiac vein and in some cases from marginal or posterolateral venous branches. Occasionally, an enlarged Thebesian valve

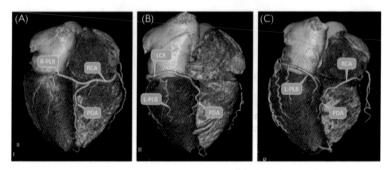

Figure 2.2.3 Representative cases of coronary dominance.

(A) A case with right-dominant coronary system (80–85% of individuals), where the posterior descending artery (PDA) arises from the right coronary artery (RCA). (B) A case with a left-dominant system (15–20% of individuals). (C) A co-dominant circulation is visible, with branches supplying the posterior wall from both the left circumflex (LCx) and RCA epicardial arteries (approximately 1% of the population).

R-PLB: right posterolateral branch; L-PLB: left posterolateral branch.

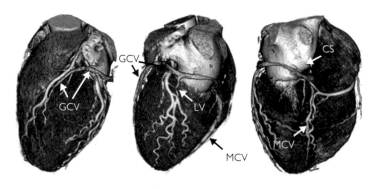

Figure 2.2.4 Anatomy of cardiac veins on three-dimensional CT images.
GCV: great cardiac vein; LV: lateral vein; MCV: middle cardiac vein; CS: coronary sinus.

at the junction of the CS with the right atrium may complicate percutaneous access to the CS.
- The GCV is the longest venous vessel of the heart. It ascends in the anterior interventricular groove and collects blood from the anterior side of the heart.
- The middle cardiac vein or posterior interventricular vein courses near to the posterior interventricular groove beside the PDA.
- The small cardiac vein courses near the right atrioventricular groove and drains directly into the coronary sinus.
- The lateral veins of the heart (also known as obtuse marginal veins) run along the left ventricle and drain into the great cardiac vein or the coronary sinus.

See Figure 2.2.4.

Diagnostic accuracy of CCTA

- The diagnostic accuracy of CCTA has been evaluated in numerous single-centre and a few multicentre studies against the gold standard of invasive coronary angiography (Table 2.2.1). Most of the data are from the era of 64-slice systems.
- Pretest probability (i.e. prevalence of coronary artery disease in the tested population) affects the predictive value of CCTA according to the Bayesian theorem: sensitivity is very high across all studies (usually ≥95%) and the negative predictive value is close to 100% in patients with low-to-intermediate pretest probability.
- Specificity (approximately 85%) and positive predictive value (70–90%) are generally lower.

Study	Sensitivity	Specificity	PPV	NPV	Non-evaluable segments (%)
Miller *et al.* (2008) • 64-slice CT • 291 patients	85	90	91	83	1
Budoff *et al.* (2008) • 64-slice CT • 230 patients	95	83	64	99	1
Meijboom *et al.* (2008) • 64-slice CT • 360 patients	99	64	86	97	0

Table 2.2.1 Multicentre diagnostic coronary CT angiography studies with 64-slice CT

PPV: positive predictive value; NPV: negative predictive value.

- The likelihood ratio (LR) gives a more accurate estimation of post-test probability independent of disease prevalence. Negative LRs are very low (<0.1), particularly for disease of the LMA and LAD.

Guideline recommendations regarding the use of CCTA

Current European recommendations recommend CCTA as a first-line imaging test for CAD, particularly in patients with low-to-intermediate pretest probability of CAD, whenever there is availability of the technique and expertise, and patient suitability criteria are met (class I recommendation; see Figure 2.2.5).

Prognostic value of coronary CT angiography findings

- The presence and extent of CAD is associated with adverse cardiovascular outcome (Figure 2.2.6).
- Besides the high diagnostic accuracy, CCTA is associated with improved cardiac outcomes when it is implemented early in the diagnostic algorithm of patients with suspected CAD (see Figure 2.2.7).
- Risk estimates based on CCTA findings may be useful to initiate appropriate secondary preventive treatment and select patients for revascularization procedures.
- Along with vessel and segment involvement scores, more detailed coronary plaque analysis with CCTA provides additional prognostic features (see Chapter 2.6 for more details).

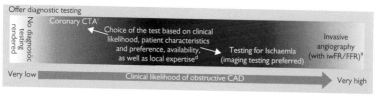

Figure 2.2.5 Recommendations for diagnostic testing in patients with suspected coronary artery disease (CAD) based on pretest probability.

2019 European Society for Cardiology guidelines for the diagnosis and management of chronic coronary syndromes.

iwFR: instantaneous wave-free ratio; FFR: fractional flow reserve.

Source: Knuuti J, Wijns W, Saraste A, et al; ESC Scientific Document Group. (2020) 2019 ESC Guidelines for the diagnosis and management of chronic coronary syndromes. *Eur Heart J*, 41(3):407–477. doi: 10.1093/eurheartj/ehz425. © European Society of Cardiology. Published with permission by Oxford University Press.

Coronary artery segmentation

Coronary segmentation provides a universal language to communicate findings derived from CT angiography (CTA). The modified segmentation scheme provided by the American Heart Association (AHA) is the most commonly used tool to facilitate interdisciplinary communication and to improve diagnosis and treatment of CAD by also reducing intra- and intermodality variability. The evaluation of lesion

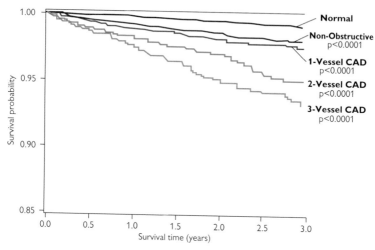

Figure 2.2.6 Follow-up of 24,775 patients undergoing ≥64-detector row coronary CT angiography, based on the CONFIRM registry.

CAD: coronary artery disease.

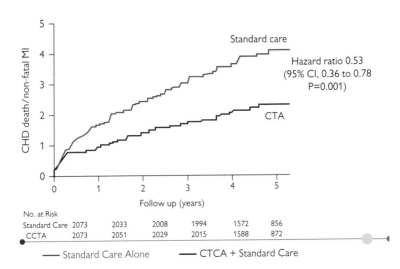

Figure 2.2.7 The SCOT-HEART 5-year follow-up data demonstrated a 47% reduction in death and myocardial infarction with diagnostic algorithm including early coronary CT angiography compared to standard care.

CHD: coronary heart disease; MI: myocardial infarction; CI: confidence interval.

location is also an important step to assess high-risk anatomy or the extent of CAD by calculating segment involvement scores. The modified AHA segmentation system was incorporated in the Society of Cardiovascular Computed Tomography (SCCT) guidelines for the interpretation and reporting of coronary CTA. The nomenclature and segmentation scheme are provided in Figure 2.2.8 and Table 2.2.2.

Reporting

Structured reporting of CCTA involves different components, including the patient's clinical history, technical aspects of image acquisition, and image interpretation. In order to improve interdisciplinary communication of CCTA findings and to guide the management of patients with stable chest pain, the Coronary Artery Disease – Reporting and Data System (CAD-RADS) has been introduced. CAD-RADS categories are based on the SCCT stenosis severity grade. The presence of modifiers (including non-diagnostic segments, stents, grafts, and plaques with adverse features) should also be considered

Structured reporting of coronary CTA should include the following aspects:

1. Clinical history
   Patient demographics, including age, sex, cardiovascular risk factors, and the nature of chest pain should be listed.

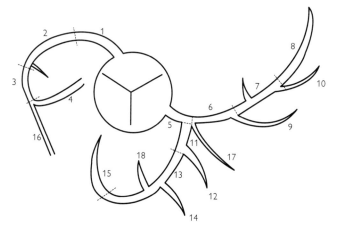

Figure 2.2.8 Axial coronary anatomy.

Coronary segmentation modified after the American Heart Association segmentation scheme used in clinical practice. Segment names are described in Table 2.2.2.

2. Indications

   Beyond the presence of coronary artery disease (CAD), clinical indications can include the evaluation of potential coronary anomalies; anatomy of the great vessels (before left ventricular assist device implantation) and cardiac chambers (patients after cardiac tamponade; congenital anomalies); evaluation of the heart valves (thrombus, calcification); and patency of coronary stents and bypass grafts.

3. Comparison

   If available, CCTA scans should be compared with prior imaging (prior CTA, single-photon emission CT, positron emission tomography, magnetic resonance imaging and echocardiography).

4. Technique and acquisition

   The imaging protocol used, including the assessment of coronary artery calcium score followed by CCTA examination (including contrast injection protocol), should be described. The nature of image acquisition (prospective electrocardiogram triggering or retrospective gating) and heart rate at the time of acquisition should also be denoted. An estimation of radiation dose should be reported (e.g. dose length product or effective dose).

5. Medication

   Administration of prior medications, including beta blockers and nitroglycerin, should be documented.

Table 2.2.2 Segment nomenclature (modified American Heart Association classification)

Segment number	Segment name	Description
1	Proximal RCA	From RCA ostium to half the distance to the acute margin of the heart
2	Mid-RCA	From the end of the proximal RCA segment to the acute margin of the heart
3	Distal RCA	From the end of mid-RCA segment to the origin of PDA
4	RCA–PDA	PDA vessel arising from RCA
16	RCA–PLB	PLB vessel arising from RCA
5	LM	From the origin of LM to bifurcation of LAD and LCx
6	Proximal LAD	From the end of LM to first large septal or diagonal branch (>1.5 mm)
7	Mid-LAD	End of proximal LAD to half of the distance to the apex
8	Distal LAD	End of mid-LAD to end of LAD
9	Diagonal 1	First diagonal branch
10	Diagonal 2	Second diagonal branch
11	Proximal LCx	End of LM to the OM1 origin
12	OM1	First obtuse marginal branch
13	Mid-distal LCx	from OM1 branch to end of LCx or PDA origin
14	OM2	Second obtuse marginal branch
15	LCx–PDA	PDA vessel arising from LCx
17	IM	From LM between LAD and LCx in case of trifurcation
18	LCX- PLB	PLB vessel arising from LCx

RCA: right coronary artery; PDA: posterior descending artery; PLB: posterolateral branches; LM: left main; LAD: left anterior descending artery; LCx: left circumflex artery; OM1: obtuse marginal 1; IM: intermediate artery.

6. Image quality

   Image quality should be checked and potential artefacts (e.g. motion, step, and blooming) should be listed (for a detailed description of artefacts, see Chapter 1.8).

7. Findings

   All coronary segments >1.5 mm in diameter should be graded for stenosis severity. Adverse plaque features, stents, and bypass grafts should be evaluated. Attention should be paid to extracardiac findings (see Chapter 3.15).

8. Interpretation
   - Total calcium score should be reported.
   - CAD-RADS category with management recommendations should be indicated.
   - Relevant extracardiac findings should be listed.

CAD-RADS categories

CAD-RADS categories are based on the SCCT stenosis grading scale (Table 2.2.3).

Interpretation of different CAD-RADS categories

- CAD-RADS 0—absence of CAD:
  - 0% maximal coronary stenosis and no plaque.
- CAD-RADS 1—minimal CAD:
  - 1–24% maximal coronary stenosis = minimal stenosis, or
  - plaque with no stenosis (positive remodelling).
- CAD-RADS 2—CAD with mild maximal stenosis:
  - 25–49% coronary stenosis = mild stenosis.
- CAD-RADS 3—CAD moderate with maximal stenosis:
  - 50–69% coronary stenosis.
- CAD-RADS 4—CAD with severe stenosis:
  - CAD-RADS 4A: 70–99% coronary stenosis;
  - CAD-RADS 4B: left main >50% stenosis or three-vessel obstructive (≥70% stenosis) disease.
- CAD-RADS 5—total coronary occlusion:
  - 100% coronary stenosis = occlusion.
- CAD-RADS N—obstructive CAD cannot be excluded:
  - non-diagnostic study.

Tips for reporting

- Category CAD-RADS 4 does not exists (it is always CAD-RADS 4A or 4B).
- Patients with no, minimal, and mild stenosis, and a non-diagnostic segment >1.5 mm, should be graded as CAD-RADS N, as CTA cannot be used to guide further management. Patients with a moderate or higher degree of stenosis should be graded as, for example, CAD-RADS 3/N, as additional evaluation (functional test or invasive coronary angiography) is needed.

Table 2.2.3 Society of Cardiovascular Computed Tomography grading scale for stenosis severity	
Degree of stenosis (%)	Terminology
0	No visible stenosis
1–24	Minimal stenosis
25–49	Mild stenosis
50–69	Moderate stenosis
70–99	Severe stenosis
100	Total occlusion

CAD-RADS modifiers

Four modifiers can be added to the CAD-RADS category (Table 2.2.4): N (non-diagnostic); S (stent); G (graft); and V (vulnerable plaque).

These are listed after the CAD-RADS category with the use of symbol/(slash).

Tips for reporting

- CAD-RADS 1/N or 2/N do not exist (non-diagnostic segments are indicated from CAD-RADS 3 and higher).
- Modifier 'V' (vulnerable plaque) denotes the presence of low attenuation plaque, positive remodelling, napkin-ring sign, and spotty calcification. If two of these features are present, modifier 'V' should be added to the CAD-RADS category.

Key teaching messages

- Coronary CCTA has recently been established as a first-line test for patients with stable chest pain and a low-to-intermediate clinical likelihood of obstructive CAD.
- CCTA is considered to be an excellent gatekeeper for invasive angiography, with high sensitivity and a negative predictive value. In patients with a high pretest likelihood, CCTA may yield false-positive results.
- In clinical practice the degree of stenosis caused by the plaque is described visually for each coronary segment (see Chapter 2.6).
  - CTA provides information on the extent of the disease (e.g. segment involvement score), plaque type (e.g. calcified, partially calcified, or non-calcified), adverse plaque features (e.g. positive remodelling, low attenuation, and napkin ring sign), or the location (e.g. high-risk anatomy, left main artery

Table 2.2.4 CAD-RADS modifiers

	Definition	Coronary CTA	Modifier
Low Attenuation plaque	Plaque <30 HU	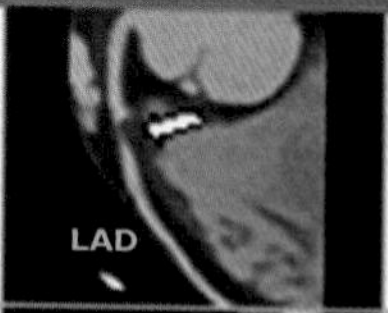 LAD	V
Positive remodeling	Outward growth of the plaque with preservation of the lumen	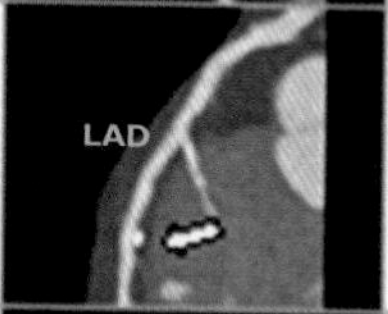 LAD	V
Napkin ring sign	Central low attenuation adjacent to the lumen and a higher "ring like" attenuation around	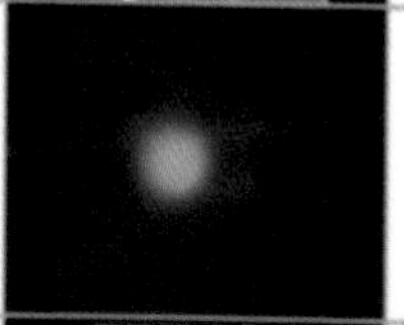	V
Spotty calcification	Small calcifications ≤3 mm and >130 HU	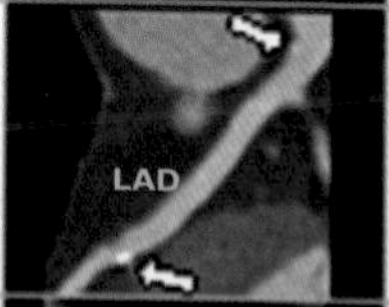 LAD	V
Stent	Always the highest stenosis degree should be reported regardless the location (stent or lumen)	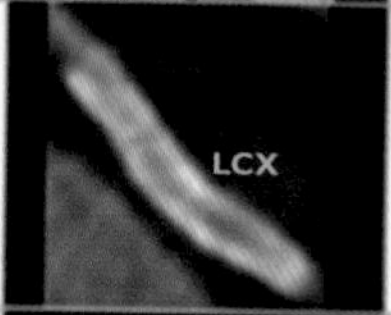 LCX	S
Graft	Always the highest stenosis degree should be reported regardless the location (graft or lumen)	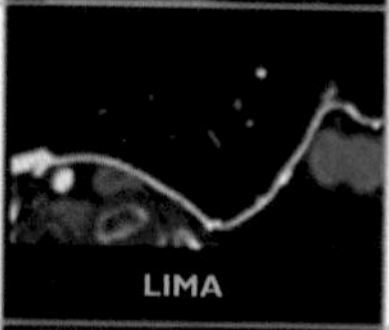 LIMA	G
Non evaluable segment	CAD RADS 0, 1, 2: CAD RADS N CAD RADS 3 etc.... CAD RADS 3/N	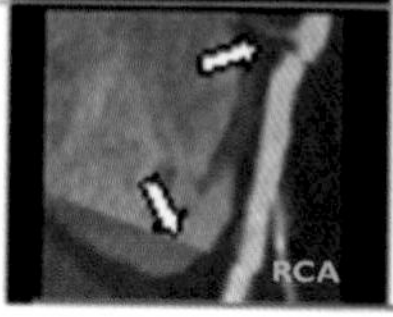 RCA	N

CTA: CT angiography; HU: Hounsfield units; LAD: left anterior descending artery; LCx: left circumflex artery; LIMA: left internal mammary artery; RCA: right coronary artery.

Key teaching messages

109

stenosis, and three-vessel disease) and severity (e.g. segment stenosis score) of CAD.

- The addition of CCTA to standard care in the evaluation of contemporary patients with stable chest pain can reduce adverse events by guiding secondary prevention therapy (e.g. lipid-lowering therapies) and identifying high-risk patients for invasive angiography.
- Structured reporting platforms and CAD-RADS classification in the reporting of CCTA findings could enhance interdisciplinary communication.

References

Budoff MJ, Dowe D, Jollis JG, Gitter M, Sutherland J, Halamert E, et al. Diagnostic performance of 64-multidetector row coronary computed tomographic angiography for evaluation of coronary artery stenosis in individuals without known coronary artery disease: results from the prospective multicenter ACCURACY (Assessment by Coronary Computed Tomographic Angiography of Individuals Undergoing Invasive Coronary Angiography) trial. J Am Coll Cardiol 2008; 52: 1724–32.

Meijboom WB, Meijs MFL, Schuijf JD, Cramer MJ, Mollet NR, van Mieghem CAG, et al. Diagnostic accuracy of 64-slice computed tomography coronary angiography: a prospective, multicenter, multivendor study. J Am Coll Cardiol 2008; 52: 2135–44.

Miller JM, Rochitte CE, Dewey M, Arbab-Zadeh A, Niinuma H, Gottlieb I, et al. Diagnostic performance of coronary angiography by 64-row CT. N Engl J Med 2008; 359: 2324–36.

Further reading

Cury RC, Abbara S, Achenbach S, et al. Coronary Artery Disease-Reporting and Data System (CAD-RADS): An expert consensus document of SCCT, ACR and NASCI: Endorsed by the ACC. JACC Cardiovasc Imaging 2016;9(9):1099–113.

Knuuti J, Wijns W, Saraste A, Capodanno D, Barbato E, Funck-Brentano C, et al. 2019 ESC Guidelines for the diagnosis and management of chronic coronary syndromes: the Task Force for the diagnosis and management of chronic coronary syndromes of the European Society of Cardiology (ESC). Eur Heart J 2020; 41: 407–77.

Chapter 2.3

How to apply coronary CT angiography in patients with stable chest pain

Tessa Genders

Teaching points

- Coronary CT angiography (CCTA) is an excellent first-line diagnostic test for patients with stable chest pain without high-risk features.
- If the pretest probability (PTP) of coronary artery disease (CAD) is low-to-intermediate, a negative CCTA reliably excludes the presence of obstructive CAD.
- CCTA with a computed fractional flow reserve can provide a comprehensive anatomical and functional assessment of CAD, which allows for selective referral to invasive coronary angiography for patients who are most likely to benefit from revascularization.

Introduction

For many years, functional tests such as exercise electrocardiogram (ECG), nuclear stress testing, and stress echocardiography have been the cornerstone modalities in the diagnostic work-up of patients with stable chest pain. However, over the past decade, CCTA has established itself as a reliable alternative and is often the preferred test.

- The 2019 European Society of Cardiology guidelines for the diagnosis and management of chronic coronary syndromes recommend CCTA as a first-line diagnostic test in patient with stable chest pain and a low-to-intermediate pretest probability of CAD.
- The UK's National Institute for Health and Care Excellence recommends CCTA as the first-line test in all patients with stable chest pain, except in those with non-anginal chest pain and a normal resting ECG.
- The 2021 American Heart Association/American College of Cardiology guidelines for the evaluation and diagnosis of chest pain recommend CCTA or ischaemia imaging in patients with stable chest pain and an intermediate-to-high pretest probability of CAD (favouring CCTA over ischaemia imaging in patients <65 years of age).

Whom to test

The first step in the diagnostic approach for a patient with chest pain is to differentiate an acute coronary syndrome (unstable angina or acute myocardial infarction (MI)) from a chronic coronary syndrome due to stable coronary artery disease (CAD). Patients are considered to have stable chest pain in the absence of the following: symptoms at rest; rapidly progressive symptoms; recent onset of moderate-to-severe symptoms; and significantly elevated troponin levels. After careful history-taking, physical examination, resting ECG, and laboratory evaluation, the PTP of CAD in a patient with stable chest pain should be considered as it determines whether to test and which test to use (Figure 2.3.1). The predictive value of a diagnostic test depends on the disease prevalence within a population. The probability of CAD in an individual patient with stable chest pain can be calculated based on age, sex, and type of chest pain (see Table 2.3.1).

Chest pain is classified as:
- Typical chest pain
  1. Substernal chest discomfort.
  2. Precipitated by exertion or emotional stress.
  3. Relieved by rest or sublingual nitroglycerin.
- Atypical chest pain: meets two of the above criteria.
- Non-anginal chest pain: meets one or none of the above criteria.

The need for diagnostic testing depends on the PTP of CAD (see Figure 2.3.2).
- PTP <5% (very low): further cardiac testing can be deferred safely.
- PTP 5–15% (low): consider non-invasive testing in the presence of cardiovascular risk factors (e.g. hypertension, hyperlipidaemia, diabetes mellitus, family history of premature CAD, smoking, or other risk factors) and other clinical parameters such as the presence of resting ECG abnormalities, left ventricular systolic dysfunction, or extensive coronary artery calcification.
- PTP 15–85% (intermediate): non-invasive testing is most useful (CCTA or ischaemia imaging should be considered).
- PTP >85% (high): direct referral to invasive coronary angiography (ICA) is reasonable, especially in the setting of severe symptoms, symptoms despite optimal medical management, or in the presence of left ventricular systolic dysfunction.

Diagnostic performance of coronary CT angiography in patients with stable chest pain

Based on a meta-analysis that included 65 studies with a total of 5332 patients with known or suspected CAD and a clinical indication for ICA, CCTA demonstrated

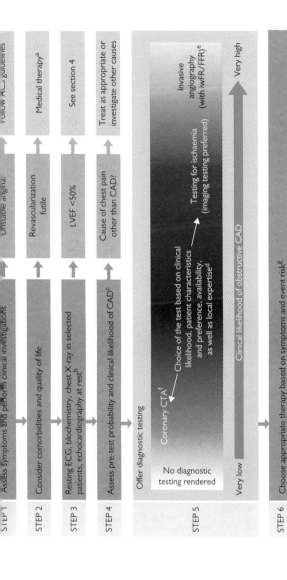

Figure 2.3.1 Approach for the initial diagnostic management of patients with chest pain.

ACS: acute coronary syndrome; ECG: electrocardiogram; LVEF: left ventricular ejection fraction; CAD: coronary artery disease; CTA: computed tomography angiography; iwFR: instantaneous wave-free ratio; FFR: fractional flow reserve. [a]If the diagnosis of CAD is uncertain, establishing a diagnosis using non-invasive functional imaging for myocardial ischaemia before treatment may be reasonable. [b]May be omitted in very young and healthy patients with a high suspicion of an extracardiac cause of chest pain, and in multimorbid patients in whom the echocardiographic result has no consequence for further patient management. [c]Consider exercise ECG to assess symptoms, arrhythmias, exercise tolerance, blood pressure response, and event risk in selected patients. [d]Ability to exercise, individual test-related risks, and likelihood of obtaining diagnostic test result. [e]High clinical likelihood and symptoms inadequately responding to medical treatment, high event risk based on clinical evaluation (such as ST segment depression, combined with symptoms at a low workload or systolic dysfunction indicating CAD), or uncertain diagnosis on non-invasive testing. [f]Functional imaging for myocardial ischaemia if coronary CTA has shown CAD of uncertain grade or is non-diagnostic. [g]Consider also angina without obstructive disease in the epicardial coronary arteries.

Source: Knuuti J, Wijns W, Saraste A, et al; ESC Scientific Document Group. (2020) 2019 ESC Guidelines for the diagnosis and management of chronic coronary syndromes. Eur Heart J, 41(3):407–477. doi: 10.1093/eurheartj/ehz425. © European Society of Cardiology. Published with permission by Oxford University Press.

Table 2.3.1 Pretest probability of obstructive coronary artery disease as recommended by the 2019 European Society of Cardiology guideline for the management of chronic coronary syndromes, based on a pooled analysis

Age	Typical chest pain (%)		Atypical chest pain (%)		Non-anginal chest pain (%)		Dyspnoea (%)	
	Men	Women	Men	Women	Men	Women	Men	Women
30–39	3	5	4	3	1	1	0	3
40–49	22	10	10	6	3	2	12	3
50–59	32	13	17	6	11	3	20	9
60–69	44	16	26	11	22	6	27	14
70+	52	27	34	19	24	10	32	12

Cells in white represent pretest probabilities <5%, light blue 5–15%, and dark blue >15%.

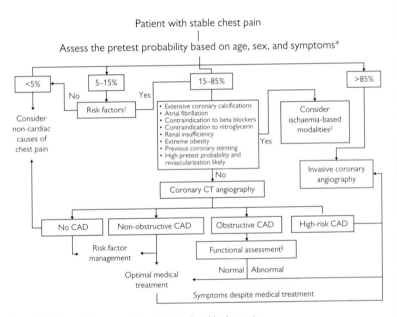

Figure 2.3.2 Diagnostic approach for patients with stable chest pain.

CT: computed tomography; CAD: coronary artery disease. *See Table 2.3.1, based on contemporary pooled analysis as recommended by the European Society of Cardiology. †Risk factors: hypertension, hyperlipidaemia, diabetes mellitus, family history of premature CAD, or smoking. ‡Nuclear stress testing, stress echocardiography, stress magnetic resonance imaging, or stress positron-emission tomography CT perfusion imaging. §Assessing the functional severity of an intermediate stenosis can be done with CT-based fractional flow reserve, CT myocardial perfusion imaging, or any other ischaemia-based imaging modality.

a sensitivity of 95% and a specificity of 79% for the diagnosis of obstructive CAD defined as the presence of >50% stenosis on ICA. Based on subgroup analysis, it was found that the positive predictive value of CCTA is ≥50% in patients with a PTP as low as 7%, and that the post-test probability of CAD is <15% with a negative CCTA in patients with a PTP of up to 67%.

Strengths and weaknesses of coronary CT angiography in stable coronary artery disease

See Table 2.3.2.

Table 2.3.2 Strengths and weaknesses of coronary CT angiography (CCTA) in stable coronary artery disease (CAD)	
Strengths	Implication
High sensitivity (>95%) and very high negative predictive value	A patient with a low-to-intermediate pretest probability and a negative CCTA can be reassured that their symptoms are not due to epicardial CAD
Direct visualization of the coronary anatomy, including vessel wall and plaque characteristics	Provides prognostic information and opportunities for risk factor optimization. Identification of high-risk CAD such as critical left main disease or triple-vessel CAD allows for a prompt referral to ICA
CT-based fractional flow reserve can provide information about the haemodynamic significance of intermediate lesions	When obstructive (but not high-risk) CAD is identified, further assessment of the haemodynamic significance of the findings should be pursued, as the mere presence of obstructive CAD is a poor predictor of ischaemia
Weaknesses	
Disease severity may be overestimated in the presence of extensive coronary calcification	In patients with extensive coronary artery calcification (either seen on prior imaging or found during CCTA), other imaging modalities should be considered
Image quality depends on technical and patient factors	Tachycardia, irregular heart rhythms, obesity, and prior coronary stents significantly reduce image quality and diagnostic performance of CCTA
The need for intravenous contrast carries the risk of CIN	In patients with renal insufficiency, the risk of contrast-induced nephropathy is increased, and alternative imaging modalities should be considered

ICA: invasive coronary angiography; CIN: contrast-induced neuropathy.

Outcomes of coronary CT angiography as a first-line diagnostic test in stable chest pain

Several randomized clinical trials (RCTs) have studied the value of CCTA in the evaluation of patients with stable chest pain.

- The PROspective Multicenter Imaging Study for Evaluation of chest pain (PROMISE) randomized 10,003 symptomatic patients without known CAD to a strategy of initial anatomical testing with CCTA or to functional testing (exercise ECG, nuclear stress testing, or stress echocardiography). The authors found no difference in the primary endpoint of death, MI, hospitalization for unstable angina, or major procedural complication at a median of 2 years of follow-up (3.3% vs. 3.0%, $P = 0.75$) but an increased rate of ICA (12.2% vs. 8.1%).
- SCOT-HEART randomized 4146 patients with chest pain to standard care plus CCTA versus standard care alone. Standard care generally included stress ECG. The primary endpoint of 'diagnostic certainty' was significantly increased, whereas the secondary endpoint including fatal and non-fatal MIs was non-significantly decreased in the CCTA arm (26 vs. 42; hazard ratio 0.62, 95% confidence interval 0.38–1.01 ($P = 0.0527$)). Subsequent 5-year follow-up of SCOT-HEART demonstrated a significantly lower rate of non-fatal MI for patients randomized to the standard care plus CCTA arm.
- A meta-analysis combining PROMISE, SCOT-HEART, and two other RCTs found that the use of CCTA versus functional stress testing did not reduce mortality or cardiac hospitalizations, but lowered the incidence of MI and increased the rates of ICA and revascularization.

Functional assessment of patients with coronary disease severity on CT angiography

- In some, but not all, studies, anatomy-based testing with CCTA increased the rates of ICA and revascularization, raising concern over unnecessary procedures.
- In patients with stable chest pain, functional testing including invasive fractional flow reserve (FFR) can be used to assess whether a lesion is flow-limiting, which predicts whether the patient will benefit from revascularization.
- CCTA can be combined with CT-based fractional flow reserve or CT perfusion imaging to improve the specificity of CCTA. The ability to assess whether an intermediate lesion is flow limiting reduces the rates of ICA and revascularization.

Further reading

Foy AJ, Dhruva SS, Peterson B, Mandrola JM, Morgan DJ, Redberg RF. Coronary computed tomography angiography vs functional stress testing for patients with suspected coronary artery disease: a systematic review and meta-analysis. *JAMA Intern Med* 2017; 177: 1623–1631.

Haase R, Schlattmann P, Gueret P, Andreini D, Pontone G, Alkadhi H, et al. Diagnosis of obstructive coronary artery disease using computed tomography angiography in patients with stable chest pain depending on clinical probability and in clinically important subgroups: meta-analysis of individual patient data. *BMJ* 2019; 365: l1945.

Juarez-Orozco LE, Saraste A, Capodanno D, Prescott E, Ballo H, Bax JJ, et al. Impact of a decreasing pre-test probability on the performance of diagnostic tests for coronary artery disease. *Eur Heart J Cardiovasc Imaging* 2019; 20: 1198–207.

Knuuti J, Wijns W, Saraste A, Capodanno D, Barbato E, Funck-Brentano C, et al. 2019 ESC Guidelines for the diagnosis and management of chronic coronary syndromes: the Task Force for the diagnosis and management of chronic coronary syndromes of the European Society of Cardiology (ESC). *Eur Heart J* 2020; 41: 407–77.

Chapter 2.4

CT-based fractional flow reserve

Domenico Mastrodicasa

Teaching points

- CT-derived fractional flow reserve (CT-FFR) is a postprocessing technique that utilizes the principles of computational fluid dynamics to compute catheter-based FFR from coronary CT angiography (CCTA).

- CT-FFR analysis is helpful when the CCTA reveals stenosis of unclear haemodynamic significance and the results are expected to alter clinical management.

- A coronary lesion is considered to be flow limiting when the corresponding CT-FFR is ≤0.80.

- Adequate beta-blockade and sublingual nitrates are crucial to ensure high image quality and high diagnostic accuracy of CT-FFR.

- CT-FFR should be measured 1–2 cm distal to the lower end of the coronary stenosis.

- CT-FFR is not feasible in stented vessels or bypass grafts.

- Currently, a single solution for remotely performed CT-FFR (HeartFlow, Inc.) is clinically available. Several on-site solutions for CT-FFR calculations are being developed by various manufacturers but are not yet clinically available.

Principles of CT-derived fractional flow reserve

- The fractional flow reserve (FFR) is the pressure ratio between the coronary artery (distal to a stenosis) and the aortic root during maximal microvascular dilation.

- Traditional FFR is measured during invasive coronary angiography and requires infusion of adenosine to induce hyperaemia.

- CT-derived FFR (CT-FFR) is a postprocessing technique using coronary CT angiography (CCTA) to compute FFR non-invasively and inform treatment decisions.

- CT-FFR applies the principles of computational fluid dynamics to the patient-specific anatomical three-dimensional model of the coronary tree extracted from an individual high-resolution CCTA. The flow simulations (Navier–Stokes equations) rely on physiological principles to estimate resting blood flow (based on myocardial mass), coronary branch flow (based on Murray's law), and the effects of maximal hyperaemia.

- CT-FFR can be computed and displayed at any point along the coronary vessels.
- CT-FFR does not require the administration of adenosine or specific changes in the standard CCTA protocol.

CT-derived fractional flow reserve (FFR) versus invasive FFR

- CT-FFR correlates with invasive FFR (r = 0.82) with a small systematic underestimation (mean difference 0.03) and slight overestimation of haemodynamic severity.
- Reported sensitivity and specificity for the detection of FFR-positive lesions are 91.2% and 93.5%, respectively.
- If compared to a binary reference (invasive FFR ≤0.80) the probability of discordance increases for values closer to the threshold. CT-FFR results between approximately 0.70 and 0.85 should be considered with more caution, and all results should be interpreted in the individual clinical context.

Clinical use of CT-derived fractional flow reserve

- Stable chest pain and suspected coronary artery disease (CAD), in the presence of potentially significant lesions on CCTA, generally >40% diameter stenosis, when the results are expected to alter clinical management (see Figure 2.4.1).

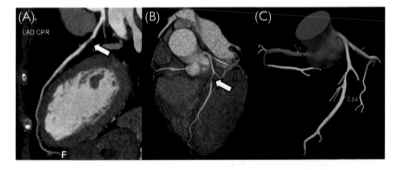

Figure 2.4.1 Coronary CT angiography of a 57-year-old woman with typical angina (Agatston score 0).

(A) Curved multiplanar reformation (CPR) and (B) three-dimensional (3D) volume rendering of the left anterior descending artery (LAD) shows moderate (50–69% diameter stenosis), potentially obstructive stenosis just distal to the first diagonal branch (Coronary Artery Disease – Reporting and Data System (CAD-RADS) 3; arrow). (C) 3D coronary tree with colour overlay showing CT-derived fractional flow reserve values. A value of 0.84 was calculated 10–20 mm distal to the stenosis, indicating a non-obstructive lesion. No further testing was needed.

- Exclusion of haemodynamically significant coronary stenosis in patients presenting with chest pain in the Emergency Department—after an acute coronary syndrome has been ruled out.

CT-derived fractional flow reserve contraindications

- Contraindications to CCTA.
- Inadequate CCTA quality.
- Acute coronary syndrome (not ruled out) or clinical instability.
- Recent history of myocardial infarction (<4 weeks).
- History of surgical or percutaneous coronary revascularization. After percutaneous coronary intervention, CT-FFR may be possible in the non-stented vessels.
- Coronary anomalies and/or congenital heart disease.
- Coronary occlusion.

Severe coronary calcifications complicate accurate delineation of the coronary lumen, which affects both visual interpretation and flow simulations. The presence of calcifications does not preclude CT-FFR; however, overall accuracy will gradually decrease with higher calcium scores.

CT scanner requirements and patient preparation

- The feasibility of a CT-FFR analysis depends on high-quality CCTA images.
- CCTA should be performed on a 64-slice CT scanner or more advanced system.
- The administration of beta-blockers and nitroglycerin is strongly recommended to obtain a heart rate <65 beats per minute, to reduce cardiac motion artefacts, and to optimize coronary artery visualization.

Interpretation of CT-derived fractional flow reserve results

- In general, a coronary lesion is considered to be flow limiting when the corresponding CT-FFR is ≤0.80. However, for more detailed clinical decision-making, see Table 2.4.1.
- CT-FFR should be measured 1–2 cm downstream to the distal end of the coronary stenosis of interest (Figures 2.4.2 and 2.4.3).
- Even in the absence of coronary atherosclerosis, CT-FFR values gradually decrease from proximal to distally. Distal CT-FFR measurements should not be used for decision-making regarding proximal coronary stenoses.
- CT-FFR should be interpreted while looking at the original CCTA findings to relate the anatomical CCTA findings with lesion-specific CT-FFR values and consideration of all the available clinical information.

Table 2.4.1 CT-derived fractional flow reserve (CT-FFR) threshold for clinical decision-making

CT-FFR	Likelihood of flow limitation coronary stenosis*	Clinical decision-making
≥0.80	Low	• Optimal medical treatment • No further downstream testing required
0.75–0.80	Borderline-possible, 'grey zone'	• Additional integration with clinical and imaging factors is required (i.e. symptoms, plaque morphology, and lesion location)
<0.75	High	• Consider invasive angiography and revascularization • In small vessels, distal lesions or side branches: consider optimal medical therapy instead of referral to invasive angiography

*Because of fundamental methodological differences between techniques that test myocardial ischaemia, a degree of discordance close to a binary threshold for haemodynamic significance will be unavoidable.

• CT-FFR is not contraindicated in the presence of calcifications, although manual or automatic corrections of the lumen segmentation are needed to account for the blooming artefact. Extensive coronary calcification increases the uncertainty of the CT-FFR results.

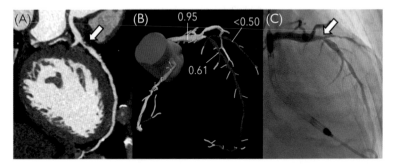

Figure 2.4.2 Coronary CT angiography of a 75-year-old man with heart failure (left ventricular ejection fraction 23%; Agatston score 309).

(A) Curved multiplanar reformation of the left anterior descending artery shows a moderate-to-severe (70–99%) stenosis in the proximal segment caused by a mostly non-calcified plaque (Coronary Artery Disease – Reporting and Data System (CAD-RADS) 4; arrow). (B) FFR$_{CT}$ three-dimensional model shows a CT-derived fractional flow reserve (CT-FFR) value of 0.61, indicating a haemodynamically significant lesion. (C) Subsequently, the patient underwent invasive coronary angiography to have a stent placed.

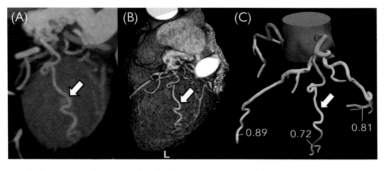

Figure 2.4.3 Coronary CT angiography of a 72-year-old woman with dyspnoea on exertion (Agatston score 161).

(A) Maximum intensity projection and (B) volume rendering of the ramus intermedius (RI) show a convoluted course on the left ventricle surface and no stenosis. (c) FFR_{CT}, three-dimensional model of the left anterior descending artery, RI (arrow), and circumflex arteries reveals a distal CT-derived fractional flow reserve (CT-FFR) value of 0.89, 0.72, and 0.81, respectively. The CT-FFR in the RI gradually decreases along the vessel and goes below the 0.80 threshold in the distal end. It is not recommended that the low distal CT-FFR measurement is used for clinical decision-making in the absence of lesion-specific pressure loss.

CT-derived fractional flow reserve report

• The results of CT-FFR must always be evaluated in the clinical context of the patient, considering symptoms, coronary anatomy, suitability of revascularization, and patient preferences (Table 2.4.2).

Table 2.4.2 When and how to report CT-derived fractional flow reserve (CT-FFR) findings	
CCTA and CT-FFR findings	Recommendations on reporting
Minimal (1–24%) or mild (25–49%) stenosis	CT-FFR generally not necessary, but may be considered for borderline lesions in the proximal vessels
Moderate (50–69%) and severe (>70% to 99%) stenosis	Provide CT-FFR values for all lesions (see Figures 2.4.1 and 2.4.2)
Serial coronary lesions	CT-FFR should be reported 10–20 mm distal to each lesion. If not possible, then provide CT-FFR values and the distance between stenosis and the site of the CT-FFR measured
CT-FFR ≤0.80 in the distal coronary tree in the absence of lesion-specific pressure loss	If CT-FFR values are reported, adequate context should be provided to avoid misinterpretation

- Report the presence of a low, borderline, or high likelihood of haemodynamic significance (Table 2.4.1) of the lesions identified in the impression of the original CCTA report.
- Ideally, the CCTA and CT-FFR reports are combined in a single uniform report that will most clearly relate anatomical and functional information.
- Given the time gap between CCTA and CT-FFR results, a preliminary CCTA report may be initially released. An addendum could be later integrated in the original CCTA report when the CT-FFR results are available.

Clinical availability and European guidelines

- To date, HeartFlow Analysis (HeartFlow, Redwood City, CA, USA) is the only US Food and Drug Administration-approved CT-FFR technique.
- Since 2017, the National Institute for Health and Care Excellence's (NICE) chest pain guidelines have recommended HeartFlow Analysis as a safe approach with high diagnostic accuracy to determine the impact of a coronary stenosis on blood flow in patients with recent-onset, stable chest pain. NICE established that CT-FFR may avoid the need for invasive investigations and be potentially cost-saving.
- The 2019 European Society of Cardiology guidelines on chronic coronary syndromes classified CCTA as a Class 1 recommendation for diagnosing CAD in symptomatic patients. CT-FFR may be used as an add-on to CCTA to improve clinical decision-making.

Further reading

Coenen A, Kim YH, Kruk M, Tesche C, De Geer J, Kurata A, et al. Diagnostic accuracy of a machine-learning approach to coronary computed tomographic angiography-based fractional flow reserve: result from the MACHINE Consortium. *Circ Cardiovasc Imaging* 2018; 11: e007217.

Cook CM, Petraco R, Shun-Shin MJ, Ahmad Y, Nijjer S, Al-Lamee R, et al. Diagnostic accuracy of computed tomography-derived fractional flow reserve: a systematic review. *JAMA Cardiol* 2017; 2: 803–10.

Knuuti J, Wijns W, Saraste A, Capodanno D, Barbato E, Funck-Brentano C, et al. 2019 ESC Guidelines for the diagnosis and management of chronic coronary syndromes: the Task Force for the diagnosis and management of chronic coronary syndromes of the European Society of Cardiology (ESC). *Eur Heart J* 2020; 41: 407–77.

National Institute for Health and Care Excellence. Chest pain. Available at: https://cks.nice.org.uk/topics/chest-pain/ (accessed 22 June 2022).

Nørgaard BL, Fairbairn TA, Safian RD, Rabbat MG, Ko B, Jensen JM, et al. Coronary CT angiography-derived fractional flow reserve testing in patients with stable coronary artery disease: recommendations on interpretation and reporting. *Radiol Cardiothorac Imaging* 2019; 1: e190050.

CT myocardial perfusion and scar imaging

Koen Nieman and Gianluca Pontone

> **Teaching points**
>
> - Stress myocardial perfusion imaging using vasodilator-mediated hyperaemia allows for the identification of inducible myocardial ischaemia.
> - Static perfusion protocols can be performed on most cardiac CT systems and will demonstrate reduced myocardial enhancement in a qualitative manner.
> - Dynamic perfusion protocols require dedicated CT systems but can quantify the myocardial blood flow.
> - Late-enhancement CT imaging can demonstrate acute or chronic myocardial infarction.
> - Currently, myocardial perfusion and scar imaging are not widely applied in clinical practice.

125

Introduction

The identification of inducible myocardial ischaemia and viability are important for the diagnosis, risk stratification, and management of coronary artery disease (CAD). Similar to other perfusion imaging techniques, cardiac CT can visualize differences in myocardial blood flow during induced hyperaemia to indicate haemodynamically significant CAD. Based on the same principles as late gadolinium enhancement by magnetic resonance imaging (MRI), cardiac CT can demonstrate myocardial scar.

Myocardial perfusion imaging

- Myocardial blood flow is regulated by the (vasoconstrictive) resistance in the small coronary vessels and can be increased up to fourfold to meet increased demand.
- Even in the presence of obstructive CAD, at rest, adequate perfusion will be maintained through autoregulation of the peripheral resistance, unless severe ischaemia and resting angina are present.

Table 2.5.1 Vasodilators for CT myocardial perfusion imaging

	Adenosine	Regadenoson	Dipyridamole
Mechanism	Adenosine receptor A2A agonist	Selective adenosine receptor A2A agonist	Blocks reuptake of endogenous adenosine
Dose	140 µg/kg/min, 3–6 min (continue during scan)	0.4 mg	140 µg/kg/min, 4 min
Duration of action	Immediate onset	Peaks at 1–4 min	Effect peaks at 7–15 min
Half-life	<5 s	30 min	30–45 min
Side effects	Chest discomfort, bronchospasm, AV block, sinus arrhythmia	Dyspnoea, headache, and flushing	Chest discomfort, bronchospasm, AV block
Contraindications	Bronchospasm, second- or third-degree AV block or sick sinus syndrome (unless protected by pacemaker)	Second- or third-degree AV block or sick sinus syndrome (unless protected by pacemaker). Caution for bronchospasm	Bronchospasm, second or third-degree AV block or sick sinus syndrome (unless protected by pacemaker)

AV: atrioventricular

- During exercise or pharmacological vasodilation blood flow to myocardial territories supplied by obstructed coronary vessels cannot sufficiently increase.
- Lower myocardial blood flow results in reduced enhancement on CT images after contrast injection.
- Myocardial perfusion imaging (MPI) by CT (MPI$_{CT}$) generally requires intravenous vasodilators (Table 2.5.1):
  - stimulation of the adenosine receptors causes hyperaemia (A2A receptor), atrioventricular conduction delay (A1), and bronchospasm (other);
  - regadenoson selectively stimulates the A2A receptor;
  - side effects include a slight increase in heart rate and a slight decrease in blood pressure, chest discomfort and flushing (both more with adenosine), dyspnoea (more with regadenoson), headache, ST segment changes, dizziness, and nausea;
  - severe complications (myocardial infarction (MI), bronchospasm) are rare.
  - theophylline or aminophylline are an antidote to vasodilators and expedite the normalization of side effects.

Scan techniques

- *Static* perfusion imaging (Figure 2.5.1): acquisition of one data set to capture instantaneous differences in myocardial attenuation during the first pass of contrast medium (Figure 2.5.2).

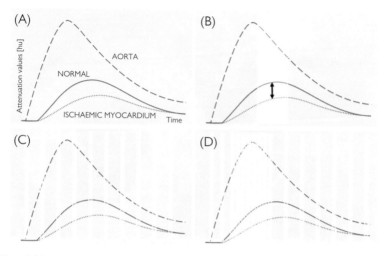

Figure 2.5.1 (A) Enhancement (CT attenuation values) in the aorta, and the normal and ischaemic myocardium during the first pass of a contrast medium. (B) For static perfusion imaging a single data set is acquired and the attenuation difference between normal and ischaemic myocardium can be assessed visually. Dynamic perfusion imaging by shuttle mode on a (C) dual-source CT system and (D) using a varying sample rate on a wide detector array CT system for repeated sampling and quantitative perfusion parameters.

HU: Hounsfield units.

Figure 2.5.2 Static stress myocardial perfusion imaging.

(A) Critical stenoses at the proximal left anterior descending artery (LAD). (B) Dominant left circumflex artery (LCx) and (C) right coronary artery (RCA) free of relevant stenoses. (D–G) Left ventricular short-axis images (D, E) and long-axis images (F, G) showing, after adenosine administration, stress myocardial perfusion defects at the mid-to-apical anteroseptum and anterior walls. (H, I) Internal carotid artery with fractional flow reserve showing no relevant stenoses at the RCA and dominant LCx, and critical stenoses at the proximal LAD.

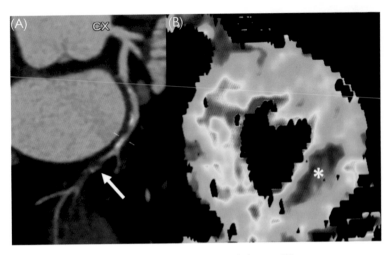

Figure 2.5.3 Dynamic CT myocardial perfusion imaging using dual-source CT system.

(A) CT angiography shows diffuse disease of the dominant left circumflex branch. (B) The myocardial blood flow map shows a blue area (*) of low myocardial blood flow in the inferolateral wall consistent with the perfusion territory of the left circumflex branch (CX).

- Scan protocol similar to coronary CT angiography (CCTA), with a comparable radiation dose.
- Timing of the scan: scans are performed using bolus tracking and visual assessments to time image acquisition
- Dual-energy techniques can be applied to enhance the iodine concentration and contrast between the ischaemic and normal myocardium.
- *Dynamic* perfusion imaging: acquisition of multiple low-resolution scans to plot the regional myocardial enhancement during first-pass over 30–35 seconds, from which quantitative measures of myocardial perfusion can be calculated (Figure 2.5.3).
  - Correction of beam hardening and motion/displacement is essential for accurate and consistent sampling of the myocardial attenuation.
  - Current *dual-source CT systems* with a limited longitudinal range apply a shuttle mode technique for alternated acquisition of the cranial and caudal sections, and a net sampling rate of 1:4 heart cycles (Figure 2.5.3).
  - *Wide-array CT systems* that cover the entire left ventricle use a stationary axial scan mode. The sampling rate is potentially every heart

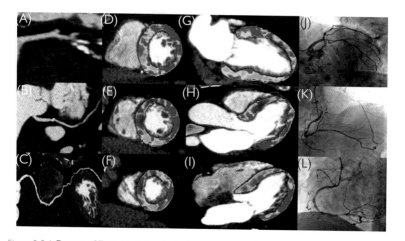

Figure 2.5.4 Dynamic CT myocardial perfusion imaging using a wide-detector CT system.

(A) Chronic proximal left anterior descending artery (LAD) occlusion. (B) Moderate stenosis at the mid-left circumflex artery (LCx). (C) Right coronary artery (RCA) severe stenoses at proximal and distal level; moreover, eterocoronary retrograde filling of the LAD from the posterior descending artery (PDA) is described. (D–I) Left ventricle short-axis (D, E, F) and long-axis (G, H, I) images showing, after adenosine administration, stress myocardial perfusion defects at septum from base to apex, at the inferior wall from base to apex, and mid-to-apical anterior wall. (J–L) Internal carotid artery showing proximal LAD occlusion and moderate stenosis at the mid LCx (J), and significant stenoses of the RCA at the proximal and distal level, with retrograde filling of the LAD from the PDA, with the latter vessel affected by proximal severe stenosis.

cycle, but can be selectively decreased to limit radiation exposure (Figure 2.5.4).
See Table 2.5.2.

Patient requirements

- No contraindications to iodine or vasodilators.
- Irregular rhythm, left ventricular dyssynchrony (left bundle branch block), inability to perform breath hold, an uncooperative patient, and prolonged circulation time (heart failure, valvular regurgitation) all reduce perfusion imaging performance.
- Dynamic MPI_{CT} relies on spatial consistency between the samples, and despite correction algorithms a regular rhythm and a complete breath hold are important for optimal image quality.

	Static mode	Dynamic mode
Table 2.5.2 Static and dynamic myocardial perfusion imaging protocols		
Scanner	64-slice CT and beyond	• Dual-source CT (second-generation or beyond) • Wide-detector CT (complete coverage)
Scan mode	ECG-synchronized axial or spiral scan mode	• Shuttle mode (dual-source CT) • Stationary mode (wide-detector CT)
Scan time	One to several heart cycles	25–35 s
Radiation dose	Similar to CCTA	5–10 mSv
Source CT data	CT angiogram acquired over 1 or more cycles, additional cardiac phases depending on scan protocol	Series (10–15 time points) of low-resolution volumetric data sets
Output	CTA	Myocardial blood flow maps or other functional parameters
Interpretation	• Qualitative assessment • Indexed attenuation values relative to epicardial or remote myocardium	• Absolute blood flow measures • Indexed measures relative to remote myocardium
Challenges	• Scan timing • Beam-hardening artefacts	• Scanner requirements and radiation dose • Displacement artefacts

ECG: electrocardiogram; CCTA: coronary CT angiography; CTA: CT angiography;

Interpretation techniques

- Qualitative (static MPI_{CT}): visual identification of territories with lower attenuation.
- Semi-quantitative (static MPI_{CT}): attenuation ratio between segment/layer of interest and remote myocardium.
- Quantitative (dynamic MPI_{CT}): calculation of regional myocardial blood flow from (deconvoluted) time-attenuation curves relative to the arterial input function (sampled in the aorta). Because global myocardial blood flow (MBF) values vary between individuals, scanners, and scans, there is no agreed MBF threshold that indicates myocardial ischaemia. Relative MBF values (compared to remote myocardium) show better consistency.
- Direct correlation between MPI_{CT} and angiographic disease severity on CCTA.
- Based on meta-analyses the sensitivity and specificity of static MPI_{CT} is 87% and 71% versus 94% and 76% for dynamic MPI_{CT}.

Myocardial injury imaging

Myocardial scar secondary to prior infarction may be identified in patients with known or unknown CAD. Features of myocardial scar that differentiate it from healthy myocardium include the following:

- acute infarct—reduced myocardial blood flow (microvascular occlusion) and myocyte damage;

- chronic scar—low myocardial blood flow (decreased demand), increased interstitial space, wall thinning and ventricular remodelling, fatty infiltration, and calcifications;

- thrombus may be present (Table 2.5.3).

Acute myocardial infarction

- CT angiography (CTA; first-pass): often well-defined perfusion defect with attenuation values as low as non-enhanced myocardium in case of complete vessel occlusion.

  - Reconstruction of thicker slices, narrow-window display settings or thin-slab minimum intensity projections may be required to appreciate subtle myocardial defects (Figure 2.5.5).

  - Beam hardening artefacts at the interface of the contrast-enhanced left ventricle cavity and the myocardium can cause false defects. Comparison of different cardiac phases can help distinguish true (static) perfusion defects from false beam-hardening artefacts.

  - If available, regional hypokinesia may be evident on multiphasic reconstructions.

- Postcontrast studies (late enhancement): infarcted myocardium will be brighter due to delayed contrast washout. If reperfusion is not achieved, late acquired

Table 2.5.3 Cardiac CT imaging features in acute and chronic myocardial infarction

	Calcium scan (non-contrast)	CT angiography (first-pass)	Post-contrast CT (late-enhancement)
Acute infarct		Hypoattenuation (low flow), wall motion abnormalities (multiphase reconstructions)	Hyperattenuation (bright), hypoattenuation (dark core), thrombus
Chronic scar	Fatty replacement, calcifications (cardiac enlargement)	Wall thinning/dilatation, hypoattenuation (reduced flow; fatty replacement), calcifications, thrombus	Hyperattenuation (bright), thrombus

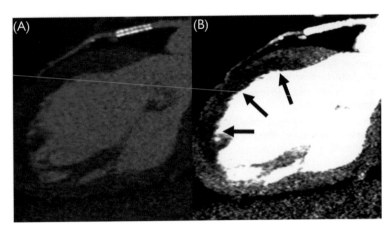

Figure 2.5.5 (A) CT angiography after primary percutaneous coronary intervention of the proximal left anterior descending coronary artery. (B) By appropriately windowing the images a large perfusion defect (arrows) emerges, suggesting poor reflow of the dependent myocardium.

images can show a dark core, also called microvascular obstruction or no-reflow, associated with poor functional outcome (Figure 2.5.6).

Chronic ischaemic scar

- CTA: (subendocardial) hypoenhancement secondary to lower perfusion of the fibrotic scar tissue, as well as replacement by fat tissue.
  - Chronic perfusion defects are subtler and often limited to the endocardial border, although attenuation values can be very low (<0 Hounsfield units) in case of fatty replacement (Figure 2.5.7).

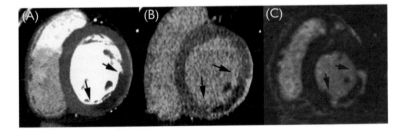

Figure 2.5.6 (A) CT angiography of a patient several days after an inferolateral myocardial infarction (between arrows) shows decreased myocardial blood flow. (B) A repeat CT scan 10 minutes after contrast injection shows persistent low flow (dark between arrows) surrounded by bright myocardium. (C) Late-enhancement magnetic resonance imaging, acquired during systole, similarly shows a dark area of no reflow within an area of bright infarction.

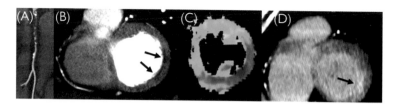

Figure 2.5.7 Patient with (A) a chronic occlusion of the right coronary artery and (B) a thin endocardial rim of low attenuation on CT angiography (arrows). (C) Dynamic myocardial perfusion shows very low (deep blue) myocardial blood flow. (D) Late CT, with incomplete coverage of the inferior wall, shows enhancement of the inferolateral wall, confirming myocardial scar (arrow).

- Additional findings include wall thinning, regional/global left ventricular dilatation, thrombus, and calcifications.
- Late-enhancement imaging: hyperenhancement (increased interstitial space) but no microvascular obstruction in the chronic phase (Figure 2.5.8).
  - Chronic infarcts show less iodine accumulation than acute injuries.
- Fatty replacement and calcification may be visible on non-enhanced acquisitions.
- These findings may be noted on unrelated (non-gated) CT scans of the chest/abdomen.

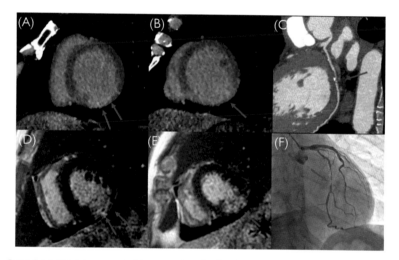

Figure 2.5.8 Late enhancement of the posterolateral wall, indicating prior myocardial infarction.

(A, B) Late CT scan (8 minutes after iodinated contrast administration) demonstrates well the presence of transmural myocardial fibrosis (hyperdense myocardial area, red arrows), confirmed on (D, E) cardiac magnetic resonance imaging (red arrows), showing ischaemic late gadolinium enhancement on the posterolateral left ventricular wall. During the same CT, coronary anatomy was evaluated with the identification of subocclusive stenosis on the left circumflex artery (C, blue arrow), which was subsequently confirmed at invasive coronary angiography (F, blue arrow).

Source: Courtesy of Professor Daniele Andreini and Dr Edoardo Conte.

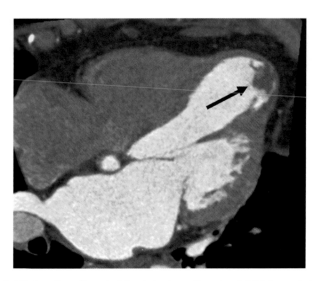

Figure 2.5.9 CT of a patient with a prior left anterior descending artery (LAD) infarct, apical remodelling and wall thinning, and an associated thrombus (arrow).

Complications

Structural complications of MI include thrombus formation (Figure 2.5.9) and rupture of the ventricular septum or free wall rupture (Figure 2.5.10).

Late-enhancement scan protocol

- Larger contrast volumes improve contrast between the infarcted and normal myocardium.
- Low tube voltage (kVp) or dual-energy imaging increases myocardial contrast.
- Reconstruction and/or interpretation of thick slices to decrease noise.

See Table 2.5.4.

Table 2.5.4 Late-enhancement myocardial imaging	
Contrast volume	Large (100–150 ml)
Timing	5–7 min
Scan mode	Axial scan mode preferred
Scan range	Limited to the myocardium
Tube voltage	Low (80 kVp if possible)
Image reconstruction	Thicker slices and smooth kernels to reduce noise

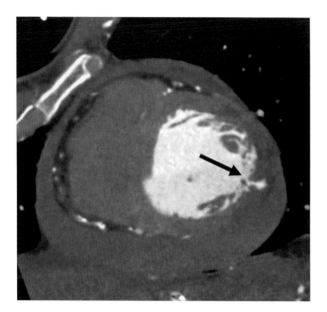

Figure 2.5.10 CT angiography of a patient with a subacute lateral infarct. There is a pericardial effusion caused by a rupture of the infarcted myocardium (arrow).

Limitations

- Late-enhancement imaging contrast between normal and abnormal myocardium is lower than MRI.

- Delineation of the endocardial border may be difficult owing to enhancement of the blood.

- Transmural infarct size and expected functional recovery (after revascularization) are difficult to quantify.

- Overall, cardiac CT is considered as a second-line technique for MI and viability.

Further reading

Danad I, Szymonifka J, Schulman-Marcus J, Min JK. Static and dynamic assessment of myocardial perfusion by computed tomography. *Eur Heart J Cardiovasc Imaging* 2016; 17: 836–44.

Lardo AC, Cordeiro MA, Silva C, Amado LC, George RT, Saliaris AP, et al. Contrast-enhanced multidetector computed tomography viability imaging after myocardial infarction: characterization of myocyte death, microvascular obstruction, and chronic scar. *Circulation* 2006; 113: 394–404.

Singh A, Mor-Avi V, Patel AR. The role of computed tomography myocardial perfusion imaging in clinical practice. *J Cardiovasc Comput Tomogr* 2020; 14: 185–94.

Atherosclerotic plaque imaging

Márton Kolossváry

- Besides stenosis assessment, coronary CT angiography allows visualization of the vessel wall and therefore compositional assessment of atherosclerotic plaques.

- Qualitative plaque features are used to describe plaque composition in routine clinical practice, which have added value in patient risk stratification.

- Segmentation of the atherosclerotic lesions permits volumetric and textural (radiomic) analyses; however, these techniques are not used routinely in clinical practice.

In the past, coronary CT angiography (CCTA) was used as a gatekeeper for invasive coronary angiography (see Chapter 2.2). However, CCTA is capable of not only depicting coronary stenosis, but also the coronary wall, which allows the visualization, characterization, and quantification of atherosclerosis.

Coronary stenosis assessment

In clinical practice the degree of coronary stenosis is described by visual assessment at the site of the narrowest luminal obstruction caused by the plaque as compared to the closest proximal reference vessel diameter without any plaque (Figure 2.6.1).
   Note:

- For clear communication of the results, adding the diameter stenosis range after the semi-quantitative stenosis category is recommended.

- For details on concise reporting please refer to Chapter 2.2.

Quantitative stenosis measurements

Following segmentation of the coronary lumen (please see Chapter 2.1 for further details), computer software is capable of quantifying the degree of stenosis caused by a given plaque. Usually, two metrics are used:

- *diameter stenosis*—the minimal luminal diameter at the location of the most severe narrowing divided by the luminal diameter at the closest proximal reference point, where there is no plaque;

Qualitative plaque stenosis categories

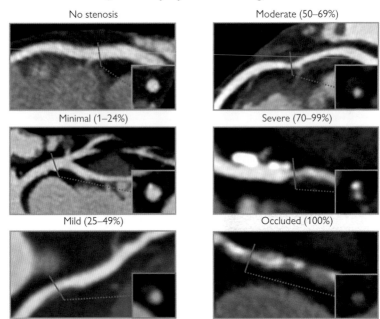

Figure 2.6.1 Multiplanar reconstructions and cross-sections of given stenosis categories.

- *area stenosis*—the minimal luminal area at the location of the most severe narrowing divided by the luminal area at the closest proximal reference point, where there is no plaque.

Note:

- Guidelines do not endorse the use of quantitative stenosis assessment in routine clinical practice, as it is not currently reproducible or accurate.

Compositional plaque assessment

Compositional plaque assessment aims to evaluate the probability of future acute clinical events. On non-contrast CT, coronary calcium score is able to quantify the degree of calcification present in the coronary arteries. This surrogate marker of plaque burden is one of the strongest independent predictors of major adverse cardiac events (MACE; for details see Chapter 2.1). However, with the use of intravenous contrast agents, CCTA is able to visualize and characterize plaque composition.

Qualitative methods

Clinically, the degree of calcification is used to describe the composition of the plaque. Based on the most recent guidelines, the degree of calcification (Figure 2.6.2) should be classified as:

- non-calcified;
- predominant non-calcified;
- predominant calcified;
- calcified.

Qualitative compositional assessment–degree of calcification

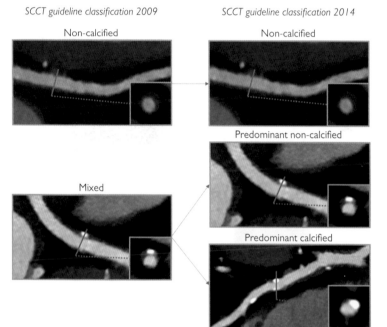

Figure 2.6.2 Multiplanar reconstructions and cross-sections of given plaques with different degrees of calcification.

SCCT: Society of Cardiovascular Computed Tomography.

As looking only at the degree of calcification is a crude estimate of plaque structure, other methods to encompass fine structural features have also been proposed. The plaque attenuation pattern scheme further divides non-calcified and partially calcified plaques based on the spatial heterogeneity of the non-calcified plaque portions (Figure 2.6.3).

- Homogeneous: non-calcified plaque areas have a homogeneous appearance (similar Hounsfield unit (HU) values).
- Heterogeneous: non-calcified plaque areas have a heterogenous appearance (different HU values). These plaques can also show the napkin ring sign, which is defined in the next list.

Adverse plaque features aim to identify morphologies that increase the risk of later MACE. These features are:

- *napkin ring sign* (described as a plaque cross-section with a central area of low attenuation apparently in contact with the lumen, while the whole structure is surrounded by a ring-shaped higher-attenuation plaque tissue);
- *low attenuation* (plaque with any or a given proportion of voxels under a specific HU threshold, which is usually 30 HU);

Qualitative compositional assessment – plaque attenuation pattern

Classification of non-calcified and partially calcified plaques

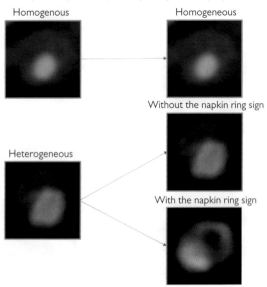

Homogenous

Homogeneous

Without the napkin ring sign

Heterogeneous

With the napkin ring sign

Figure 2.6.3 Representative cross-sections of plaques showing different plaque attenuation patterns.

- *positive (outward) vessel remodelling* (remodelling index, defined as vessel cross-sectional area at the level of maximal stenosis divided by the average of the proximal and distal reference sites' cross-sectional areas to be ≥1.1);
- *spotty calcification* (a calcified speckle surrounded by non-calcified plaque tissue, which has a density of >130 HU and a diameter of <3 mm).

These imaging biomarkers derived from CCTA have been shown to increase the hazard of MACE, above and beyond stenosis and calcification.

Note:
- Evaluation of adverse plaque characteristics is highly subjective and therefore these markers suffer from inter- and intrareader variability.

Ultrastructural information from CCTA may be combined with biological signals from other imaging modalities (e.g. radionuclide imaging tracers of inflammatory plaque activity) to provide a more comprehensive assessment of plaque vulnerability (Figure 2.6.4). Such hybrid imaging approaches are currently just experimental and await clinical validation.

Semi-quantitative methods

Several semi-quantitative methods have been proposed, which provide a patient-based summary of atherosclerotic plaque burden, while not requiring segmentation of the coronary vessels. Most of these only summarize stenosis information; however, some also incorporate plaque composition and location.

- Segment stenosis score: each segment is assigned a score between 0 and 5 based on stenosis category (see Figure 2.6.1). These scores are then added together to provide a patient- based summary.
- Segment involvement score: each segment is assigned 0 or 1 depending on whether there is a plaque present. These scores are then added together to provide a patient- based summary.
- Leaman score: for each segment, the stenosis scores are weighted based on how much blood flows through that segment, based on literature data. The CCTA adaptation also weights the scores based on the degree of calcification.

Quantitative methods

After segmentation (see Chapter 2.1 for further details), the voxels between the inner and outer vessel wall contours are considered to be plaque. This permits the quantification of plaque volume (in mm^3). These voxels then can be categorized into different plaque components based-on HU values. Many cut-off values and methods of calculation are present in the literature.

Note:
- Acquisition settings (i.e. kV and mAs), patient characteristics (i.e. body mass index), contrast protocols, scanners, and software all potentially affect HU values, and therefore limit the reproducibility of quantitative results.

Usually, the volumes are categorized into non-calcified and calcified plaque volume. A part of non-calcified plaque volume: low-attenuation non-calcified plaque volume

Qualitative compositional assessment - high risk plaque features

Napkin ring sign

Low attenuation

Positive remodelling

Spotty calcification

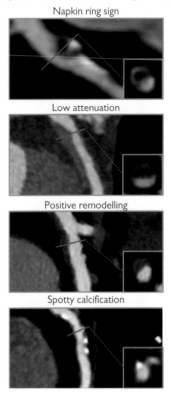

Figure 2.6.4 Multiplanar reconstructions and cross-sections of high-risk plaque features.

is much researched (conventional cut-off: <30 HU) as it has been shown to correlate with later MACE.

While volumetric plaque quantification has been shown to be additive regarding patient prognostication, it discards all spatial information. As many different morphologies may have the same volumes, volumetric plaque quantification contains limited data regarding plaque morphology. This has led to the emergence of new technologies, such as radiomics, which quantifies the spatial interplay of the voxels to describe concepts such as heterogeneity using mathematical formulas (see Chapter 3.16 for further details). Spectral imaging and photon-counting image acquisition techniques may further improve plaque assessment in the future.

Note:
• Due to time constraints and the limited literature data, quantitative plaque composition assessment is currently not done in routine clinical practice.

Further reading

Kolossvary M, Szilveszter B, Merkely B, Maurovich-Horvat P. Plaque imaging with CT—a comprehensive review on coronary CT angiography based risk assessment. *Cardiovasc Diagn Ther* 2017; 7: 489–506.

Kolossvary M, Kellermayer M, Merkely B, Maurovich-Horvat P. Cardiac computed tomography radiomics: a comprehensive review on radiomic techniques. *J Thorac Imaging* 2018; 33: 26–34.

Leipsic J, Abbara S, Achenbach S, Cury R, Earls JP, Mancini GJ, et al. SCCT guidelines for the interpretation and reporting of coronary CT angiography: a report of the Society of Cardiovascular Computed Tomography Guidelines Committee. *J Cardiovasc Comput Tomogr* 2014; 8: 342–58.

Maurovich-Horvat P, Ferencik M, Voros S, Merkely B, Hoffmann U. Comprehensive plaque assessment by coronary CT angiography. *Nat Rev Cardiol* 2014; 11: 390–402.

Saremi F, Achenbach S. Coronary plaque characterization using CT. *AJR Am J Roentgenol* 2015; 204: W249–60.

Chapter 2.7

Stents and grafts

Sujana Balla and Koen Nieman

Teaching points

- Metal stents cause artefacts that negatively affect interpretation of the coronary lumen, thereby limiting the utility of cardiac CT to larger stents (>3 mm diameter) in optimally performed studies.
- Cardiac CT can identify bypass graft disease with high accuracy, although interpretation of the distal coronary arteries can be challenging in patients with diffuse coronary disease.

Coronary stents

Background

- An estimated 1.5 million coronary interventions are performed annually in Europe.
- Conventional stents have struts made of stainless steel or alloys containing cobalt, platinum, or chromium. Bioresorbable scaffolds made of polylactic-L-acid lack metal struts (Figure 2.7.1).
- Complications after stenting include in-stent restenosis and thrombosis.

Challenges of stent imaging

- Metal stents cause artefacts that interfere with in-stent lumen interpretation (Figure 2.7.2).
- Blooming: high X-ray attenuation by the metal combined with the limited spatial resolution and image filtering increases the apparent size of the struts.
- Beam hardening: disproportional absorption of lower-energy X-ray photons by the metal raises the mean potential of the remaining beam, causing low absorption and a dark shadow behind the stent.
- Artefact severity depends on stent features and scan techniques (Table 2.7.1).
- Metal artefacts worsen with motion, causing streak artefacts.

Optimization of data acquisition and reconstruction

- Optimization of image quality reduces high-density artefacts (Table 2.7.2).
- Lowering the heart rate to minimize motion artefacts is critical in patients with stents.

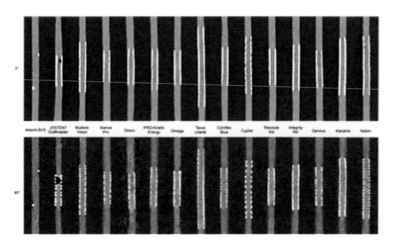

Figure 2.7.1 *In vitro* stents.

Series of 3 mm coronary stents scanned *in vitro* under stationary conditions. The stents are stainless steel (JOSTENT, Taxus, Cypher, Genous, Nobori), cobalt–chromium alloys (Xience Pro, Orsiro, PRO-Kinetic Energy, Coroflex Blue, Resolute Integrety RX, Kaname), platinum–chromium alloys (Omega), and poly-L-lactic acid (Absorb BVS). At 0 degrees (along the z-axis) the distinction of struts is lower than at 90 degrees (in-plane).

Reproduced from Gassenmaier T, Petri N, Allmendinger T, et al. Next generation coronary CT angiography: in vitro evaluation of 27 coronary stents. *Eur Radiol.* 2014;24(11):2953-61. doi: 10.1007/s00330-014-3323-6 with permission from Springer.

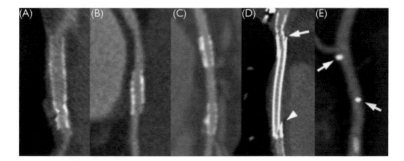

Figure 2.7.2 Coronary stents.

Examples of interpretable CT scans of patent grafts in (A) large and (B, C) smaller coronary arteries and (D) a bypass graft. (A) Distal tapering increases metal density and the blooming effect of the stent. (C) Residual calcified plaque increases the density of the stent. (D) Density depends on the type of stent and increases where devices overlap. (D) Stack artefacts (arrows). (E) Bioresorbable scaffold made of polylactic acid is undetectable on CT, before and after resorption, except for two metal indicators at the edges of the device (arrows).

Table 2.7.1 Favourable conditions for imaging stented coronary arteries

Stent	Alloys containing metals of lower atomic mass, thin struts (low alloy density), non-metal and/or resorbable scaffolds, large stent diameter, no overlapping stents, no complex bifurcation stenting with multiple stent layers, devices located proximally in coronary segments with limited motion radius, no severe calcifications in the vessel wall
Patient	Smaller body size, regular rhythm with slow rate, adequate cooperation and able to hold breath, stent positioned parallel to the imaging plane
Acquisition	High tube voltage, sufficient tube current, high temporal resolution, fewer samples by wider detector coverage
Reconstruction	Iterative reconstruction with sharp filters, thin overlapping slices

- A high tube potential (120 kVp) decreases metal artefacts but generally increases radiation dose.
- Iterative reconstruction, sharp kernels, and thin slices reduce blooming, sharpen edges, and improve in-stent lumen visualization, although increased image noise can be a trade-off (Figure 2.7.3).

Table 2.7.2 Scan considerations after revascularizations

	Coronary stents	Bypass grafts
Preparation	Heart rate modulation and other measures to optimize image quality	• Review surgical report if available • Heart rate modulation
Acquisition	• Higher tube voltage (120 kVp) to decrease metal artefacts • Consider wider exposure window for reconstruction of different cardiac phases	• Higher tube voltage (120 kVp) in case of calcified coronary disease and decrease artefacts from surgical clips • Extended scan range to include the proximal bypass grafts • Fast scan protocols and a caudocranial scan direction in patients unable to maintain a long breath hold (postoperative)
Reconstruction	Thin slices and sharper kernels	Thin slices and sharper kernels for calcified coronary branches
Image display and interpretation	• Longitudinal and short-axis multiplanar reformations • If available, compare different phases to distinguish artefacts from in-stent restenosis	• Double-oblique multiplanar reformations and maximum intensity projections to depict longer graft segments. • 3D volume rendering can provide an overview of the surgical configuration

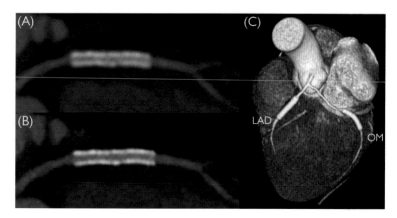

Figure 2.7.3 Convolution kernels.

Blooming artefacts caused by highly attenuating alloys combined with limited spatial resolution increase the apparent size of stents (C). (A) Using a standard reconstruction kernel, the lumen within the stent is interpretable only in the centre of the vessel. (B) Dedicated, sharp reconstruction kernels reduce the blooming effect and improve assessment of stented coronary arteries.

LAD: left anterior descending artery; OM: obtuse marginal branch.

Interpretation of stented coronary arteries

- Stent patency is based on enhancement of the lumen in the stent.
- Distinction between subtle in-stent restenosis and beam hardening artefacts is difficult but can be improved by comparison of different cardiac phases (Figure 2.7.4).

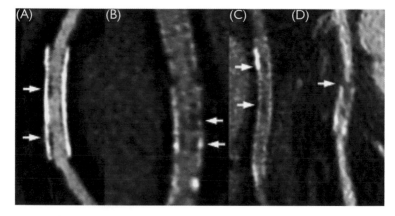

Figure 2.7.4 **Stent disease.**

(A) Large-diameter stent with subtle neointimal hyperplasia. (B) Large-diameter stent with moderate restenosis. (C) Severe in-stent restenosis within a smaller stent. (D) Small stent with severe obstruction extending beyond the top edge of the stent.

- Distal coronary opacification does not rule out stent occlusion.
- CT-derived fractional flow reserve has not been validated in stented vessels and its accuracy is expected to be negatively affected by metal artefacts.

Diagnostic performance of CT angiography in stents

- According to meta-analyses, CT angiography (CTA) has a sensitivity of 90% and specificity of 91% for in-stent restenosis, after the exclusion of up to 40% of non-assessable stents.
- Diagnostic performance is lower in unselected cohorts without the exclusion of non-assessable stents.
- The multisociety 2010 US appropriate use criteria consider CT 'appropriate' for asymptomatic patients with prior percutaneous coronary intervention (PCI) of the left main coronary artery or stents with a diameter ≥3 mm.
- Coronary CTA is classified as 'uncertain' for symptomatic patients with stents with diameters <3 mm.

Coronary artery bypass grafts

Background

- Coronary artery bypass grafting (CABG) is performed in 62/100,000 Western Europeans annually.
- There is a substantial venous graft failure rate of up to 50% at 5 years; arterial graft survival is much higher.
- Graft failure is roughly divided as technical (early), thrombosis (intermediate), graft atheroma (late), or progressive coronary disease (late after surgery).

Types and configuration of grafts

- Arterial grafts: internal mammary arteries (IMA) proximally left *in situ* or as free grafts, radial arteries, and gastroepiploic arteries (uncommon).
- Saphenous vein graft: larger diameter than arterial grafts, fewer surgical clips.
- Single grafts: (multiple) separate grafts each with single end-to-side coronary anastomoses.
- Sequential/jump grafts: (multiple) side-to-side and terminal end-to-side anastomoses.
- Y grafts: free graft proximally connected to other graft, for instance free radial artery from left IMA.

See Figure 2.7.5.

Challenges of CT imaging after bypass graft surgery

- Metal surgical material (clips; sternal sutures): beam hardening and streak artefacts (Figure 2.7.6).

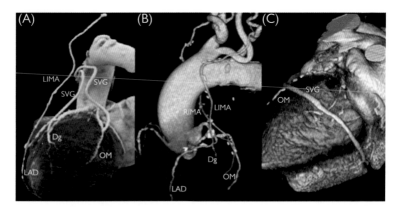

Figure 2.7.5 Three-dimensional (3D) graft anatomy by CT.

Single grafts (A): 3D reconstruction of a left internal mammary artery (LIMA) anastomosed to the LAD, and single vein grafts (SVG) anastomosed to the diagonal (Dg) and obtuse marginal branches (OM). (B) Total arterial revascularization: LIMA anastomosed first to a diagonal branch and then the LAD, and the right internal mammary artery (RIMA) anastomosed to the obtuse marginal branch. (C) Sequential graft: long saphenous vein graft with anastomoses to the obtuse marginal, posterolateral, and posterior descending branches.

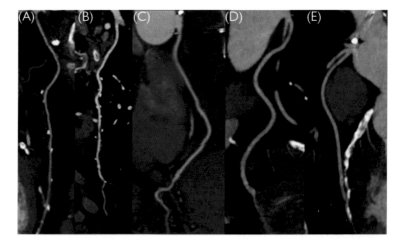

Figure 2.7.6 Patent grafts.

(A) Curved multiplanar reformation of a left internal mammary artery (LIMA) with bright vessel clips anastomosed to the left anterior descending artery (LAD). (B) Patent LIMA anastomosed to a LAD with native run-off disease. (C) Patent saphenous vein graft from the aorta to the posterior descending artery of the right coronary artery. (D) Vein graft, originating together with another vein graft, distally anastomosed to an obtuse marginal branch of the left circumflex artery. (E) Vein graft anastomosed to a diagonal branch of a severely atherosclerotic LAD.

- Evaluation of native coronary branches is difficult in the presence of diffuse, calcified coronary disease.
- Understanding the functional significance of graft disease.
- Early after surgery (<1 month), fluids in the chest may reduce image quality and chest discomfort may interfere with patient's ability to breath hold.

Clinical indications

- Identification of early complications after bypass graft surgery.
- 2010 appropriate use criteria consider CTA for graft patency 'appropriate' in symptomatic patients but 'uncertain' >5 years and 'inappropriate' <5 years post-CABG in asymptomatic patients.
- Prior to redo thoracotomy to assist in surgical planning via depiction of grafts and other structures.

Optimization of data acquisition and reconstruction

- Grafts have a larger diameter and lower motion radius, and are therefore relatively easy to image even with older CT scanners.
- The scan range needs to be cranially extended to include the proximal grafts and origin of the IMA.
- A slightly longer delay between the arrival of contrast in the aorta and scan start may avoid potentially incomplete enhancement of long, large-diameter grafts and coronary run-offs.
- Assessment of graft stenosis, particularly at the level of the coronary anastomosis, improves from better scanner equipment and adequate patient preparation (heart rate control).
- Assessment of the coronary arteries, distal run-offs, and non-bypassed coronary branches is challenging, and optimal image quality is critical.

Interpretation of bypass grafts

- Retrieve the surgical report of the number, type, and configuration of grafts.
- Review aortic root and ascending aorta, and the arch branches in case of *in situ* IMA grafts.
- Review surgical complications: pericardial effusion, pneumonia, pleural effusion, haemothorax, and mediastinitis.
- Graft patency: continuous, homogenous enhancement of the graft lumen with smooth edges. Particular attention to proximal and distal coronary anastomoses.
- Processing tools: axial slice scroll for the identification of grafts, gross anatomy, and patency. Volume rendering for three-dimensional graft visualization can be helpful. Double-oblique multiplanar reformations positioned along the course of the grafts to assess graft status. Thin-slab maximum intensity projections are useful in the absence of metal clips for assessment of small vessels. Curved multiplanar reformations along the graft coronary lumen to transmit findings (Figure 2.7.7).

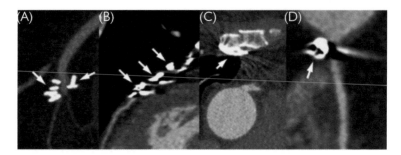

Figure 2.7.7 Graft artefacts.

(A) Clearly depicted vascular clips near the anastomosis. (B) Vascular clips around the left internal mammary artery close to the left anterior descending artery anastomosis creating severe beam-hardening artefacts in combination with cardiac motion. (C) High-density artefacts caused by a sternal wire. (D) Artefacts caused by an indicator at the aortic anastomosis obscures the proximal graft .

- Considerations for occluded grafts:
  - in case of complete graft occlusion only a low-attenuation 'shadow' of the graft may be discerned with opacification of only the proximal graft stump (Figure 2.7.8);
  - in case of a collapsed graft (early) after surgery, the course of the graft may no longer be identified;
  - there is often opacification of the distal coronary branch either through residual antegrade coronary flow or retrograde flow via collaterals;
  - myocardial ischaemia and viability should be considered, as not all occluded grafts cause myocardial ischaemia and revascularization may not benefit the patient.
- Beyond 5 years post-CABG anginal symptoms are equally likely to be caused by progression of native coronary disease, and therefore coronary run-offs and non-grafted branches should be evaluated.
- Uncommon CABG complications: tethering, inappropriate anastomoses, external compression, and aneurysm formation.
- Prior to redo-thoracotomy: patency and location of grafts crossing the midline. Proximity of grafts and other cardiac structures to the sternum.
- Evaluation of the coronary segments proximal to an (occluded) graft may benefit PCI planning.

Diagnostic performance of CTA

- Good at assessing grafts, including distal anastomosis ranges.
- For the detection of graft disease (>50% stenosis), it has a sensitivity of 98%, a specificity of 96%, a positive predictive value of 94%, and a negative predictive value 99%.
- Slightly higher sensitivity for the detection of occlusions than for stenosis.

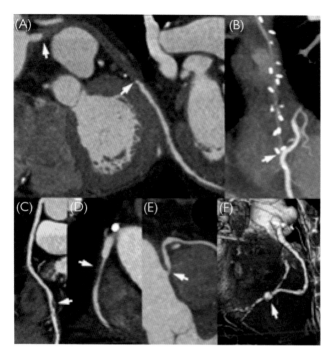

Figure 2.7.8 Graft disease.

(A) Complete occlusion of a venous graft between the anastomosis at the aorta and the first coronary anastomosis, and patency of the distal graft. (B) Functional occlusion (arrow) of a left internal mammary artery graft anastomosed to the left anterior descending artery. (C) Moderate stenosis of a venous graft. (D) Long segment of graft stenosis . (E) Kinking of a venous graft between the aorta and the pulmonary artery. (F) Graft aneurysm at the site of anastomosis with the RCA .

Further reading

Hamon M, Lepage O, Malagutti P, Riddell JW, Morello R, Agostini D, Hamon M. Diagnostic perform-ance of 16- and 64-section spiral CT for coronary artery bypass graft assessment: meta-analysis. *Radiology* 2008; 247: 679–86.

Sun Z, Almutairi AMD. Diagnostic accuracy of 64 multislice CT angiography in the assessment of cor-onary in-stent restenosis: a meta-analysis. *Eur J Radiol* 2010; 73: 266–73.

Taylor AJ, Cerqueira M, Hodgson J, Mark D, Min J, O'Gara P, et al. ACCF/SCCT/ACR/AHA/ASE/ ASNC/NASCI/SCAI/SCMR 2010 Appropriate Use Criteria for Cardiac Computed Tomography. A Report of the American College of Cardiology Foundation Appropriate Use Criteria Task Force, the Society of Cardiovascular Computed Tomography, the American College of Radiology, the American Heart Association, the American Society of Echocardiography, the American Society of Nuclear Cardiology, the North American Society for Cardiovascular Imaging, the Society for Cardiovascular Angiography and Interventions, and the Society for Cardiovascular Magnetic Resonance. *J Am Coll Cardiol* 2010; 56: 1864–94.

Chapter 2.8

Coronary anomalies

Andrew Chang, Ian Rogers and Koen Nieman

> **Teaching points**
> - Cardiac CT accurately depicts variant and anomalous coronary anatomy.
> - Anomalies that involve a coronary trajectory between the aorta and pulmonary artery are associated with myocardial ischaemia and sudden death.

Introduction

Coronary artery anomalies (CAAs) are found in approximately 1–2% of the population. Although most CAAs are benign, approximately 20% manifest with a spectrum of clinical significance—some are detected upon work-up of non-specific anginal symptoms, while others are associated with myocardial infarction or sudden cardiac death in otherwise healthy young people. Many CAAs are isolated primary anomalies, but they can be associated with other congenital heart diseases.

Coronary anomalies can be classified as:

1. Anomalies of origin.
2. Anomalies of termination.
3. Abnormal body/course of the vessel.

Anomalies of origin

Anomalous coronary arteries may originate from inappropriate levels of the aortic root, inappropriate sinuses, inappropriate chambers/vascular structures, or from abnormally conjoined/separated parent coronary arteries. Clinically more important, however, is the subsequent course of the aberrant artery—in particular a course between the aorta and pulmonary artery (PA), potentially leading to compression and myocardial ischaemia.

Origin from inappropriate aortic root level
High coronary take-off

- Coronary ostia >1 cm above the sinotubular junction (Figure 2.8.1).
- Associated with myocardial ischaemia and sudden cardiac death in rare cases.
- Although often an isolated anomaly, it can be secondary to aortic root ectasia.

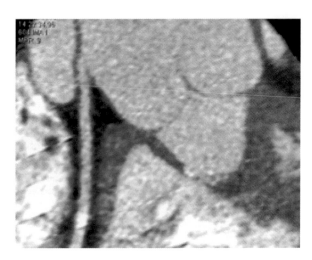

Figure 2.8.1 High take-off of the coronary artery.

Low take-off
- Low coronary ostia down to the level of the aortic valve attachment.
- Risk of accidental injury/obstruction during aortic valve replacement surgery/ transcatheter aortic valve implantation.

Commissural origin
- Coronary ostia within 5 mm of a commissure between two aortic valve cusps.
- In patients with triangular septum between the commissure and aorta, or with small proximal coronaries, this condition may be associated with sudden cardiac death.

Origin from inappropriate sinus of Valsalva

The left main coronary artery (LMCA) usually originates from the left posterior aortic sinus and the right coronary artery (RCA) from the right anterior aortic sinus. However, aberrant RCAs can arise from the left sinus, while the LMCA, left anterior descending (LAD), or circumflex can arise from the right (Figure 2.8.2). They may also arise from the non-coronary sinus (Figure 2.8.2B, P). A slit-like orifice, an acute take-off angle, an interarterial course (between the aorta and PA), and/or a short course within the aortic wall (intramural course) are risk factors for compression with subsequent ischaemia and are considered features of 'malignancy'.

Left main coronary artery from the right anterior sinus
- The LMCA arising from the right sinus can run between the aortic root and pulmonary artery (Figure 2.8.2A), anterior to the PA (Figures 2.8.2C and 2.8.3), retroaortically (Figure 2.8.2D), or inferiorly through the myocardial septum (Figure 2.8.2F).

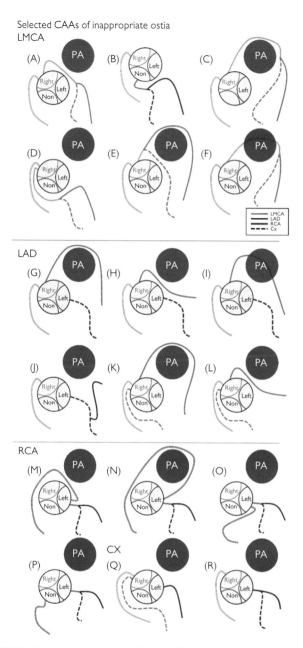

Figure 2.8.2 Selected coronary artery anomalies arising from inappropriate ostia, arranged by aberrant coronary artery.

(a–f) Left main coronary artery (LMCA). (g–l) Left anterior descending artery (LAD). (m–r) Right coronary artery (RCA).

PA: pulmonary artery; Cx: circumflex.

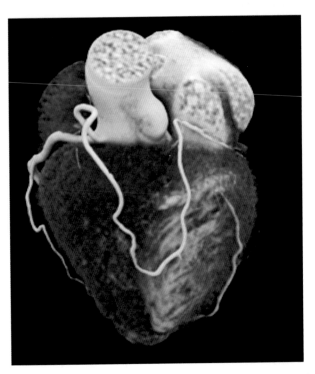

Figure 2.8.3 Left main coronary artery arising from right ostium with course around the right ventricular outflow tract.

- Anomalous LMCAs (and branches) between the aorta and PA/right ventricular (RV) outflow tract are at risk of external compression by aortic dilation during exercise, which can cause myocardial ischaemia, infarction, angina, syncope, ventricular tachyarrhythmias, or sudden cardiac death. An abnormally acute take-off angle and close proximity to the aortic wall predisposes to haemodynamic disruption.

LAD from right anterior sinus
- LAD from the right sinus (Figure 2.8.2G–L). Occasionally, only the distal RCA branches arise from the right sinus and the proximal portion originates (normal) from the LMCA.
- External compression of an anomalous LAD between the aortic root and PA can cause ischaemia (Figure 2.8.2H, I, L).

RCA from left anterior sinus
- RCA arising from the left sinus can run between the aortic root and PA (Figures 2.8.2M and 2.8.4), anteriorly around the PA (Figure 2.8.2N), or retroaortically (Figure 2.8.2O).

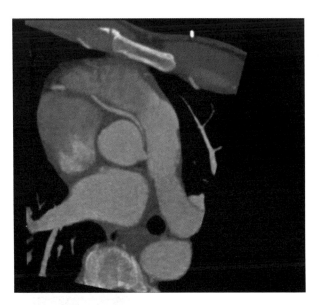

Figure 2.8.4 Malignant course of the right coronary artery between the aorta and the pulmonary artery.

Course of artery continues posterior to the right ventricular outflow tract.

- An RCA course between the aortic root and PA may cause myocardial ischaemia but is less frequently associated with severe complications than an LMCA or LAD with this course. The RCA may also run within the aortic wall, and have abnormally acute take-off angles, increasing the potential for obstruction or extrinsic compression.

Circumflex artery from the right anterior sinus
- The left circumflex (LCx) originates from the right sinus or the RCA (Figure 2.8.2Q) and typically courses behind the aorta.
- This most common CAA is usually benign.

Origin from abnormal common coronary arteries
Absent left main coronary artery

- The LAD and LCx arise from separate ostia, usually from the left sinus (Figure 2.8.5).
- Benign, but may be more common in patients with aortic valve disease.

Single coronary artery
- One coronary artery arising from any of the three sinuses and branching in a variety of directions including retroaortically, anteriorly, retrocardiac, through the septum, or between the aortic root and the PA (Figure 2.8.6).

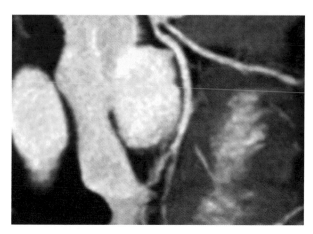

Figure 2.8.5 Absent left main coronary artery.
Note the left anterior descending artery and left circumflex artery arising from separate ostia.

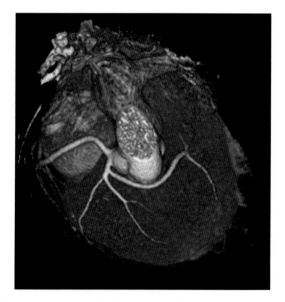

Figure 2.8.6 Single coronary artery (arising from right ostium).

- Associated with tetralogy of Fallot, pulmonary atresia, or persistent truncus arteriosus. Options for coronary collateralization are limited.

Anomalous posterior descending artery origin
- Rarely, the posterior descending artery (PDA) originates from the first septal branch, with the LAD substituting the distal PDA course by wrapping around the left ventricular (LV) apex.

Split right coronary artery
- Two separate arteries in the RCA distribution. The second RCA may have a separate ostium in the right sinus or arise from the other RCA. The second RCA can be mistaken for a high, large RV branch.

Split left anterior descending artery
- Two separate arteries running in the LAD distribution. The second LAD may arise as a distinct branch of the LMCA, from a separate ostium in any of the three sinuses, or as a branch of the RCA. It can also be a branch of the other LAD. The longer of the two vessels, wrapping around the LV apex, is labelled the 'long' LAD (the other is labelled the 'short' LAD).

Ectopic origin of first septal branch
First septal branch arising from the LMCA, RCA, or their branches instead of the LAD (rare).

Absent coronary artery
- For example, absent LCx and large, dominant RCA that crosses the crux to supply the lateral wall.
- Associated with truncus arteriosus or pulmonary atresia.

Origin from inappropriate chamber or vessel
Anomalous origin from pulmonary artery

- Coronary artery arising from the PA trunk (Bland–White–Garland syndrome), or branches (Figure 2.8.7). Blood from the contralateral coronary artery reaches the anomalous artery via enlarged collaterals with reversal of flow in the anomalous artery and drainage into the PA.
- Clinical significance: anomalous LMCA from the pulmonary artery (ALCAPA) results in baseline ischaemia due to deoxygenated blood supplying the left coronary distribution. There is increased risk of atherosclerosis. ALCAPA can present as myocardial ischaemia or heart failure in infants. If robust RCA collaterals form, it can present in adulthood, sometimes as sudden cardiac death. Anomalous RCA from the PA (ARCAPA) is rarer and usually asymptomatic. In 50% of cases, ARCAPA is associated with aortic stenosis, ventricular septal defect, tetralogy of Fallot, or aortopulmonary window. Extensive collaterals and coronary dilatation are typically found.

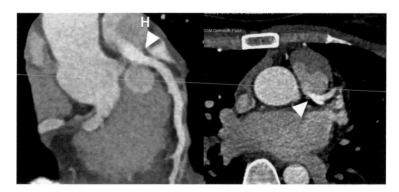

Figure 2.8.7 Anomalous left coronary artery from the pulmonary artery (ALCAPA).

Anomalous origin from a ventricle
- Coronary arteries can arise from the LV or RV (rare). A coronary origin from the LV can result in retrograde flow during diastole, while those originating from the RV can demonstrate retrograde flow during both systole and diastole.
- Associated with pulmonary atresia. Retrograde flow can cause ischaemia.

Other anomalous origins
- Coronary arteries rarely originate from the aortic arch, innominate artery, RCA, internal mammary artery, bronchial artery, subclavian artery, or descending aorta.

Anomalies of termination

Coronary artery fistulae

- Distal coronary communication with the RV, right atrium, pulmonary artery (Figure 2.8.8), coronary sinus (Figure 2.8.9), superior vena cava, pulmonary vein, left atrium, or LV.
- Large fistulae to right heart chambers can cause RV volume overload, while those to the LV can cause LV overload. Large, dilated fistulae are at risk of potentially catastrophic rupture. Small fistulae are relatively common and may be clinically silent. Occasionally, a coronary steal phenomenon through the fistula may cause myocardial ischaemia.
- Full characterization may require adequate opacification of their draining structures (e.g. PA or RV). Fistulous coronary arteries may become dilated, thin-walled, and exhibit atherosclerotic changes, thrombosis, or fibrosis.

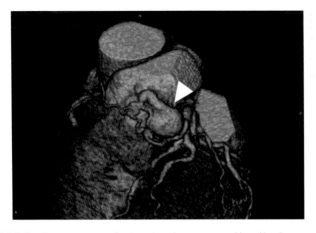

Figure 2.8.8 Left main coronary artery fistula to the pulmonary artery. Note dilated, tortuous segments.

Anomalies of coronary body or course

Congenital ostial stenosis or atresia

- Premature ostial termination and absence of a coronary artery, which may arise from an inappropriate sinus (extremely rare).
- Primary due to embryological occlusion (sometimes with pulmonary atresia) or secondary to Kawasaki disease, Takayasu arteritis, atherosclerosis, or syphilitic aortitis. Often there are extensive collaterals, but cardiac ischaemia may develop.

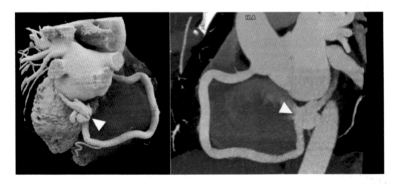

Figure 2.8.9 Right coronary artery fistula to the coronary sinus.

- Ostial stenosis or atresia may be mistaken for atherosclerotic LMCA occlusion but will not have atherosclerotic changes such as calcium or arterial plaque. It may also be mistaken for a single coronary artery. Atretic origins are marked by ostial dimples.

Hypoplastic coronary artery

- Main branches with a diameter <1.5 mm (without compensatory branches or collaterals) are hypoplastic.
- Associated with ischaemia and sudden cardiac death. May be seen with anomalous LMCA origin or LV hypoplasia.

Coronary ectasia or aneurysm

- Coronary diameter ≥1.5 times larger than adjacent segments is considered ectatic or aneurysmal (Figure 2.8.10).
- Prevalence: 20–30% of aneurysms are congenital. Secondary causes: atherosclerosis (most common), Kawasaki disease (Figure 2.8.11), Takayasu arteritis, syphilis, connective tissue disorders, polyarteritis nodosa, and iatrogenic trauma.
- Increased risk of spontaneous thrombosis and myocardial infarction.

Myocardial bridging

- Coronary arteries usually run epicardially aside from their distal ends. In myocardial bridges the coronary artery is partially or fully covered by myocardium (Figure 2.8.12), which may lead to dynamic compression during exertion. The LAD is most frequently affected and is clinically significant.
- Prevalence: 20–25% of the population by CT—higher in pathological studies.

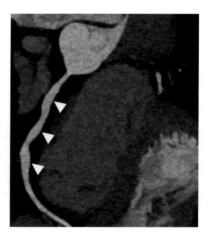

Figure 2.8.10 Ectatic right coronary artery, likely due to atherosclerosis.

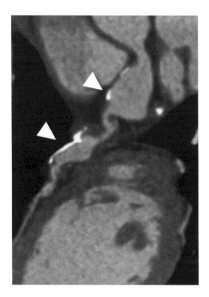

Figure 2.8.11 Aneurysmal coronary segments from Kawasaki disease.
Note the multiple aneurysms with secondary calcifications.

- Although usually asymptomatic, long or deep bridges can be associated with exercise-induced ischaemia and endothelial spasm. Coronary artery segments proximal to the bridge are more prone to atherosclerosis from turbulent backflow. Association with sudden cardiac death is unclear.
- The number, length, and depth of bridge segments can be reported. A high composite myocardial bridge muscle index is associated with anginal symptoms.

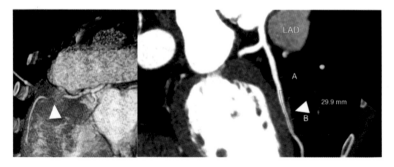

Figure 2.8.12 Myocardial bridge.
LAD: left anterior descending artery.

Subendocardial coronary course

- Rarely, coronary arteries may course subendocardially.

Coronary crossing

- In exceedingly rare cases, major coronaries or their branches may crossover one another. These vessels may have abnormal ostia.

Further reading

Angelini P. Coronary artery anomalies: an entity in search of an identity. *Circulation* 2007; 115: 1296–305.

Pandey NN, Sinha M, Sharma A, Rajagopal R, Bhambri K, Kumar S. Anomalies of coronary artery origin: evaluation on multidetector CT angiography. *Clin Imaging* 2019; 57: 87–98.

Saade C, Fakhredin RB, El Achkar B, Ghieh D, Mayat A, Abchee A, et al. Coronary artery anomalies and associated radiologic findings. *J Comput Assist Tomogr* 2019; 43: 572–83.

Chapter 2.9

CT for suspected acute coronary syndrome

Admir Dedic and Murat Arslan

Teaching points

- Low-to-intermediate-risk patients with an inconclusive work-up are most suited for coronary CT angiography.
- Patient preparation and adequate heart-lowering measures are crucial.
- Patients with no coronary plaque have an excellent prognosis and can safely be discharged to home after careful examination of other emergent conditions.
- Patients with obstructive coronary artery disease, especially in combination with corresponding myocardial hypoenhancement, deserve expedited investigation with invasive angiography.

Introduction

Efficient and reliable evaluation of patients suspected of having non-ST elevation acute coronary syndrome (NSTE-ACS) remains a challenging task that is presented daily to physicians in emergency departments (EDs) worldwide. The differential diagnosis is broad, encompassing life-threatening disease, as well as benign, self-terminating conditions (Table 2.9.1). Standard clinical evaluation typically incorporates a patient history, physical examination, and the results of serial electrocardiograms (ECGs) and cardiac biomarkers. The primary goal of this evaluation is to identify low-risk patients who can be safely discharged, and to identify those in whom the symptoms are most likely due to a myocardial infarction. However, the initial work-up is often not conclusive, as up to 30% of patients are neither discharged nor diagnosed with NSTE-ACS. Coronary CT angiography (CCTA) provides visualization of the coronary artery tree, myocardium, and surrounding organs in a matter of minutes, without the need to provoke ischaemia. Its negative predictive value surpasses all non-invasive tests, approaching 100%, and the positive predictive value is reasonable. Implementing early CCTA improves the efficiency of the standard clinical work-up in low-to-intermediate-risk patients. New high-sensitivity troponin assays have recently been introduced that detect smaller amounts of myocardial injury in less time. Experiences thus far in EDs show that patients with serial low values have an excellent prognosis and can be discharged safely without the need of further testing. Because of a decrease in specificity, there is now a substantial group of patients with detectable or slightly elevated troponins, often not demanding immediate action, for whom CCTA may provide guidance.

Table 2.9.1 Differential diagnoses of acute coronary syndromes in the setting of acute chest pain

Cardiac	Pulmonary	Vascular	Gastrointestinal	Orthopaedic	Other
Myopericarditis; cardiomyopathies[a]	Pulmonary embolism	Aortic dissection	Oesophagitis, reflux, or spasm	Musculoskeletal disorders	Anxiety disorders
Tachyarrhythmias	(Tension)-Pneumothorax	Symptomatic aortic aneurysm	Peptic ulcer, gastritis	Chest trauma	Herpes zoster
Acute heart failure	Bronchitis, pneumonia	Stroke	Pancreatitis	Muscle injury/ inflammation	Anaemia
Hypertensive emergencies	Pleuritis			Costochondritis	
Aortic valve stenosis			Cholecystitis	Cervical spine pathologies	
Takotsubo cardiomyopathy					
Coronary spasm					
Cardiac trauma					

Bold: common and/or important differential diagnoses. [a]Dilated, hypertrophic and restrictive cardiomyopathies may cause angina or chest discomfort.

Source: Roffi, M., et al., 2015 ESC Guidelines for the management of acute coronary syndromes in patients presenting without persistent ST-segment elevation: Task Force for the Management of Acute Coronary Syndromes in Patients Presenting without Persistent ST Segment Elevation of the European Society of Cardiology (ESC). *Eur Heart J* 2016. 37(3): p.267–315. Table reproduced with the permission of the publisher.

Special considerations in patients with acute chest pain

- Generally, the heart rate (HR) is higher and more variable due to psychological or physical stress and a higher symptomatic drive. Adequate lowering and stabilization of the HR with a beta-blocker is crucial. Consider anxiolytics and practice the breath hold in advance. Prospective ECG-gated scanning is preferred, although a retrospective ECG-gated scan might be preferable in patients with high and variable HRs despite medication.
- Consider non-coronary, but potentially life-threatening, conditions.
- Non-enhanced imaging for calcium imaging is generally not accepted in acute chest pain, because of a higher probability of significant non-calcified plaque or embolic coronary events. Also, alternative causes for acute chest pain (pulmonary embolism, aortic dissection) will be missed without contrast enhancement.

Patient selection

According to European Society of Cardiology guidelines, CCTA should be considered as an alternative to invasive angiography to exclude acute coronary syndrome (ACS) when there is a low-to-intermediate likelihood of coronary artery disease (CAD) and when cardiac troponin and/or ECG are inconclusive.

- High clinical suspicion despite serial low (hs)-troponin values (Figure 2.9.1). Unfavourable risk profile, ECG changes, typical progressive symptoms, or symptoms at rest.

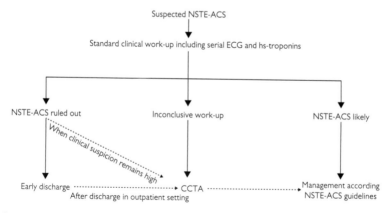

Figure 2.9.1 Patient selection.
NSTE-ACS: non-ST elevation acute coronary syndrome; CCTA: coronary CT angiography.

- Inconclusive work-up with slightly elevated (hs)-troponins without a characteristic rise or fall pattern in combination with a normal or non-diagnostic ECG.
- Low-risk patients who have been discharged might be scheduled to undergo CCTA in an outpatient setting.

In addition, patient characteristics should be suitable for adequate data acquisition (Chapter 1.4).

Coronary CT angiography results and recommendations

- No stenosis or plaque—associated with a very favourable prognosis, further assessment for CAD not needed. Consider other aetiologies.
- Non-obstructive CAD—associated with a favourable prognosis, further in-hospital assessment for CAD generally not needed. Consider risk modulation and pharmacotherapy with outpatient follow-up. In-hospital evaluation should be considered if clinical suspicion remains high, there are persistent symptoms, or in the presence of high-risk plaque features (Figure 2.9.2).

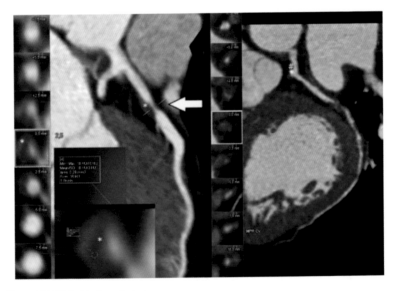

Figure 2.9.2 High-risk plaque feature.

White arrow indicates positive remodeling.
*Low-attenuation plaque. #Spotty calcification.

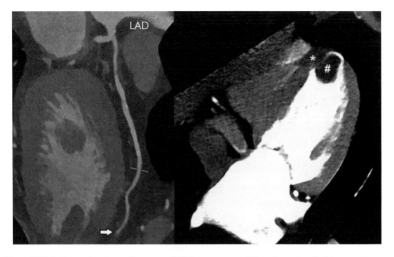

Figure 2.9.3 Left anterior descending artery (LAD) on coronary CT angiography of a 64-year-old woman presenting with acute chest pain triggered by an emotional event.

Echocardiographic findings mimic Takotsubo cardiomyopathy. Blunt termination very distally is easily overlooked (especially when using automated curved multiplanar reformation images) that is caused by plaque rupture and distal embolization of the proximal plaque. Note the apical left ventricular thrombus on the right panel. The white arrow points to the blunt termination of the distal LAD.
*Regional myocardial hypoenhancement. #Apical left ventricular thrombus.

- Pitfalls: obstructive disease in small segments (<2 mm diameter) or distal embolization following a plaque rupture (Figure 2.9.3). Always interpret together with the clinical picture, ECG findings, and biomarker results.
- Obstructive CAD—NSTE-ACS is more likely and the patient should be admitted and receive guideline recommended therapy. Higher stenosis grade or acute occlusions, especially in combination with regional myocardial hypoenhancement (Figure 2.9.4) make NSTE-ACS very likely. Consider invasive angiography in these cases, also in the presence of obstructive three-vessel disease or obstructive left main CAD (or its equivalent). Stress testing may be considered in the absence of elevated troponins.
- Significant non-cardiac findings (Figure 2.9.5)—treatment according to underlying cause.

Triple-rule-out protocol

In some patients with acute chest pain standard clinical evaluation does not produce a clear working diagnosis. When additional diagnoses besides ACS are considered, such as aortic dissection or pulmonary embolism, a triple-rule-out scan may be

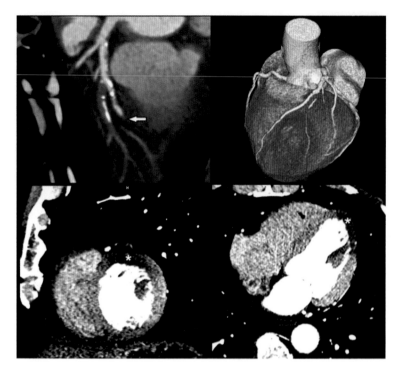

Figure 2.9.4 Acute occlusion of diagonal branch with corresponding regional myocardial hypoenhancement.

The white arrow points to acute occlusion of the diagonal branch.

*Regional myocardial hypoenhancement.

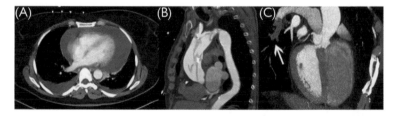

Figure 2.9.5 Collateral findings causing acute chest pain.

(A) Pericarditis with pericardial effusion. (B) Aortic dissection. (C) Pulmonary embolism.

considered for assessment of the coronary arteries, thoracic aorta, and pulmonary arteries with a single examination. These protocols are associated with higher radiation and contrast agent doses than a dedicated CCTA protocol, because of the wider thoracic coverage and opacification of both the right- and left-side circulations. Even more so than a dedicated CCTA protocol, image quality is highly dependent on local expertise, CT scanner technology, adequate patient preparation, contrast agent injection technique, and timing of image acquisition. Therefore, appropriate patient selection is crucial.

Conclusions

CCTA has proven to be a valuable tool in suspected NSTE-ACS. Thorough patient preparation and adequate HR-lowering measures are crucial. Low-to-intermediate-risk patients with an inconclusive work-up are most suited for CCTA. Patients with no coronary plaque have an excellent prognosis and often can be safely discharged after careful examination of other emergent conditions. Patients with obstructive CAD, especially in combination with corresponding myocardial hypoenhancement, deserve expedited investigation with invasive angiography.

Further reading

Hoffmann U, Truong QA, Schoenfeld DA, Chou ET, Woodard PK, Nagurney JT, et al. Coronary CT angiography versus standard evaluation in acute chest pain. *N Engl J Med* 2012; 367: 299–308.

Roffi M, Patrono C, Collet J-P, Mueller C, Valgimigli M, Andreotti F, et al. 2015 ESC Guidelines for the management of acute coronary syndromes in patients presenting without persistent ST-segment elevation: Task Force for the Management of Acute Coronary Syndromes in Patients Presenting without Persistent ST-Segment Elevation of the European Society of Cardiology (ESC). *Eur Heart J* 2016; 37: 267–315.

Nieman K, Hoffmann U. Cardiac computed tomography in patients with acute chest pain. *Eur Heart J* 2015; 36: 906–14.

Twerenbold R, Boeddinghaus J, Mueller C. Update on high-sensitivity cardiac troponin in patients with suspected myocardial infarction. *Eur Heart J* 2018; 20(suppl_G): G2–10.

Wnorowski AM, Halpern EJ. Diagnostic yield of triple-rule-out CT in an emergency setting. *AJR Am J Roentgenol* 2016; 207: 295–301.

Chapter 2.10

Graft vasculopathy
in transplanted hearts

Andrea Bartykowszki

Teaching points

- Cardiac allograft vasculopathy (CAV) is among the top causes of death 1 year post-heart transplantation (HTX).
- CAV causes diffuse narrowing of the coronary lumen and has a different appearance to atherosclerotic plaque formation.
- Annual or biannual assessment of coronary status is recommended after HTX.
- The absence of innervation of the transplanted hearts warrants special considerations during coronary CT angiography.
- Normal radiomorphological appearance of the heart after transplantation may vary.

Introduction

Cardiac allograft vasculopathy (CAV) is among the top causes of death at 1 year and beyond after heart transplantation (HTX). Heart transplant recipients do not experience typical ischaemia-related symptoms; therefore, regular (annual or biannual) screening for CAV is indicated. Invasive coronary angiography (ICA) is considered to be the gold standard method to diagnose the disease. However, at experienced centres, coronary CT angiography (CCTA) can be an alternative to ICA to detect the vasculopathy.

The absence of parasympathetic and sympathetic innervation of the transplanted hearts results in higher resting heart rate (HR), minimal HR variability, and the inefficiency of beta-blocker therapy.

Lesion characteristics

- CAV is characterized by diffuse luminal narrowing caused by concentric intimal hyperplasia (Figure 2.10.1).

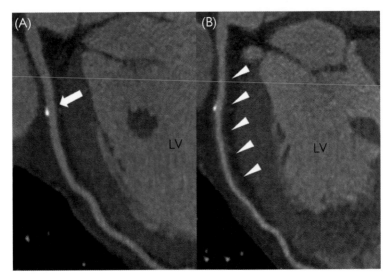

Figure 2.10.1 Manifestation of cardiac allograft vasculopathy during follow-up CT.

(A) Follow-up CT 2 years after heart transplantation. Minimal stenosis is visible, caused by a partially calcified lesion on the mid-segment of the left anterior descending artery (LAD; white arrow). Calcification may indicate pre-existing coronary atherosclerosis. (B) Follow-up CT 3 years after heart transplantation. Diffuse luminal narrowing is visible on the proximal and mid-segment of the LAD caused by non-calcified lesions (white arrowheads).

LV: left ventricle.

- In most cases, lesions initially involve the distal segments of the coronary tree and then spread proximally.
- The composition of the lesions differs from atherosclerotic plaques as calcium depositions are unlikely. The presence of calcification usually indicates pre-existing coronary artery disease.

Scan technique

- The general settings are similar to standard CCTA.
- There are special considerations because of the higher resting HR (Table 2.10.1).

Table 2.10.1 How to set up your scanner for imaging heart transplantation (HTX) patients	
Scanner type	• Dual-source CT (second-generation or beyond) • Wide-detector CT for larger coverage
Scan mode	• Prospectively ECG-triggered scan mode preferred • In case of HR >80 bpm triggering on the systolic phase of the RR cycle, widening of the acquisition to 40–80% of the RR cycle is suggested
Scan settings	Similar to standard CCTA, but perform a non-enhanced scan only to determine adequate scan range (coronary calcium score is not interpretable in HTX patients)
Contrast volume	A bolus of 60–70 ml iodinated contrast media injected at a rate of 4–5 ml/s
Tube voltage	100–120 kV adjusted to the patient's body mass index
Challenges	• High resting HR despite premedication • Postoperative cardiac appearance

ECG: electrocardiogram; HR: heart rate; bpm: beats per minute; CCTA: coronary CT angiography.

Patient preparation

• Premedication with beta-blockers is usually ineffective, or the effect is diminished or delayed.

• The selective sinus node I(f) channel inhibitor ivabradine can be an alternative during HR control (see Chapter 1.4).

• Nitroglycerin premedication is always necessary when contraindications are not present.

• Screening of renal function is important, as heart transplant recipients frequently have renal insufficiency.

Interpretation and reporting

• According to the Society for Cardiovascular Computed Tomography (SCCT) guidelines for the interpretation and reporting of CCTA, coronary lesions should be reported (see Chapter 2.2).

• There is a wide range of normal cardiac appearance after transplantation, depending on the operation technique used. Atrial anastomoses can be created by using a bi-atrial, or more recently, a bi-caval technique.

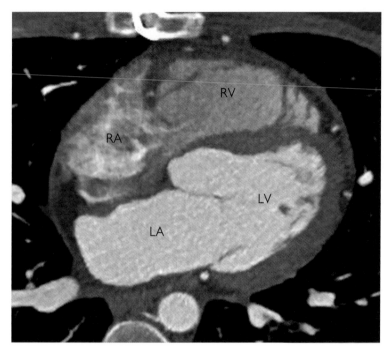

Figure 2.10.2 Clockwise rotation of the heart after cardiac transplantation.
LA: left atrium; LV: left ventricle; RA: right atrium; RV: right ventricle.

- With the bi-atrial (Lower and Shumway) technique the posterior wall of the recipient's left and right atria are preserved, and anastomosis is created with the anterior wall of the donor's atria. This method results in the enlargement of both atria.
- With the bi-caval technique the recipient's right atrium and almost all of the left atrium are removed, with only the posterior wall of the left atrium remaining, which is then anastomosed to the donor's left atrium. This approach results in moderate enlargement of the left atrium, and a clockwise rotation of the transplanted heart (Figure 2.10.2).
- The size discrepancy between the recipient and the donor's great vessels can results in the appearance of a pseudostenosis/dilatation (Figure 2.10.3).
- Surgical soft tissue patches around the vessel anastomoses are also frequently visible and may be mistaken for pseudoaneurysms (Figure 2.10.3).

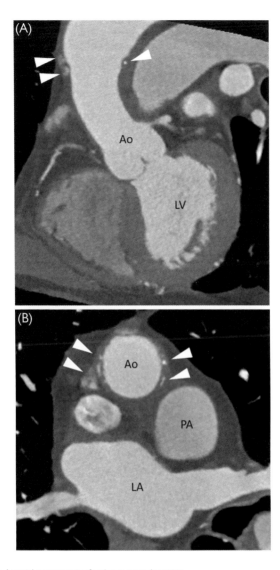

Figure 2.10.3 Arterial anastomosis after heart transplantation.

(A) Size discrepancy between the donor and the recipient aorta (Ao). (B) Cross-section at the level of the aortic anastomosis. Surgical soft tissue around the anastomosis (white arrowheads).

LA: left atrium; LV: left ventricle; PA: pulmonary artery.

Further reading

Badano LP, Miglioranza MH, Edvardsen T, Colafranceschi AS, Muraru D, Bacal F, et al. European Association of Cardiovascular Imaging/Cardiovascular Imaging Department of the Brazilian Society of Cardiology recommendations for the use of cardiac imaging to assess and follow patients after heart transplantation. *Eur Heart J Cardiovasc Imaging* 2015; 16: 919–48.

Bastarrika G, Rábago G. Cardiac CT in the setting of heart transplantation. In: Schoepf UJ (ed.) *CT of the Heart—Contemporary Medical Imaging.* New York: Humana Press, 2019, pp. 391–406.

Chapter 3.1

Ventricular volume and function

Richard A.P. Takx and Csilla Celeng

Teaching points

- Accurate measurement of left (LV) and right (RV) ventricular volume, mass, and function (including global and regional wall motion, as well as thickening) is feasible with cardiac CT.
- Retrospective electrocardiogram gating is the most common method for functional analysis. Tube current modulation allows for a significantly lower radiation dose.
- Quantification is based on endo- and epicardial contours.
- RV volume requires homogeneous enhancement of the cavity.

CT image acquisition

- Traditionally, retrospective electrocardiogram (ECG) gating is used for the acquisition of functional data sets.
- Retrospective ECG gating without dose modulation generates high-quality images of the hearth throughout the cardiac cycle. Nevertheless, it is accompanied by a high radiation dose at around 12 mSv (Figure 3.1.1; see also Chapter 1.5).
- Alternatively, functional information can be acquired retrospectively at 20% tube current within an adjustable part of the cardiac cycle (i.e. ECG tube current modulation), while 100% tube current can be used selectively for the evaluation of the coronary artery tree. This results in a significantly lower radiation dose (Figure 3.1.1).
- Contrast enhancement for ventricular function can be achieved using different protocols such as a triphasic or an individualized split-bolus technique. It is important to limit the contrast media dose while obtaining sufficient contrast opacification of the left ventricle (LV; and right ventricle (RV)). For LV functional analysis there is no need to amend the standard coronary angiography protocol.
- Ideally, images should be obtained at 10% (5% with the latest-generation scanners) of the RR interval, with a 512 × 512 matrix, and a slice thickness/increment of 0.9 mm/0.45 mm.

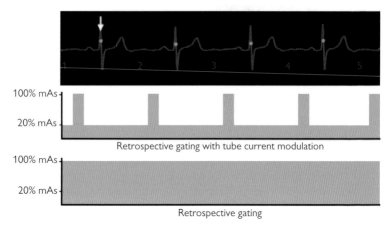

Figure 3.1.1 Different CT acquisition methods with electrocardiogram gating for function.

Quantification

• In order to extract functional information, endocardial contours have to be traced by postprocessing software in end systole (ESV) and end diastole (EDV) for both ventricles. Delineation is usually performed (semi-) automatically, but contours should be visually inspected and corrected if needed.

• Ejection fraction (EF; in %) is calculated as (EDV − ESV)/EDV × 100

• Epicardial contours of the LV will provide information on mass and wall motion.

• Papillary muscles are usually considered as part of the LV cavity (Figure 3.1.2).

• Most software packages provide measurement of ESV, end-EDV, stroke volume, EF, myocardial mass, and wall motion.

• If needed, these values can be indexed for body surface area.

Left ventricular volume and function

• CT functional analysis can evaluate global ventricular function, as well as regional wall motion and thickening (Figures 3.1.3 and 3.1.4).

• In those with acute coronary syndrome, LV function—especially regional wall motion—has prognostic and treatment implications.

• In patients with heart failure, valvular disease, and cardiac devices (e.g. LV assist device), accurate assessment of LV function is important.

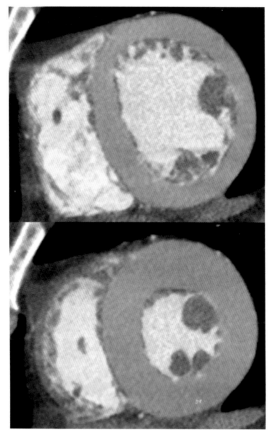

Figure 3.1.2 Short-axis images in end diastole (above) and end systole (below), with automatically segmented left ventricular (LV) muscle (green), LV cavity (red), and right ventricular cavity (blue).

- Beta-blockers are often administered for heart rate control prior to coronary CT angiography; however, their use could impact on measurements due to negative inotropic effects.
- Age- and sex-specific reference intervals for the LV and RV have to be considered (for normal reference values see Chapter 3.2).

CT has been compared to other techniques (echocardiography, single photon emission CT (SPECT), cardiac magnetic resonance) in small studies, showing good agreement for volumes and EF. Volumes tend to be overestimated with CT than with echocardiography and/or SPECT, but this has little impact on EF.

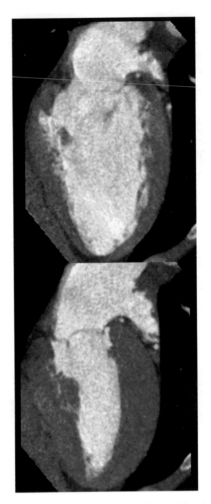

Figure 3.1.3 Vertical long-axis view of the left ventricle in end diastole (above) and end systole (below).

Right ventricular volume and function

- The RV is often overlooked. It requires sufficient contrast opacification (preferably >250 Hounsfield units (HU)) of the RV cavity (Figure 3.1.5) using an appropriate contrast injection protocol.

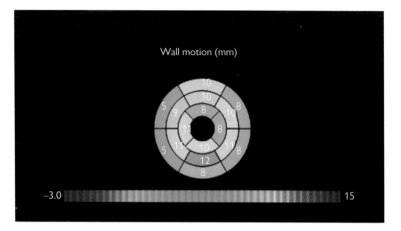

Figure 3.1.4 Left ventricle wall motion (mm).

- RV function is important in those with pulmonary hypertension, pulmonary embolism, right-sided heart failure, and arrhythmogenic RV cardiomyopathy.
- The RV has a complex three-dimensional shape (Figure 3.1.6).
- For normal reference intervals of RV volumes and EF see Chapter 3.2.

Ventricular mass

- Chronic volume and pressure overload can result in increased ventricular mass (Figure 3.1.7), which has been associated with an increased risk of cardiovascular morbidity and mortality.
- As a result, hypertrophy has been incorporated into clinical guidelines for the management of heart failure, and adequate blood pressure control is recommended for patients, to prevent symptomatic heart failure.
- CT allows for accurate measurement of LV mass (for normal reference values, see Chapter 3.2), although the reproducibility of RV mass is less reliable owing to the thin free wall and trabeculation.

Segment models

- Global and regional LV function can be scored according to standard myocardial segmentation models (Figure 3.1.8).

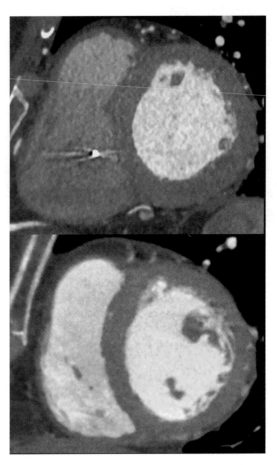

Figure 3.1.5 Insufficient right ventricle (RV) cavity opacification (above; Hounsfield units (HU) = 130) and good RV contrast opacification (below; HU = 430).

- Myocardial segments are numbered in reference to both the long- and short-axis.
- Motion can be graded as normokinesia, hypokinesia, akinesia, and dyskinesia.
- Segments can be allocated to an artery; this depends on individual coronary anatomy.

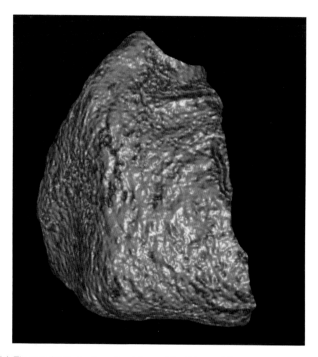

Figure 3.1.6 The complex three-dimensional shape of the right ventricle.

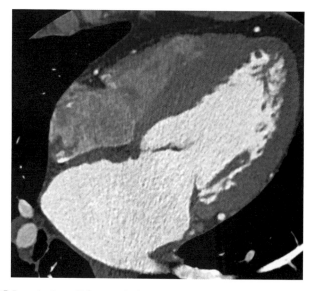

Figure 3.1.7 Example of septal left ventricular (LV) hypertrophy on a four-chamber view with a LV mass of 137 g/m² and an interventricular septum wall thickness of 21 mm.

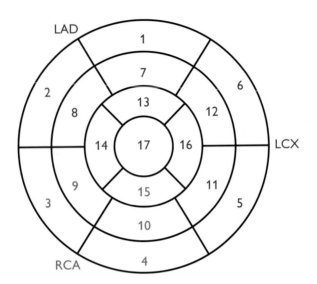

Figure 3.1.8 Segment model adapted from Peng *et al.* (2016).
LAD: left anterior descending artery; LCx: left circumflex artery; RCA: right coronary artery.

Reproduced from Peng P, Lekadir K, Gooya A, Shao L, Petersen SE, Frangi AF. A review of heart chamber segmentation for structural and functional analysis using cardiac magnetic resonance imaging. *MAGMA*, 2016;29(2):155–95. doi: 10.1007/s10334-015-0521-4 with permission from Springer (Creative Commons Attribution 4.0 International License (http://creativecommons.org/licenses/by/4.0/)).

Further reading

Authors/Task Force members; Elliott PM, Anastasakis A, Borger MA, Borggrefe M, Cecchi F, et al. 2014 ESC Guidelines on diagnosis and management of hypertrophic cardiomyopathy: the Task Force for the Diagnosis and Management of Hypertrophic Cardiomyopathy of the European Society of Cardiology (ESC). *Eur Heart J* 2014; 35: 2733–79.

Cerqueira M, Weissman NJ, Dilsizian V, Jacobs AK, Kaul S, Laskey WK, et al. Standardized myocardial segmentation and nomenclature for tomographic imaging of the heart. A statement for healthcare professionals from the Cardiac Imaging Committee of the Council on Clinical Cardiology of the American Heart Association. *Circulation*. 2002; 105: 539–42.

Dupont MV, Dragean CA, Coche EE. Right ventricle function assessment by MDCT. *AJR Am J Roentgenol* 2011; 196: 77–86.

Peng P, Lekadir K, Gooya A, Shao L, Petersen SE, Frangi AF. A review of heart chamber segmentation for structural and functional analysis using cardiac magnetic resonance imaging. *MAGMA* 2016; 29: 155–95.

Petersen SE, Aung N, Sanghvi MM, Zemrak F, Fung K, Paiva JM, et al. Reference ranges for cardiac structure and function using cardiovascular magnetic resonance (CMR) in Caucasians from the UK Biobank population cohort. *J Cardiovasc Magn Reson* 2017; 19: 18.

Takx RA, Moscariello A, Schoepf UJ, Barraza Jr JM, Nance Jr JW, Bastarrika G, et al. Quantification of left and right ventricular function and myocardial mass: comparison of low-radiation dose 2nd generation dual-source CT and cardiac MRI. *Eur J Radiol* 2012; 81: e598–604.

Chapter 3.2

Normal dimensions on cardiac CT

Giuseppe Muscogiuri

> **Teaching points**
>
> • Beyond the evaluation of coronary arteries, cardiac CT acquisition after the administration of iodine contrast agent allows the evaluation of cardiac and surrounding cardiovascular structures. In order to assess atrial and ventricular thickness, volumes, and function, an acquisition, including the entire cardiac cycle, is required.
>
> • The normal dimensions of cardiac structures may vary considerably based on age, sex, and cardiac cycle. Reference values are derived from large databases of 'normal' patients and allow identification of the pathological dimension for any given age, sex, and cardiac cycle.
>
> • Publications with reference values from cardiac CT are scarce. Therefore, the majority of reference values are adopted from somewhat larger magnetic resonance imaging (MRI) databases, as CT and MRI dimensions are closely correlated.

189

The left and right atria

The function of the left atrium (LA) and right atrium (RA) is to drain the pulmonary and systemic blood, respectively. They are volume-compliant cardiac chambers; hence, their dimensions may vary not only according to age and sex, but also on individual filling conditions (e.g. hypo- or hypervolaemia). Reference values for LA and RA dimensions are given in Table 3.2.1.

• To image both the LA and RA, a triphasic injection protocol (contrast agent bolus followed by a mixed bolus of contrast agent and saline solution) is required (see also Chapter 1.10).

• Measurement of atrial dimensions should be performed in ventricular systole.

The measurement of atrial area and volume should be performed with four-chamber multiplanar reconstruction (Figure 3.2.1).

Table 3.2.1 Atrial dimensions for males and females classified by age

	16–20 years		21–30 years		31–40 years		41–50 years		51–60 years		>60 years	
	Males	Females	Males	Females	Males	Females	Males	Females	Males	Females	Males	Females
LA (mm²)	23 (17–32)	24 (23–24)	24 (20–32)	19 (13–27)	22 (15–32)	19 (12–22)	22 (12–29)	21 (14–27)	23 (16–35)	21 (17–2)	22 (14–28)	21 (14–29)
LA$_i$ (mm²/m²)	12 (8–14)	11 (8–14)	13 (11–16)	10 (8–13)	12 (10–16)	12 (10–13)	11 (7–15)	13 (11–15)	11 (9–16)	11 (9–15)	11 (7–15)	13 (12–15)
RA (mm²)	19 (14–24)	18 (15–24)	22 (17–29)	19 (15–24)	20 (17–28)	17 (13–21)	21 (14–26)	19 (12–27)	23 (15–30)	20 (17–26)	21 (14–27)	20 (16–24)
RA$_i$ (mm²/m²)	10 (8–14)	13 (13–13)	11 (9–15)	10 (9–11)	11 (9–14)	11 (10–13)	10 (8–14)	12 (10–14)	12 (9–15)	11 (9–13)	11 (7–14)	13 (12–13)

Data in brackets are the 95% confidence intervals. LA: left atrium; i: indexed; RA: right atrium.

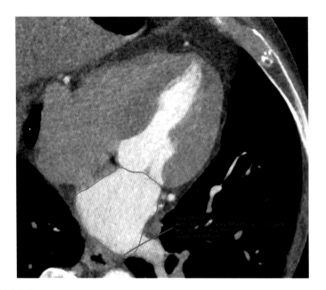

Figure 3.2.1 A 74-year-old man with suspected coronary artery disease. Evaluation of left atrium surface on multiplanar reconstruction with a four-chamber view in ventricular systole.

Ventricular volumes, mass, and function

The evaluation of biventricular volumes, mass, and function can be important in some patients undergoing coronary CT angiography (CCTA; particularly if echocardiography and magnetic resonance imaging (MRI) failed or was contraindicated). Reference values for right (RV) and left ventricular (LV) volumes and ejection fractions (EFs) are given in Tables 3.2.2 and 3.2.3, and for LV mass in Table 3.2.2.

- To image both the LV and RV, a triphasic injection protocol (contrast agent bolus followed by a mixed bolus of contrast agent and saline solution) is required in order to reach enough contrast attenuation for both ventricles (see also Chapter 1.10).

- The scan protocol needs to include the entire cardiac cycle, with the usual scan parameters of standard CCTA (see also Chapter 1.5).

- A potential influence of limited temporal resolution, use of beta-blockers and nitrates, and high rate infusion contrast agent on ventricular volumes and function measurements should be considered.

- The measurements of LV and RV volumes should be performed on a predefined stack of consecutive short-axis slices from base (valvular plane) to apex, as shown in Figure 3.2.2.

Table 3.2.2 Left ventricle indexed normal volumes and mass for males and females classified according to age

	16–20 years		21–30 years		31–40 years		41–50 years		51–60 years		>60 years	
	Males	Females	Males	Females	Males	Females	Males	Females	Males	Females	Males	Females
EDV$_i$ (ml/m^2)	89 (74–111)	81 (67–99)	94 (76–111)	83 (66–98)	90 (66–108)	81 (61–96)	76 (61–106)	83 (63–94)	80 (66–106)	72 (55–92)	78 (55–106)	71 (51–91)
ESV$_i$ (ml/m^2)	31 (20–44)	30 (23–36)	38 (27–51)	30 (16–43)	34 (27–48)	28 (13–40)	26 (18–34)	31 (23–41)	30 (14–45)	25 (12–35)	29 (13–47)	24 (14–35)
SV$_{i,i}$ (ml/m^2)	55 (43–70)	51 (43–63)	59 (45–76)	53 (49–57)	57 (39–69)	53 (38–72)	50 (40–66)	52 (35–71)	54 (42–74)	48 (39–60)	49 (36–63)	47 (30–58)
EF (%)	64 (57–76)	63 (55–71)	61 (55–69)	65 (56–76)	63 (54–71)	65 (57–78)	66 (56–74)	62 (55–71)	64 (53–75)	66 (54–79)	64 (54–75)	66 (55–79)
Mass$_i$ (g/ m^2)	73 (48–93)	58 (44–73)	71 (53–95)	52 (31–73)	69 (51–93)	56 (45–73)	72 (53–94)	60 (42–73)	69 (53–95)	57 (40–73)	66 (51–95)	49 (38–73)

Data in brackets are the 95% confidence intervals. EDV: end diastolic volume; ESV: end systolic volume; SV: stroke volume; EF: ejection fraction; Mass: ventricular mass; i: indexed.

Ventricular volumes, mass, and function

Table 3.2.3 Right ventricle indexed normal volumes and mass for males and females classified according to age

	16–20 years		21–30 years		31–40 years		41–50 years		51–60 years		>60 years	
	Males	Females	Males	Females	Males	Females	Males	Females	Males	Females	Males	Females
EDVi (ml/m²)	88 (62–109)	81 (67–99)	92 (68–112)	83 (66–98)	91 (70–111)	78 (58–100)	88 (60–109)	76 (56–98)	81 (66–107)	71 (50–89)	79 (61–106)	69 (45–88)
ESVi (ml/m²)	34 (24–45)	30 (23–36)	39 (22–57)	30 (16–43)	39 (24–52)	25 (16–31)	31 (20–44)	27 (18–41)	34 (18–45)	26 (15–38)	28 (15–44)	25 (17–36)
SVi (ml/m²)	53 (39–70)	51 (43–63)	57 (45–77)	53 (49–57)	53 (40–63)	53 (38–74)	49 (37–70)	49 (30–66)	54 (40–82)	45 (35–61)	51 (38–70)	44 (28–58)
EF (%)	61 (52–70)	63 (55–71)	60 (52–70)	65 (56–76)	58 (53–72)	67 (56–74)	61 (50–71)	63 (50–73)	61 (52–78)	66 (53–72)	65 (35–77)	64 (55–70)

Data in brackets are the 95% confidence intervals. EDV: end diastolic volume; ESV: end systolic volume; SV: stroke volume; EF: ejection fraction; i: indexed.

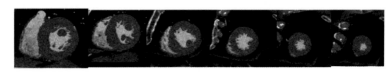

Figure 3.2.2 A 66-year-old man with suspected coronary artery disease and hypertensive heart disease.

Image shows the detection of endocardial left ventricle contours (green) in diastolic phase in order to measure end diastole.

- Compared to echocardiography, cardiac CT tends to overestimate the EF.
- Compared to MRI, cardiac CT shows a slightly lower EF.

Left ventricular myocardial thickness

A hypertrophic phenotype can be the result of several underlying cardiac diseases such as hypertrophic cardiomyopathy, storage disease, infiltrative cardiomyopathy, or hypertensive heart disease. Conversely, myocardial thinning can be indicative of ischaemic or non-ischaemic dilated cardiomyopathy. Reference values for LV wall thickness are given in Table 3.2.4.

- To opacify both the LV and the RV a triphasic injection protocol (contrast agent bolus followed by a mixed bolus of contrast agent and saline solution) is required (see also Chapter 1.10).
- Myocardial thickness is measured in diastole from a mid-ventricular short-axis reconstruction of the LV (see Figure 3.2.3).

Aortic root and ascending aorta

The aortic root is composed of the aortic anulus, the sinus of Valsalva, and the sinotubular junction (see also Chapters 3.3 and 3.9. Dilatation of these structures may be encountered with aortic valve disease, arterial hypertension, and/or connective tissue disorders, and may prompt pre-emptive surgery. Reference values for aortic dimensions are given in Tables 3.2.5 and 3.2.6.

- Evaluation of the aortic root and ascending aorta included in the scan volume should be routinely performed during CCTA.
- The acquisition protocol is the same used for CCTA.

Images should be reconstructed using multiplanar reconstruction from axial planes perpendicular to the long axis of the vessel (Figure 3.2.4; see also Chapter 3.9). The aortic anulus should be measured in systole (see Chapter 3.3), while the aortic sinus, sinotubular junction, and ascending aorta should be measured in diastole.

Table 3.2.4 Normal left ventricular wall thickness for males and females classified according to age

	16–20 years		21–30 years		31–40 years		41–50 years		51–60 years		>60 years	
	Males	Females	Males	Females	Males	Females	Males	Females	Males	Females	Males	Females
IVS (mm)	9 (8–11)	9 (7–10)	9 (7–11)	8 (7–10)	9 (8–11)	8 (7–10)	10 (8–11)	8 (6–10)	10 (7–11)	9 (7–10)	10 (8–11)	9 (6–10)
PW (mm)	8 (6–10)	7 (5–9)	8 (5–10)	8 (7–9)	9 (7–10)	8 (6–9)	9 (7–10)	7 (6–9)	8 (6–10)	7 (6–9)	8 (6–10)	7 (4–9)

Data in brackets are the 95% confidence intervals. IVS: interventricular septum; PW: posterior wall.

Aortic root and ascending aorta

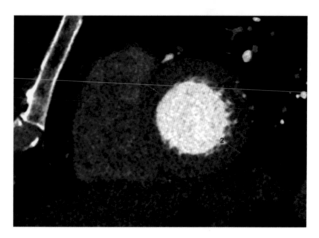

Figure 3.2.3 A 73-year-old man with suspected coronary artery disease.

Evaluation of left ventricle myocardial thickness on multiplanar reconstruction in a short-axis view.

- Specifically, the aortic sinus should be measured from cusp to commissure (Figure 3.2.5) because it is more reproducible; this method should be specified in the report.

Pulmonary veins

Pulmonary veins drain the oxygenated blood from the lung into the left atrium. Pulmonary veins often represent foci of arrhythmias that need to be treated with radiofrequency. Ostial stenoses of the pulmonary veins are potential complications of radiofrequency ablation.

The scan protocol to image pulmonary veins is the same as standard CCTA, except that ECG triggering is not mandatory (exception: patients in atrial fibrillation).

- Volume-rendering reconstruction is useful in order to obtain a multiplanar view of the pulmonary veins (Figure 3.2.6).
- The most common anatomical patterns of pulmonary vein anatomy are (in order of prevalence): four pulmonary veins (two per side); three pulmonary veins with a left common trunk; and five pulmonary veins (with an additional right intermediate vein (see also Chapter 3.7)).
- Normal pulmonary vein ostial measurements are listed in Table 3.2.7.

Table 3.2.5 Aortic root dimensions in systole for males and females classified according to age

	20–29 years		30–39 years		40–49 years		50–59 years		60–69 years		70–79 years	
	Males	Females	Males	Females	Males	Females	Males	Females	Males	Females	Males	Females
Cusp-Comm (mm)	33 (26–40)	29 (21–36)	32 (26–38)	29 (23–34)	33 (29–37)	32 (26–37)	34 (24–44)	30 (26–33)	34 (24–44)	31 (27–34)	35 (29–41)	30 (28–33)
Cusp-Commi (mm/m²)	17 (14–20)	17 (13–20)	16 (13–19)	18 (15–20)	16 (14–18)	18 (13–23)	17 (13–21)	18 (15–21)	18 (14–21)	18 (15–21)	18 (16–20)	19 (17–20)
Aortic root (cm²)	9 (5–13)	7 (3–10)	8 (4–12)	6 (4–9)	9 (67–12)	8 (6–10)	10 (3–16)	7 (5–9)	10 (7–13)	7 (5–9)	10 (6–14)	8 (6–9)
Aortic rooti (cm2/m²)	4 (3–6)	4 (2–6)	4 (2–6)	4 (3–5)	4 (3–6)	5 (3–6)	5 (2–8)	4 (3–5)	5 (3–7)	4 (3–6)	5 (4–7)	5 (4–5)

Data in brackets are the 95% confidence intervals. Cusp-Comm: cusp-commissure; i: indexed.

Pulmonary veins

Table 3.2.6 Ascending and descending thoracic aorta in diastole

	Males	Females
Mid-ascending (mm)	28 (27–29)	28 (27–29)
Mid-ascending (mm/m^2)	14 (14–15)	16 (16–17)
Mid-descending (mm)	21 (20–22)	20 (19–21)
Mid-descending (mm^2/m^2)	10 (10–11)	11 (11–12)
Diaphragm (mm)	20 (19–20)	19 (18–19)
Diaphragm (mm/m^2)	10 (10–10)	11 (10–11)

Data in brackets are the 95% confidence intervals.

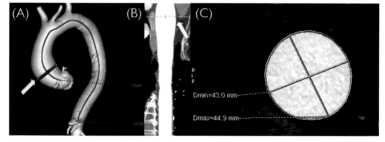

Figure 3.2.4 A 55-year-old woman with known history of bicuspid aortic valve.

Three-dimensional volume rendering of thoracic aorta showing the plan of ascending aorta measurement (A, arrow). The same plan is shown on aortic reconstruction (B, arrow) and multiplanar reconstruction (C).

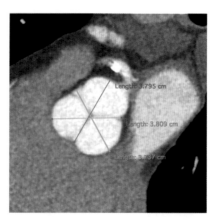

Figure 3.2.5 A 65-year-old man underwent CCTA for the evaluation of coronary artery disease.

Measurements of Cusp-Commissure of the aortic sinus were performed with multiplanar reconstruction.

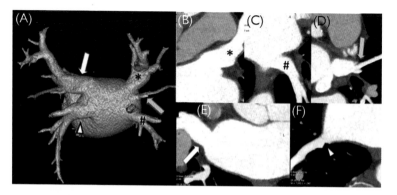

Figure 3.2.6 An 80-year-old man underwent cardiac CT angiography for suspected coronary artery disease.

Three-dimensional volume rendering showing (A) the left atrium and (B–F) multiplanar reformatted pulmonary veins. Images show (A, E) right upper pulmonary vein (white arrow), (A, F) right inferior pulmonary vein (arrowhead), (A, B) left superior pulmonary vein (asterisk), (A, C) left inferior pulmonary vein (hashtag), and (A, D) accessory left inferior pulmonary vein (blue arrow).

Pericardium

The pericardium, composed of serous and fibrous layers, contains the heart and the proximal part of great vessels (see also Chapter 3.13).

The average normal thickness of pericardium ranges between 1 and 2 mm in normal patients (Figure 3.2.7).

For the evaluation of pericardium, CT can be acquired either with or without administration of an iodine-based contrast agent.

• Acquisition without the administration of a contrast agent can provide information on pericardial thickness and the presence of pericardial calcification and/or pericardial effusion.

• Acquisition of CCTA after the administration of contrast agent allows for the evaluation of pericardial disease, as well as presence of septal bounce

Table 3.2.7 Normal pulmonary vein ostial measurements	
Right superior pulmonary vein	11.4–12.4 mm
Left superior pulmonary vein	9.6–10.5 mm
Right inferior pulmonary vein	12.3–13.1 mm
Left inferior pulmonary vein	9.0–9.9 mm

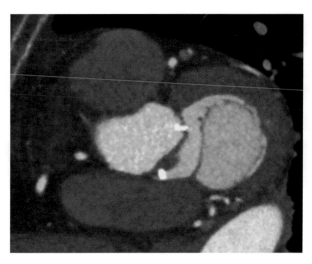

Figure 3.2.7 A 66-year-old man underwent coronary CT angiography for suspected coronary artery disease.

Evaluation of pericardial thickness on multiplanar reconstruction on short-axis.

Pulmonary arteries

Pulmonary arteries drain the deoxygenated blood from the right chambers to the lung.

While narrowing of coronary arteries is often associated with congenital heart disease, the dilatation of pulmonary arteries can be due to pulmonary hypertension, as well as congenital heart disease.

Table 3.2.8 Normal pulmonary artery values			
		Males	Females
Pulmonary artery diameters (mm)	Main	26 (25–27)	22 (22–23)
	Right	20 (20–21)	18 (17–19)
	Left	20 (20–21)	19 (18–20)
Indexed pulmonary artery diameters	Main	13 (13–14)	14 (13–14)
	Right	10 (10–11)	10 (10–11)
	Left	10 (10–11)	11 (10–12)
Data in brackets are the 95% confidence intervals.			

Often, evaluation of the pulmonary arteries in CCTA it is not optimal; however, tailored injection of a contrast agent can allow for the evaluation of pulmonary arteries (see also Chapter 3.9). Table 3.2.8 provides normal reference values for pulmonary artery diameter.

Further reading

Acquaro GD, Camastra G, Monti L, Lombardi M, Pepe A, Castelletti S, et al. Reference values of cardiac volumes, dimensions, and new functional parameters by MR: A multicenter, multivendor study. *J Magn Reson Imaging* 2017; 45: 1055–67.

Burman ED, Keegan J, Kilner PJ. Aortic root measurement by cardiovascular magnetic resonance: specification of planes and lines of measurement and corresponding normal values. *Circ Cardiovasc Imaging* 2008; 1: 104–13.

Maffei E, Messalli G, Martini C, Nieman K, Catalano O, Rossi A, et al. Left and right ventricle assessment with Cardiac CT: validation study vs. cardiac MR. *Eur Radiol* 2012; 22: 1041–9.

Chapter 3.3

Aortic valve disease

Giuseppe Muscogiuri

> **Teaching points**
>
> - Aortic valve calcium score can be used in combination with clinical and echocardiographic criteria.
> - CT can provide information about the anatomy of the valve and aortic root, and information of surrounding cardiovascular structure and coronary arteries for the estimation of stenosis severity.
> - Correct evaluation of anatomy can be helpful in guiding the therapeutic management of aortic valve disease

How to set up your scanner for aortic valve scanning

- It is highly recommended that CT images without contrast are acquired using prospective electrocardiogram (ECG) gating in aortic stenosis (AS).
- Patients that are undergoing CT angiography for the evaluation of aortic valve pathology can be prepared administrating nitrates and beta blockers, only if they are not contraindicated.
- Tube voltage and tube current should be adapted based on the habitus of patient.
- Fastest gantry rotation time, based on the scanner technology, should be used in order to minimize motion artefact.
- Field of view (FoV) should be based on the clinical need. It is suggested that a small FoV is used if acquisition is focused on the aortic valve, while a larger FoV comprising the ascending aorta and the aortic arch should be considered in the presence of an associated dilated aorta.
- Injection of contrast agent should be tailored in order to achieve a iodine delivery rate approximately of 1.6–2 g/s. The volume of contrast agent depends on the scanner's capability (usually 50–70 ml of iodine contrast agent followed by saline at the same flow rate).
- For the evaluation of the aortic root and definition of the aortic valve morphology, an acquisition using ECG-gating, including the entire cardiac cycle, is required. Evaluation of the thoracic aorta is highly recommended in specific pathologies and can be useful for surgical planning.
- Reconstruction for the assessment of lung disease is highly recommended.

How to report the CT findings

- Multiplanar reconstruction (MPR) of the aortic valve can provide information on the morphology or valve. MPR can be achieved by finding a plane that is parallel to the aortic valve on both a three-chamber view and long axis of the aorta.
- MPR of aortic bulb, parallel to the aortic valve, is helpful for the evaluation of bulb dimensions. It is suggested that the dimensions of bulb, measuring cusp commissure, are evaluated in order to reduce variability (see Chapter 3.2).
- Measurements of the sinotubular junction can easily be achieved on a reformatted plan, parallel to the sinotubular junction.

Bicuspid aortic valve

The bicuspid aortic valve (BAV) is the most common congenital cardiac malformation, affecting 1–2% of the population. It is often associated with AS, aortic regurgitation (AR), dilatation of ascending aorta, or aortic coarctation. BAV can be classified into three types:

1. Type 0 (no raphe)—lateral cusp or anterior–posterior cusp.
2. Type 1 (one raphe)—based on the fusion of cusps, it is further divided into three categories: left–right (fusion between left and right cusps; the most common); right cusp–non-coronary (fusion between right and non-coronary cusp; less common); left cusp–non-coronary (fusion between left and non-coronary cusp; uncommon)
3. Type 2 (two raphe)—this type can be observed with left–right and right–non-coronary fusion.
   - The presence of raphe is commonly associated with a dilatation of the aortic root (Figure 3.3.1).
   - Coronary CT angiography (CCTA) can detect BAV with a sensitivity and specificity of 94% and 100%, respectively, if compared to echocardiography.
     - The European Society of Cardiology suggest surgery in patients with an aortic root diameter of ≥55 mm or ≥50 mm if there are other coexisting risk factors such as aortic coarctation, systemic hypertension, a family history of dissection, or increased aortic diameter >3 mm/year measured at the same level with the same imaging technique.
     - Preoperative information regarding the coronary arteries can be extremely helpful for correct surgical planning.
     - Evaluation of aortic root anatomy can be extremely useful for correct surgical planning.
     - In patients with BAV, search for/exclude coarctation, aortic aneurysm, patent ductus arteriosus, Turner or Marfan syndrome, coronary anomalies, and ventricular/atrial septal defect.

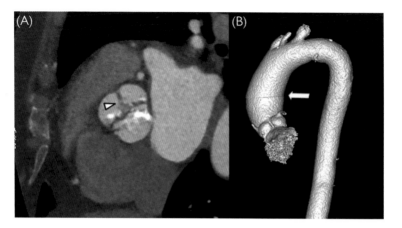

Figure 3.3.1 Sixty-five-year-old woman with a known history of bicuspid aortic valve (BAV).

Multiplanar CT image of the aortic valve shows a calcified aortic valve with partial fusion of the left cusp and non-coronary cusp (A, arrowhead). Beyond BAV, the patient has dilatation of the ascending aorta (B, arrow).

Aortic stenosis

AS is characterized by the narrowing of the aortic valve due to congenital heart disease or due to senile degeneration. Beyond echocardiography, CT can provide useful for information regarding the anatomy of the valve and surrounding structures.

- Aortic valve calcium score is recommended in low-flow low-gradient aortic stenosis when echocardiography evaluation is inconclusive (Figure 3.3.2).
- Aortic calcification can be evaluated on ECG-gated CT images without the administration of contrast agent using a low-dose CT protocol. Agatson scores of ≥2000 in men and ≥1200 in women are suggestive of severe AS (Table 3.3.1).
- Evaluation of left ventricle outflow tract anatomy can be easily assessed using CT with thin thickness.
- Using CCTA, it is possible to evaluate the morphology of the aortic valve (bicuspid or tricuspid aortic valve).

The evaluation of aortic stenosis using CT allows for the evaluation of the coronary arteries for the correct evaluation of significant coronary artery disease and location of the coronary ostia

Aortic regurgitation

Aortic regurgitation is defined by leakage of the aortic valve causing a diastolic regurgitant volume in the left ventricle cavity during diastole and is primarily assessed

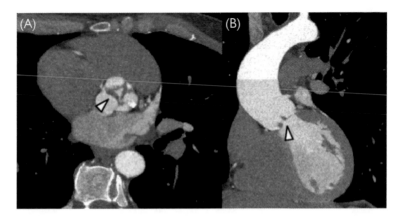

Figure 3.3.2 An 85-year-old patient with moderate aortic regurgitation.
(A, B) Uncomplete closure and thickening of aortic valve is shown (arrowhead).

by echocardiography. Aortic regurgitation is mostly caused by aortic root dilatation, or, less commonly, as a sequela of infection, and connective tissue disease.

Evaluation of aortic regurgitation using CT can be helpful in the assessment of valve anatomy and evaluation of the mechanism causing the AR, as well as the surrounding cardiovascular structures

As described in the previous section for AS, the acquisition of both diastole and systole can be helpful in the evaluation of aortic valve anatomy. The same CT parameters as AS can be used for the evaluation of AR; however, the thoracic aorta will not be acquired if it is not clinically indicated.

- CT can give important clues about the aetiology of AR: aortic root dilation, cusp retraction, incomplete cusp adaptation, cusp prolapse, cusp perforations, calcification, masses/vegetations, etc.

- Aortic regurgitation can be assessed using CT, after MPR is executed in diastole.

- CT allows for the quantification of AR severity by direct planimetry of aortic regurgitant orifice area in a diastolic frame. However, it is important to consider that the amount of regurgitation recorded cannot be accurate owing to the low

Table 3.3.1 Likelihood of severe aortic stenosis based on aortic valve calcium score (using Agatston score)		
	Men	Women
Severe aortic stenosis very likely	≥3000	≥1600
Severe aortic stenosis likely	≥2000	≥1200
Severe aortic stenosis unlikely	<1600	<800

Table 3.3.2 Severity of aortic regurgitation by planimetry of regurgitant orifice area on CT	
Mild	< 25 mm²
Moderate	25–75 mm²
Severe	>75 mm²

resolution of CT compared to magnetic resonance imaging and echocardiography (Table 3.3.2 and Figure 3.3.3).

• In case of surgical planning beyond anatomical evaluation of the valve, it is recommended that the coronary arteries and thoracic aorta are evaluated.

Aortic endocarditis and related infective complications

Aortic endocarditis could occur in native or prosthetic valves, and may lead to the development of valvular regurgitation, rupture of the left ventricle free wall, or affect the conducting system.

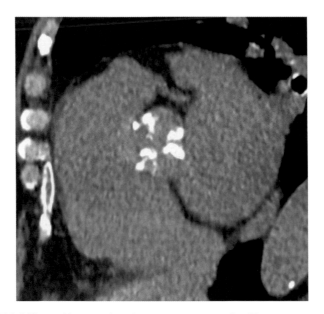

Figure 3.3.3 A 77-year-old woman who underwent non-contrast cardiac CT.
The aortic valve is heavily calcified (arrow). Calcium score was 1450.

Despite the key role of echocardiography (particularly transoesophageal echocardiography (TOE)) in the diagnosis of vegetation caused by endocarditis, CT can provide additional information and can be fundamental in planning the surgical approach. Specifically in prosthetic valve endocarditis (PVE), the diagnostic yield of echocardiography may be lower and CT may offer additional value (often in combination with fluorodeoxyglucose positron emission tomography or white blood cell single photon emission CT). (For more detailed information on PVE see Chapters 3.6 and 3.8.)

- Echocardiography (particularly TOE) is superior to CT for the detection of small vegetations or leaflet perforations; however, CT is superior for paravalvular abscesses or pseudoaneurysms.
- CCTA can be fundamental in gathering evidence of massive vegetation or in the case of emergency surgery, allowing for the assessment of both valve and coronary artery anatomy.
- In native endocarditis, CCTA can be helpful in the evaluation of valvular perforation, thickening and perivalvular abscess, pseudoaneurysm, or fistula.
- In patients undergoing transcatheter aortic valve replacement, it is possible to evaluate perivalvular complications using CT.
- In patients with endocarditis, embolic complications have been described in the thorax, abdomen, and brain. Adapting the FOV and scan range, and timing of the image acquisition to cover these parts of the body should be considered.

Aortic valve pseudoaneurysm after surgery

Aortic pseudoaneurysm is defined as a partial dehiscence of the suture line and left ventricle outflow tract. Pseudoaneurysm is defined as a rupture of the mitral-aortic fibrosa with the pseudoaneurysm wall composed of fibrous tissue.

The CT parameters are the same described earlier; however, similar to endocarditis the images can be acquired in both systole and diastole for the evaluation of rocking vegetation.

- CT allows for depiction of the gap between the prosthetic valve and left ventricle outflow tract.
- CT can be extremely important for evaluation of the coronary arteries before surgical evaluation.

Further reading

Baumgartner H, Falk V, Bax JJ, De Bonis M, Hamm C, Holm PJ, et al. 2017 ESC/EACTS Guidelines for the management of valvular heart disease. *Eur Heart J* 2017; 38: 2739–91.

Borger MA, Fedak PWM, Stephens EH, Gleason TG, Girdauskas E, Ikonomidis JS, et al. The American Association for Thoracic Surgery consensus guidelines on bicuspid aortic valve-related aortopathy: full online-only version. *J Thorac Cardiovasc Surg* 2018; 156: e41–74.

Ternacle J, Clavel M-A. Assessment of aortic stenosis severity: a multimodality approach. *Cardiol Clin* 2020; 38: 13–22.

CT prior to transcatheter/surgical aortic valve replacement

Marco Guglielmo

Assessment of aortic stenosis severity: calcium score of the aortic valve

- See Chapter 3.3.

Aortic annulus

- Aortic annulus is defined as a virtual ring that connects the three lowest points of attachment of the aortic valve cusps ('hinge points') to the left ventricle outflow tract (LVOT) wall.
- Accurate aortic annulus measurement is crucial for choosing the correct size of prosthesis.
- Aortic annulus is usually not circular, but rather elliptical in shape. Two-dimensional echocardiography typically measures the shorter diameter of the oval aortic annulus, while three-dimensional imaging such as cardiac CT

Table 3.4.1 Practical tips: how to set up your scanner for a pre-transcatheter aortic valve replacement scan	
Patient preparation	• Use of nitrates is contraindicated in patients with severe aortic stenosis. Beta-blocker use is not recommended (except in selected cases with careful clinical oversight) • In patient with severe renal impairment, IV hydration can be considered before cardiac CT (see Chapter 1.10; fast anatomic coverage and low kilovoltage (70–80 kV) may reduce the amount of contrast agent injected)
Scan range	The scan volume must extend at least from the subclavian arteries to the superficial femoral arteries at the level of the femoral head
Scan protocol—scan strategy	In principle, two different approaches are possible. 1. Two-scan strategy: cardiac ECG-triggered acquisition of the aortic root and heart followed by a separate non-ECG-gated CTA of the thorax, abdomen, and pelvis 2. Single-scan strategy: ECG-synchronized data acquisition of the thorax followed by a non-ECG-synchronized CTA of the abdomen and pelvis (higher radiation dose)
ECG triggering	Image acquisition, including the entire cardiac cycle (retrospective gating or prospective gating with large window including systolic frames), is recommended
Contrast injection protocol	• Biphasic injection protocol • Flow rate 4–6 ml/s • Bolus tracking with peak contrast in the ascending aorta
Image reconstruction	Reconstructed slice width <1 mm for the aortic root and <1.5 mm for the peripheral vessels). A 64-slice or higher-end scanner is required

IV: intravenous; ECG: electrocardiogram; CTA: CT angiography.

Box 3.4.1 CT report for preprocedural transcatheter aortic valve implantation assessment	
Aortic valve	Morphology (tricuspid/bicuspid), calcifications (location, extent), calcium score (if discordant Doppler parameters)
Aortic annulus	Maximum/minimum diameters, area, calcifications
Left ventricular outflow tract	Calcification locations and extent (especially large, protruding calcifications)
Coronary obstruction risk	Small sinus of Valsalva (<30 mm), low coronary ostia from the annular plant (<12 mm), highly calcified aortic cusps
Aorta	Width of aortic sinus, ascending aorta, aortic arch, descending aorta, elongation with kinking of the aorta, dissection, large thrombi protruding into the lumen, exophitic plaques
Fluoroscopic projection	Optimal C-arm angulations providing an orthogonal view of the aortic annular plane
Peripheral arterial anatomy	Minimal vessel diameters, tortuosity, and calcifications
Coronary arteries	Rule out significant coronary stenosis if adequate image quality

measures both the smaller and larger diameter of the aortic annulus and is more accurate for annulus sizing.

Multioblique reconstruction of the aortic anulus

- Data set is manipulated manually or to obtain an orthogonal plane on the centreline of the aorta, immediately below the lowest insertion points of the aortic cusps (Figure 3.4.1). Dedicated software applications allow an anatomical segmentation with a semi-automatic identification of the aortic annulus.
- Owing to the dynamic changes of the aortic annulus during the cardiac cycle, all data set phases should be reviewed. An image of sufficient quality showing the larger aortic annulus should be used. Usually, a systolic image should be used but, in case of septal hypertrophy, the aortic annulus may be larger in diastole. Moreover, image quality should be preferred over cardiac phase selection and diastolic images may be of better quality, providing more reliable measurements.
- Three measurements of the aortic annulus may be obtained (Figure 3.4.2):
  - maximum and minimum diameter, mean diameter;
  - maximum area;
  - circumference (for accurate perimeter measurements, the 'spline' technique: manual segmentation points connected by a cubic spline interpolation) should be preferred over manual contour or polygon drawing techniques.
- For individual sizing recommendations consult each manufacturer's product sizing sheets.

Aortic valve

- The presence of calcifications is important to ensure prosthesis anchorage, but severe calcifications may hamper the apposition of the prosthesis to the aortic root, leaving gaps between the prosthetic frame and the aortic root that result in paravalvular aortic regurgitation. A qualitative scale from 1 to 4 can be used to define calcifications (Figure 3.4.3).

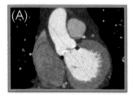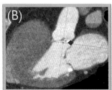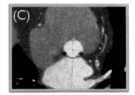

Figure 3.4.1 (A, B) The data set is manipulated to obtain (C) an oblique axial plane exactly aligned with the three most caudal points of the aortic cusps.

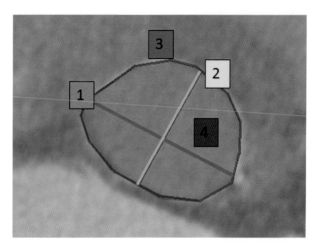

Figure 3.4.2 Aortic annulus measurements.

1 (orange): maximum diameter; 2 (yellow): minimum diameter; 3 (blue): perimeter; 4 (purple): area.

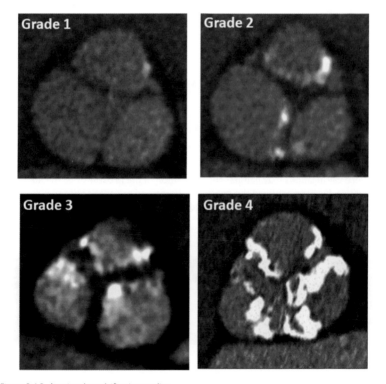

Figure 3.4.3 Aortic valve calcification grading.

Grade 1: no or minimal calcifications; grade 2: mildly calcified (small isolated spots); grade 3: moderately calcified (multiple larger spots); grade 4: heavily calcified (extensive calcification of all cusps).

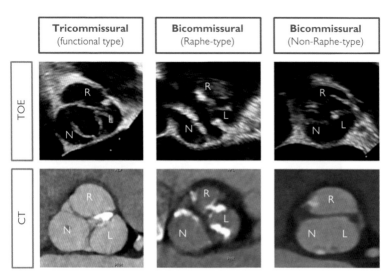

	Tricommissural (functional type)	Bicommissural (Raphe-type)	Bicommissural (Non-Raphe-type)
TOE			
CT			

Figure 3.4.4 Bicuspid valve classification according to Jilaihawi *et al.* (see Further Reading). R: right coronary cusp; L: left coronary cusp; N: non-coronary cusp; TOE: transoesophageal echocardiography.

- Bicuspid aortic valves may be associated with an increased risk of paravalvular aortic regurgitation, reduced implantation success, and a higher risk of pacemaker implantation after transcatheter aortic valve implantation (TAVI).
- Bicuspid aortic valves (Figure 3.4.4) can be classified as: (1) tricommissural (one commissure completely fused between two cusps); (2) bicommisural raphe-type (two cusps are fused by a fibrous or calcified ridge); and (3) bicommisural non raphe-type (two cusps completely fused from their basal origin by no visible ridge).
- The risk of paravalvular aortic regurgitation increases with severe raphe calcification. For a more detailed discussion on bicuspid aortic valves see Chapter 3.3.

Annular and subannular calcifications

- The presence, location, and extent of annular and subannular (LVOT) calcifications should be described (Figure 3.4.5). In particular, large protruding calcifications can increase the risk of annular rupture during valve deployment and should be mentioned in the report. Moreover, subannular severe calcifications increase the risk of atrioventricular blocks and the need for pacemaker implantation.

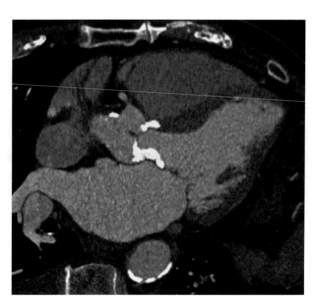

Figure 3.4.5 Annular and subannular calcifications protruding in the left ventricular outflow tract.

Reducing the risk of coronary obstruction

- Features that increase the risk of coronary obstruction during TAVI include:
  - low coronary ostia (distance from the annular plane <12 mm);
  - shallow sinus of Valsalva and narrow sinotubular junction;
  - long and heavily calcified cusps (Figure 3.4.6);
  - use of balloon-expandable valves;
  - valve-in-valve TAVI.
- The coronary heights should be measured perpendicularly from the annular plane (Figure 3.4.6A).

Assessment of the aorta

- It is recommended that aortic diameters are measured in diastolic data sets.
- The width of the aortic sinus should be measured on a transverse double-oblique plane parallel to the annular plane. Preferably, three cusp-to-commissure measurements should be performed.

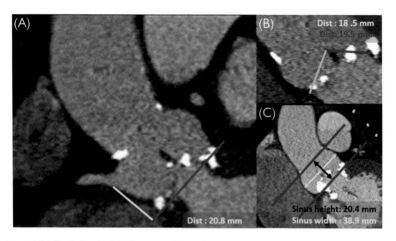

(A) Dist : 18.5 mm
Dist : 19.5 mm

(C) Sinus height: 20.4 mm
Sinus width : 38.9 mm

Dist : 20.8 mm

Figure 3.4.6 Predicting the risk of coronary obstruction.

(A) Coronary heights. (B) Cusp lengths. (C) Sinus of Valsalva dimension.

- The width of the sinotubular junction, ascending aorta, aortic arch, and descending aorta should be measured on transverse double-oblique planes orientated orthogonally to the long axis of the aorta.
- Massive elongation with kinking of the aorta, dissection, large thrombi protruding into the lumen, and exophytic plaques should be described.
- Severe calcifications of the ascending aorta or 'porcelain' aorta may pose a risk for embolization during aortic cross-clamping for surgical aortic valve replacement (SAVR).
- Coronary artery bypass grafts and their course underneath the sternum should be reported if they are at risk for laceration during sternotomy for SAVR.
- The relationship/distance of the ascending aorta and aortic valve to the right-sided thoracic wall should be reported if SAVR via a minimally invasive right thoracotomy approach is contemplated (Figure 3.4.7).

Fluoroscopic projection

- During transcatheter implantation, it is important to use a fluoroscopic projection that provides an exactly orthogonal view onto the aortic annular plane.
- CT allows (either manually or through dedicated software) identification of the angulation of the C-arm that will provide the desired view during the implantation procedure.

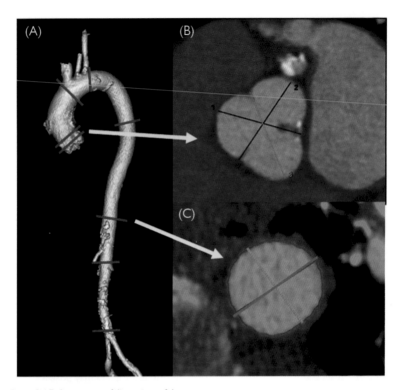

Figure 3.4.7 Assessment of dimensions of the aorta.

(A) Volume rendering of the aorta with standard points of measurements (red). (B) Width of the aortic sinus; three cusp-to-commissure measurements are performed. In the other locations, (C) maximum and minimum diameters of the vessel are measured at different levels in perpendicular to the centreline plane.

- Optimal C-arm angulations should be reported as degrees left anterior oblique or right anterior oblique, with the corresponding values for cranial or caudal angulation (Figure 3.4.8).

Coronary arteries

Coronary arteries can sometimes be difficult to evaluate in TAVI patients due to the high prevalence of calcifications in this population and the contraindications to nitrates and beta-blockers. However, given its high sensitivity and negative predictive value, cardiac CT represents an excellent gatekeeper to invasive coronary angiography (ICA) in TAVI patients.

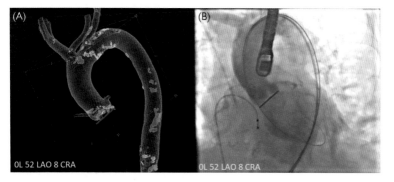

Figure 3.4.8 (A) C-arm fluoroscopic view choice. (B) Intraprocedural fluoroscopy using the predicted C-arm view.

- In the presence of adequate image quality, coronary CT angiography (CCTA) may rule out significant coronary stenosis and ICA can be excluded from the preprocedural diagnostic work-up, reducing further radiation, contrast media administration, and hospitalization costs.
- Coronary anomalies can be easily identified with CCTA—for example, an anomalous left circumflex artery from the right coronary sinus with a retroaortic course may be injured during annular SAVR.

Left ventricle

The presence of left ventricular (LV) thrombus should be excluded with cardiac CT and often represents a contraindication for CT.

Vascular access

Peripheral arterial anatomy

- Iliac and femoral arteries should be reconstructed with standard CT angiography techniques and evaluated for the following features:
  - diameters of the common iliac, external iliac, and common femoral arteries (Figure 3.4.9);
  - vessel tortuosity;
  - calcifications (a qualitative scale should be used (mild, moderate, or severe)).
- Report high bifurcation of the femoral arteries (above the mid-level of the femoral head).

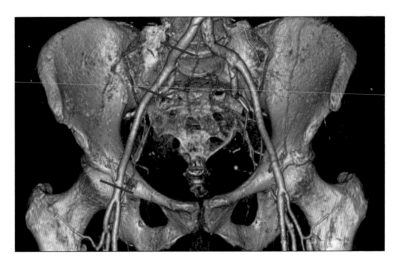

Figure 3.4.9 Ileofemoral anatomy must be evaluated and minimal vessel diameters reported.

Identification of risk factors for vascular complications

• External sheath diameter exceeding minimal artery diameter.
• Moderate/severe calcifications (particularly circular calcifications).
• Peripheral arterial disease.

Other access

• If transfemoral access is impractical, subclavian, carotid, direct aortic, transapical, or transcaval approaches may be considered. In these cases, CT can be used to measure the alternate vessels, identifying vascular pathology, tortuosity, or calcifications.
• In case of a transapical approach, CT should give information on the thoracic wall, LV apex (presence of apical thrombus), and angulation between the LVOT and LV apex, as steeper angles may complicate the procedure.
• In the case of a transaortic approach, information about the thoracic wall, lung parenchyma, and aortic wall calcification should be provided.
• In the case of minimally invasive SAVR, femoral cannulation sites for extracorporeal circulation should be evaluated.
• Embolic protection devices for transcatheter aortic valve replacement (TAVR) require meticulous examination of the aortic arch and the supra-aortic arteries, to assess anatomical suitability.

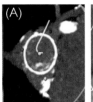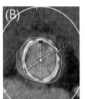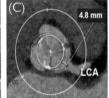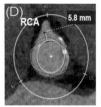

Figure 3.4.10 (A)Virtual transcatheter aortic valve to coronary distance (VTC) measurement in the presence of a stented bioprosthetic valve. (B) A circular region of interest with the dimension of the new prosthesis is drawn, (C, D) the distance between the left coronary artery (LCA), right coronary artery (RCA), and the circle represents the VTC.

Valve-in-valve transcatheter aortic valve replacement

- Implantation of a transcatheter aortic valve has become an option in the treatment of patients with a degenerated bioprosthetic valve. The rate of coronary occlusion is higher in patients with valve-in-valve implantation than TAVI in native aortic stenoses.
- In the presence of a stented bioprosthetic valve, the virtual transcatheter aortic valve to coronary distance should be measured. This measurement predicts the distance from the expanded transcatheter aortic valve frame to the coronary ostia (Figure 3.4.10).

CT features that increase the risk of coronary occlusion during valve-in-vale TAVR include:

- shallow sinus of Valsalva, and narrow and low sinotubular junction;
- low coronary ostia;
- 'stentless' or supra-annular implanted bioprosthetic valves;
- estimated distance of the virtual transcatheter heart valve to the coronary ostia <4 mm.

Extracardiac and extravascular findings

- Incidental findings can be found in >50% of all TAVR CTs.
  - Significant findings (approximately one-third of patients)—malignant tumours
  - Non-significant findings (approximately two-thirds of patients)—pleural effusion, bronchiectasis, diverticulosis, and hiatal hernia.
- Incidental CT findings should always be reported if clinically relevant. The repercussions of incidental findings, including the presence of malignancy, must be evaluated by the heart valve team on a case-by-case basis with regard to their influence on procedural success and prognosis.
  See also Chapter 3.15.

Further reading

Baumgartner H, Falk V, Bax JJ, De Bonis M, Hamm C, Holm PJ, et al. 2017 ESC/EACTS Guidelines for the management of valvular heart disease. *Eur Heart J* 2017; 38: 2739–91.

Blanke P, Weir-McCall JR, Achenbach S, Delgado V, Hausleiter J, Jilaihawi H, et al. Computed tomography imaging in the context of transcatheter aortic valve implantation (TAVI)/transcatheter aortic valve replacement (TAVR): an expert consensus document of the Society of Cardiovascular Computed Tomography. *J Cardiovasc Comput Tomogr* 2019; 12, 1–24.

Francone M, Budde RPJ, Bremerich J, Dacher JN, Loewe C, Wolf F, et al. CT and MR imaging prior to transcatheter aortic valve implantation: standardisation of scanning protocols, measurements and reporting—a consensus document by the European Society of Cardiovascular Radiology (ESCR) *Eur Radiol* 2020; 30: 2627–50.

Jilaihawi H, Chen M, Webb J, Himbert D, Ruiz CE, Rodés-Cabau J, et al. A bicuspid aortic valve imaging classification for the TAVR era. *JACC Cardiovasc Imaging* 2016; 9: 1145–58.

Chapter 3.5

Mitral valve disease

Marco Guglielmo

Teaching points

- Cardiac CT provides excellent anatomical details and can be used as an alternative method for the anatomical assessment of mitral valve (MV) apparatus and the quantification of mitral regurgitation, although echocardiography and magnetic resonance imaging remain the better techniques in this field (Table 3.5.1).
- Cardiac CT can be used for the accurate depiction of the mitral apparatus and its surrounding anatomical structures before transcatheter MV replacement (TMVR).
- Cardiac CT is the technique of choice for anatomical assessment prior to TMVR for native mitral valve disease and for failing surgical MV replacement or repair. Cardiac CT is fundamental for mitral annulus and 'neo' left ventricular outflow tract measurement before TMVR implant.

Although echocardiography remains the gold standard for assessing mitral valve (MV) diseases and their haemodynamic consequences, advanced cardiac imaging, including cardiac CT, is acquiring growing importance in the field, especially since the introduction of transcatheter MV replacement (TMVR) into clinical practice.

Anatomical assessment of the mitral valve and mechanisms of mitral regurgitation

- Echocardiography (transthoracic and particularly transoesophageal (TOE)) is the best-established technique for assessing MV disease. Cardiac CT is reserved for rare cases of patients not amenable to echocardiography or magnetic resonance imaging (MRI). Cardiac CT can provide a detailed visualization of the MV apparatus and all its components (papillary muscles, chordae tendineae, MV leaflets, mitral annulus), and can distinguish effectively between different aetiologies of mitral regurgitation (MR; functional vs. degenerative).
- MV prolapse can be identified and characterized by cross-referencing long-axis views of the MV with short-axis views of the various scallops (Figure 3.5 1). Mitroannular disjunction, an abnormal atrial displacement of the MV leaflet hinge point that frequently is associated with myxomatous bi-leaflet prolapse (Barlow disease), can be identified in systolic phases (Figure 3.5.1).

Table 3.5.1 How to set up your scanner for mitral valve imaging

Patient preparation	Beta-blocker and nitrates are not necessary (unless concomitant coronary angiography is planned)
Scan range	Consider a large field of view to include the left anterior ribcage for simulating transapical access
ECG triggering	A full cycle (0–100%) retrospective helical scan is recommended (without ECG dose modulation)
Contrast injection protocol	Triphasic contrast infection to opacify right-sided cavities (if trans-septal approach is contemplated)

ECG: electrocardiogram.

Quantification of the severity of mitral regurgitation

Quantification of MR with CT is feasible but not well established. Two methods exist:

1. Stroke volume method—a full cycle (0–100%) CT scan is required. Stroke volumes can be calculated by the difference in the ventricular end diastolic and end systolic volumes. Mitral regurgitant volume is given as the difference between the left and right stroke volumes. A few small studies have indicated a good correlation of regurgitant volume and fraction by CT with cardiac magnetic resonance and/or echocardiography.

2. In functional MRI, direct planimetry of the regurgitant orifice area on systolic frames is feasible (challenging, as MV has to be reconstructed into double oblique plane parallel to the mitral anulus that transects the narrowest mitral regurgitant orifice).

CT prior to transcatheter mitral valve repair

A large variety of transcatheter mitral repair devices are commercially available. Their appropriate use requires often detailed anatomical information on the MV apparatus and underlying structures by cardiac CT.

- Edge-to-edge mitral leaflet repair (MitraClip, PASCAL)—the gold standard technique prior to edge-to-edge repair is TOE. Cardiac CT is an alternative in patients not suitable for TOE to assess the following anatomical features: coaptation depth; coaptation length; flail gap; and flail width (Figures 3.5.2 and 3.5.3).

- Indirect mitral annuloplasty (Carillon)—coronary sinus anatomy (Figure. 3.5.4), persistent left superior vena cava, Thebesian valve, relationship between the coronary sinus and the left circumflex artery, relationship between the coronary sinus and the mitral anulus, and mitral annular calcifications.

- Direct mitral annuloplasty (Cardioband)—sizing of the mitral annulus, assessment of mitral annulus calcifications, relationship of left circumflex artery and coronary sinus with the mitral annulus, and anchor implant angle.

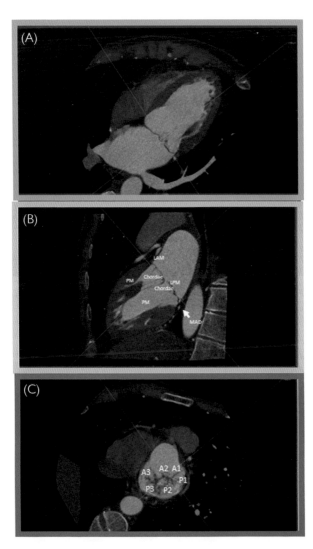

Figure 3.5.1 Bi-leaflet mitral valve prolapse.

Coronary CT angiography is able to depict the entire anatomy of the mitral valve apparatus: papillary muscles (PM), chordae tendinea, and anterior (LAM) and posterior (LPM) mitral leaflets. (A, B) Using orthogonal reformatting planes is possible to obtain an *en face* view (C) of the mitral valve, and to identify the anterior (A1, A2, A3) and posterior (P1, P2, P3) scallops of the mitral leaflets.

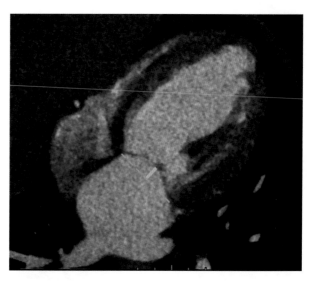

Figure 3.5.2 Patient with functional mitral regurgitation and tethering of the mitral valve leaflets. Coaptation length: red line; coaptation depth: orange line.

Cardiac CT prior to transcatheter mitral valve replacement

Cardiac CT has become the standard imaging modality to assess the suitability of a patient to percutaneous TMVR for native mitral valve disease and for failing surgical MV replacement or repair. It is fundamental for mitral annulus measurement and

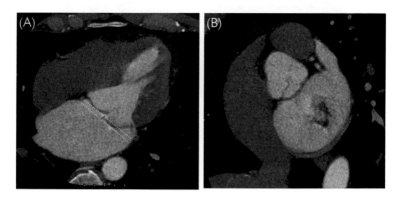

Figure 3.5.3 Mitral valve prolapse with flail of the posterior mitral leaflet. (A) Flail gap (red line). (B) Flail width (orange line).

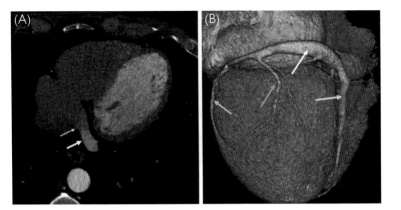

Figure 3.5.4 (A) Axial CT image showing the coronary sinus (white arrow) posterior to the left ventricle, draining into the right atrium. The Thebesian valve (yellow arrow) is seen as a thin, hypodense linear structure at the junction between the right atrium and the coronary sinus. (B) Volume-rendering image illustrating the coronary sinus (white arrow) and some of its tributary veins: the posterior interventricular vein or middle vein (yellow arrow), the posterolateral vein (light blue arrow), and the left marginal vein (green arrow).

left ventricular outflow tract (LVOT) assessment before TMVR implant. Clinically, TMVR is primarily performed using balloon-expandable Edwards SAPIEN devices (Edwards Lifesciences, Irvine, CA, USA) for valve-in-ring (ViR), valve-in-valve, or valve-in-mitral annular calcification (ViMAC) procedures, or using newer devices, including dedicated TMVR valves.

- *Mitral anular assessment with cardiac CT:* the mitral annulus is a complex, non-planar, saddle-shaped structure. It is characterized by an anterior horn, contiguous to the aortic valve (aortomitral continuity), and a posterior horn at the insertion between the posterior mitral leaflet and the atrioventricular junction. The nadirs of the saddle are at the level of the medial and lateral fibrous trigones (Figure 3.5.5).

- *Simulation of neo-LVOT:* TMVR creates a neo-LVOT between the basal segment of the interventricular septum and the anterior mitral leaflet, displaced anteriorly by the prosthesis. This is particularly relevant in ViR, ViMAC, and native TMVR procedures, where significant LVOT obstruction may occur. Neo-LVOT measurement should be done in end systole when the mitral annulus is larger and the LVOT is smaller (Figure 3.5.6).

Predictors of LVOT obstruction are:

- aortomitral angle (angle between the mitral and aortic annular planes) <110°;
- LVOT area <2.0 cm^2;
- small left ventricle size;
- hypertrophy of the basal segment of the interventricular septum and greater device protrusion into the left ventricle and device flaring.

  - Mitral annular calcification may be accurately depicted by CT. It is important to describe the presence, location, symmetry, and extension of calcifications.

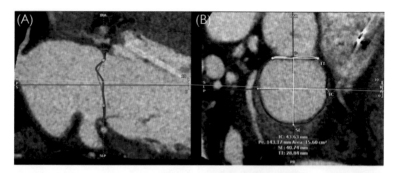

Figure 3.5.5 Using dedicated software, it is possible to identify a highly reproducible evaluation of the three-dimensional geometry of the mitral annulus, measuring the maximum area and perimeter, and the minimum and maximum diameter.

The annular contour is segmented within the three-dimensional space placing points at the insertion of the valve leaflets (A), obtaining a short-axis view of the annulus where the intercommisural (IC), septolateral (SL), and intertrigonal (TT) area and perimeter (red line) can be measured (B).

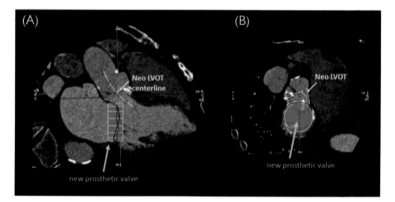

Figure 3.5.6 Dedicated three-dimensional (3D) software allows identification of the neo-left ventricular outflow tract (LVOT) by simulating the presence of the new valve that can be projected as a cylindrical volume according to the diameter and height of the prosthesis onto the mitral annulus using 3D segmentation techniques.

(A) Simulation of the presence of the proposed transcatheter mitral valve replacement prosthetic at the level of the mitral annulus (green arrow). (B) Planimetry of the neo-LVOT is performed in an orthogonal plane.

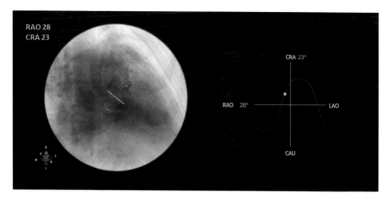

Figure 3.5.7 CT prediction of the best fluoroscopic projection for transcatheter mitral valve replacement.

Although circumferential or nearly circumferential mitral annular calcification may prevent paravalvular regurgitation creating a seal around the new valve, severe and asymmetrical calcification may hinder the TMVR implant.

Prediction of fluoroscopic angles

- Similar to transaortic valve implantation, CT has been shown to help predict a coplanar angle for coaxial deployment of the TMVR device (Figure 3.5.7).

Further reading

Blanke P, Dvir D, Cheung A, Levine RA, Thompson C, Webb JG, Leipsic J. Mitral annular evaluation with CT in the context of transcatheter mitral valve replacement. *JACC Cardiovasc Imaging* 2015; 8: 612–15.

Murphy DJ, Ge Y, Don CW, Keraliya A, Aghayev A, Morgan R, et al. Use of cardiac computerized tomography to predict neo-left ventricular outflow tract obstruction before transcatheter mitral valve replacement. *J Am Heart Assoc* 2017; 6: e007353.

Weir-McCall JR, Blanke P, Naoum C, Delgado V, Bax JJ, Leipsic J. Mitral valve imaging with CT: relationship with transcatheter mitral valve interventions. *Radiology* 2018; 288: 638–55.

CT after valve surgery/intervention

Andrea Baggiano

229

Why cardiac CT after valve surgery?

Echocardiography with a transthoracic approach (often integrated with trans-oesophageal echocardiography) remains the first-line test to assess patients with prosthetic valves. However, cardiac CT could provide additional or complementary information in many clinical settings:

- identification of the aetiology of prosthetic valve dysfunction, especially in patients with poor acoustic windows;

- identification of perivalvular complications;

- additional information for surgical planning.

How to optimize your scan protocol to assess a patient with a prosthetic valve

Advice on how to optimize the scan protocol to assess a patient with a prosthetic valve is provided in Box 3.6.1.

See also Chapter 3.14.

Box 3.6.1 How to optimize the scan protocol for patients with a prosthetic valve	
Medications	• Beta-blockers for heart rate control (clinical contraindications to be taken into consideration, such as second- or third-grade atrioventricular block, sick sinus syndrome, decompensated heart failure)
Scan parameters	• Perform native electrocardiogram (ECG)-gated scan • Use high-energy tube voltages (e.g. 120 kVp, or even 140 kVp in obese patients or when dense metallic artefacts are present) • Consider a larger field of view to include the ascending aorta (particularly after transcatheter aortic valve implantation or in patients with circulatory assist devices)
Image reconstruction	• Use sharp reconstruction kernels • Prefer iterative reconstruction algorithms to reduce radiation exposure
ECG gating	• Consider retrospective ECG gating (or prospective ECG gating with large padding into systolic frames) for optimal evaluation of leaflet motion (i.e. '4D-CTA'; particularly for valvular imaging) • Consider disabling dose modulation
Contrast protocol	• For right-sided or interatrial devices, consider triphasic injection to opacify both left and right heart chambers without streak artefacts of the superior vena cava

Pannus

• Chronic process (usually many years from surgical date) characterized by the ingrowth of fibrotic tissue (Figure 3.6.1).
• No relationship with anticoagulation therapy.
• (Semi-)circular mass curved along ring/subvalvular mass/attachment of mass to prosthetic heart valve ring/hinge points.
• Leaflet restriction common but may be absent.
• Typically, >200 Hounsfield units (HU).

Thrombus

• Irregularly shaped mass (larger than pannus), usually attached to the leaflet/hinge points (Figure 3.6.2).
• Occurs at any time point after surgery/intervention (if late, could be associated with pannus).
• Strong relationship with anticoagulation therapy.

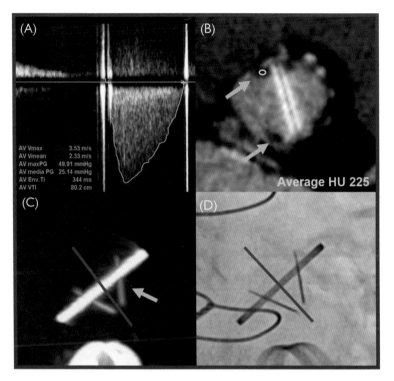

Figure 3.6.1 (A) Patient with previous aortic and mitral valve replacement with mechanical prostheses developed after 6 years increased anterograde gradients at the aortic level. (B) CT angiography showed the presence of pannus at the hinges, inducing (C) reduced anterior disc excursion, as confirmed by (D) valve fluoroscopy.
HU: Hounsfield units.

- Various mass location (sub- and supravalvular), commonly with independent motion.
- Typically, <200 HU.

Structural valve degeneration

- Usually occurs over 10–20 years.
- Long-term inflammatory/immune response.
- Prosthetic valve leaflets affected by calcifications and fibrotic tissue development (Figure 3.6.3).

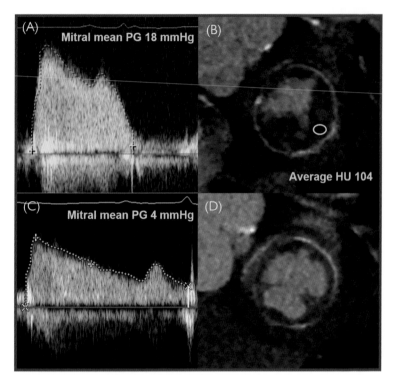

Figure 3.6.2 A patient with previous bioprosthetic mitral valve replacement who developed acute heart failure.

(A) Echocardiography proved prosthesis dysfunction, while CT angiography (CTA) showed thrombotic material affecting (B) the leaflets and surrounding atrial tissue. After anticoagulation therapy with unfractionated heparin, (C) echocardiography showed transmitral mean gradient reduction and (D) resolution of most of thrombotic material was shown on CTA.

PG: pressure gradient; HU: Hounsfield units.

- Valve dysfunction is usually induced by leaflet thickening and obstruction; tearing and ultimately detachment of the leaflets can rarely occur.

Hypoattenuated leaflet thickening

- Bioprosthetic leaflet thrombosis is usually subclinical and is described as an incidental finding.
- A layer of thrombus covers the aortic side of one or more leaflets (Figure 3.6.4).

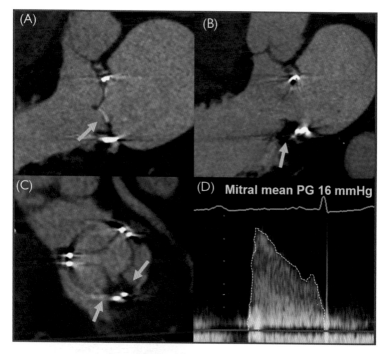

Figure 3.6.3 A patient with rheumatic disease with a previous bioprosthetic mitral valve replacement. After 10 years, the patient experienced the onset of worsening-effort dyspnoea. (A) CT angiography showed thickened and partially calcified prosthetic leaflets (arrow; modified long-axis view), and (B, C) abundant fibrotic tissue proliferation (arrow) affecting the insertion of prosthetic leaflets to the supporting ring (B, modified long-axis view; C, short-axis view). (D) These structural abnormalities (arrow) were reflected in a pathologically increased transmitral mean gradient.
PG: pressure gradient.

- Transvalvular pressure gradient is mostly within the normal range.
- The long-term clinical impact and the need for intervention are still uncertain.
- Typically, <200 HU.
- Hypoattenuated leaflet thickening is the first step in a continuous process of degenerative changes, followed by a reduction in leaflet motion, a subsequent increase in transvalvular gradients. and then the development of symptoms of valve thrombosis.

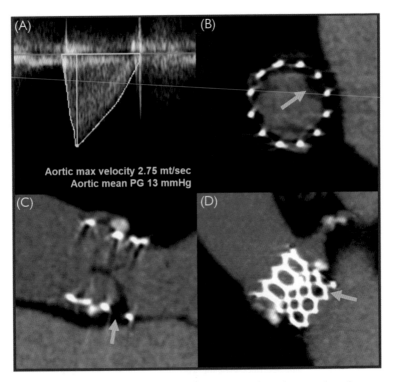

Figure 3.6.4 A patient who had a previous transcatheter aortic valve replacement showed (A) echocardiographic evidence of a stable transvalvular mean gradient. (B–D) At CT angiography, performed for coronary assessment, evidence of hypoattenuated leaflet thickening (HALT; arrows) at the aortic side of the left coronary leaflet (B, short-axis view; C, modified long-axis view; D, maximum intensity projection image showing HALT through the prosthesis struts (asterisks).

Infective endocarditis

- Vegetations are usually attached to native valve/mural endocardium, or to prosthetic material.
- Vegetations are usually in the trajectory of a regurgitant jet.
- There is no alternative anatomical explanation.
- Typically, <200 HU.
- Additional CT findings may include leaflet perforations, abscesses, and pseudoaneurysms.
- A combination with radionuclide imaging (either ^{18}F-fluorodeoxyglucose positron emission tomography or radiolabelled leukocyte scintigraphy) could be helpful in increasing the diagnostic accuracy for suspected prosthetic valve endocarditis.

For more extensive information, refer to Chapter 3.8.

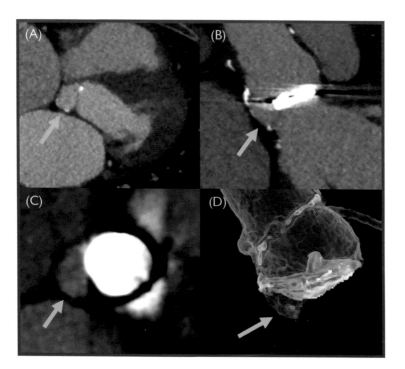

Figure 3.6.5 A patient with previous aortic valve replacement with Björk–Shiley tilting disc valve prosthesis and, later, ascending aorta replacement with tube graft.

After the development of dyspnoea, echocardiography was performed, and posterior paravalvular leakage associated with severe regurgitation was described, and then CT angiography was performed for surgical planning. (A) Axial view. (B) Modified sagittal view. (C) Valve, short-axis view. (D) Aortic volume rendering with transparency. The arrows indicate paravalvular leakage.

Pseudoaneurysm

- Contained rupture of a blood vessel or of the myocardial wall.
- Usually developed after heart surgery/intervention, infective endocarditis, myocardial infarction, or trauma.
- Transthoracic echocardiography remains the first-line test, but it has low sensitivity (insidious position of pseudoaneurysm; poor acoustic window).
- CTA provides a detailed description of the acquired cavity and relationships with other structures.

Paravalvular leakage

- Paravalvular leakage is a rare complication with either a surgical or transcatheter approach.
- Blood flows through a channel between the implanted valve and cardiac tissue as a result of a lack of appropriate sealing (Figure 3.6.5).
- It is a consequence of infective endocarditis, the presence of calcification/scar tissue at the annulus level, or technical factors during surgical procedure.
- Usually crescent, oval- or roundish-shaped, and its course may be parallel, perpendicular, or serpiginous.

Further reading

Kanjanauthai S, Pirelli L, Nalluri N, Kliger CA. Subclinical leaflet thrombosis following transcatheter aortic valve replacement. *J Interv Cardiol* 2018; 31: 640–7.

Lancellotti P, Pibarot P, Chambers J, Edvardsen T, Delgado V, Dulgheru R, et al. Recommendations for the imaging assessment of prosthetic heart valves: a report from the European Association of Cardiovascular Imaging endorsed by the Chinese Society of Echocardiography, the Inter-American Society of Echocardiography, and the Brazilian Department of Cardiovascular Imaging. *Eur Heart J Cardiovasc Imaging* 2016; 17: 589–90.

Tanis W, Habets J, van den Brink RBA, Symersky P, Budde RPJ, Chamuleau SAJ. Differentiation of thrombus from pannus as the cause of acquired mechanical prosthetic heart valve obstruction by non-invasive imaging: a review of the literature. *Eur Heart J Cardiovasc Imaging* 2014; 15: 119–29.

Chapter 3.7

Left atrium and pulmonary veins

Marco Guglielmo

> **Teaching points**
>
> Cardiac CT is able to depict accurately the anatomy of the left atrium (LA), the pulmonary veins (PVs), and the left atrial appendage (LAA); it can also rule out thrombus and can be used to guide electrophysiologically invasive procedures such as atrial fibrillation (AF) ablation or LAA closure.
>
> - The LA and its associated structures (PVs, LAA) are involved in a variety of common cardiac conditions and can be readily visualized by cardiac CT (Table 3.7.1).
> - Cardiac CT has a high sensitivity and (using appropriate delayed-phase imaging) a high specificity to detect thrombus in the LAA and is a valuable alternative to transoesophageal echocardiography (TOE).
> - Anatomical information on the LA and PVs from cardiac CT may be of value in the planning of AF ablation procedures. Additionally, electroanatomical maps of the LA facilitate safe and effective catheter manipulations in the LA.
> - Moreover, CT allows careful assessment of the shape and dimensions of the LAA prior to percutaneous LAA closure.

Ruling out thrombosis of the left atrial appendage

- Cardiac CT is an alternative to transoesophageal echocardiography (TOE) to exclude the presence of left atrium (LA) and left atrial appendage (LAA) thrombus. Although cardiac CT has a high sensitivity in detecting atrial thrombus, false-positive findings have been reported. Pectinate muscles may be hard to differentiate from thrombi by cardiac CT and blood flow dynamics can contribute to non-uniform opacification of the LAA blood pool, mimicking the presence of true filling defects. Indeed, LAA filling defects can be due to thrombus or incomplete contrast agents mixing with blood.
- A filling defect visible in the early acquisition but not the late acquisition indicates slow flow. Contrast filling defects present in both early and delayed image acquisition most likely represent thrombus (Figures 3.7.1 and 3.7.2).

Table 3.7.1 How to set up your scanner for left atrium (LA) and pulmonary vein imaging

Patient preparation	• Obtain adequate HR control by beta-blocker administration (preferably HR <65 bpm) • Nitrates are not necessary (unless concomitant coronary angiography is planned)
Scan range	• Heart to diaphragm (14–16 cm)
ECG triggering	• ECG triggered acquisition improves image quality and diagnostic accuracy
Contrast injection protocol	• Biphasic injection protocol (from 40 to 100 ml iodinated contrast depending on patient weight and renal function followed by 50 ml normal saline) • Flow rate 5 ml/s
Image acquisition	• First pass of contrast agent (bolus tracking with peak contrast in the LA) • Delayed imaging, 35–45 s after the first pass (optional). The use of double-phase cardiac CT acquisition with the analysis of late-phase images of the left atrium and LAA improves the specificity of the scan in distinguishing sluggish flow from thrombus • Tube voltage and current should be tailored for BMI according the ALARA (as low as reasonably achievable) principle.

HR: heart rate; bpm: beats per minute; ECG: electrocardiogram; LAA: left atrial appendage; BMI: body mass index.

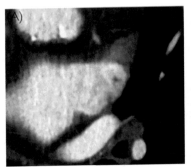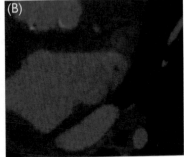

Figure 3.7.1 Left atrial appendage filling defect indicative of thrombus present in (A) early and (B) late image acquisitions.

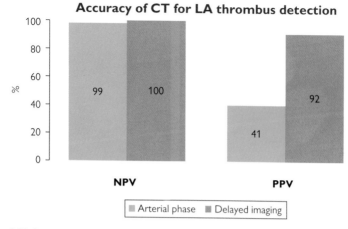

Accuracy of CT for LA thrombus detection

NPV — Arterial phase: 99, Delayed imaging: 100

PPV — Arterial phase: 41, Delayed imaging: 92

■ Arterial phase ■ Delayed imaging

Figure 3.7.2 Diagnostic accuracy for left atrium thrombus detection is significantly improved by delayed imaging with a marked increase in the positive predictive value (PPV).
NPV: negative predictive value.
Source data from Romero J, Cao JJ, Garcia MJ, Taub CC. Cardiac imaging for assessment of left atrial appendage stasis and thrombosis. *Nat Rev Cardiol.* 2014;11(8):470–80. doi: 10.1038/nrcardio.2014.77.

- The issue of radiation dose related to double acquisition to rule out LAA thrombus may be solved by dual-energy CT, a relatively recent result of the rapid advancement in scanner technology. This technology is based on acquiring images at different energy levels enabling the discrimination of different materials on the basis of their attenuation profiles. This approach helps to differentiate thrombus from slow flow with a single acquisition (Figure 3.7.3).

Ablation procedures for atrial fibrillation

- Catheter ablation (CA) is a well-established interventional therapy for restoring and maintaining sinus rhythm in patients with atrial fibrillation (AF). Pulmonary vein (PV) isolation, either by radiofrequency or cryoablation, is the most common ablation technique.
- Cardiac CT is often used for preprocedural planning of CA and for the identification of complications.
- A detailed understanding of LA anatomy is essential for a safe and effective AF ablation (Figure 3.7.4). LA imaging facilitates ablation by providing detailed anatomical description of the PVs and their abnormalities, including accessory or conjoined veins, antrum, and the remainder of the LA, enabling selection of the most suitable ablation technique prior to the procedure. PV ostia can be measured using oblique orthogonal planes (Figure 3.7.5).

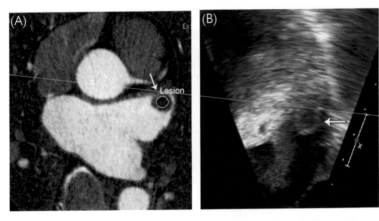

Figure 3.7.3 Dual-energy cardiac CT and transoesophageal echocardiography (TOE) images in a 79-year-old man with stroke and a left atrial appendage (LAA) thrombus.

(A) Axial CT iodine map shows a filling defect in the LAA; the mean iodine concentration within the region of interest was 1.34 mg/ml. (B) TOE image shows thrombus (arrow) in the LAA.

Reproduced from Hur J, Kim YJ, Lee HJ, et al. Cardioembolic stroke: dual-energy cardiac CT for differentiation of left atrial appendage thrombus and circulatory stasis. *Radiology.* 2012;263(3):688–95. doi: 10.1148/radiol.12111691.

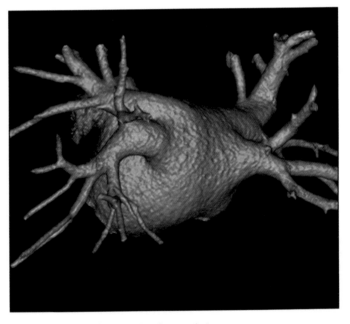

Figure 3.7.4 Left atrium and pulmonary vein volume rendering.

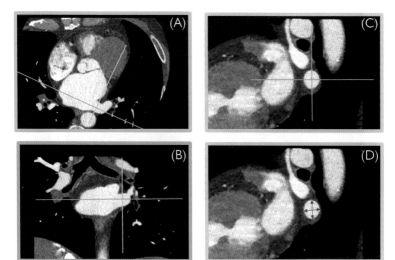

Figure 3.7.5 Pulmonary veins ostia measurement.

(A, B) The data set is manipulated using oblique orthogonal planes to obtain the ostium plane where (C, D) diameter measurements are performed.

- Preprocedural cardiac CT imaging may be used to improve ablation of AF (Figure 3.7.6).
- The image-integration cardiac CT-guided CA of AF has been shown to be superior to conventional electrophysiological-guided ablation with significantly lower recurrence rates of the arrhythmia. Moreover, preprocedural cardiac CT may provide additional information on coronary artery calcification and plaque to diagnose concomitant coronary artery disease. In addition, as cardiac CT is a three-dimensional (3D) technique that visualizes the thoracic structures that surround the heart, it is able to detect clinically significant collateral findings before the ablation procedure.
- CT can be used to detect complications after AF ablation.
  - Atrio-oesophageal fistula findings include mediastinal or pericardial free air, evidence of free communication between the oesophagus and pericardium or atrium, and inflammatory phlegmon between the oesophagus and the heart.
  - PV stenosis is a known complication of AF ablation (more common in the early days of CA, when it was performed inside the PVs; indeed, antral ablation has drastically reduced this complication) related to the thermal injury of PVs. PV stenosis can be diagnosed by CT imaging because the location and severity of PV lesions can be precisely visualized. For symptomatic patients, PV angioplasty should be considered (Figure 3.7.7).

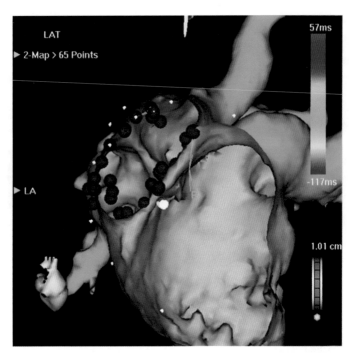

Figure 3.7.6 Three-dimensional (3D) cardiac CT volume and 3D electroanatomical mapping merge for guiding an atrial fibrillation catheter ablation procedure.
LA: left atrium.

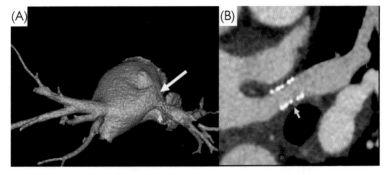

Figure 3.7.7 (A) Coronary CT angiography volume rendering showing occlusion of the left inferior pulmonary vein (white arrow) and stent of the left superior pulmonary vein (yellow arrow). (B) The normal patency of the stent is showed in the multiplanar reconstruction image.

Left atrial appendage occlusion

- Surgical or percutaneous LAA occlusion may be considered for stroke prevention in patients with AF and contraindications to long-term anticoagulant treatment. For interventional LAA closure, an accurate description of the LAA morphology and precise sizing of the diameters of the LAAs is of paramount importance before device deployment. Oversizing of the device could lead to LAA rupture and cardiac tamponade, while undersizing is related to incomplete LAA occlusion with residual peridevice blood flow and to possible device migration, dislodgement, or embolization.

- TOE and angiography are the main techniques currently used to evaluate the dimensions of the LAA before LAA occluder implantation and TOE is routinely used for procedural monitoring and follow-up after occluder positioning.

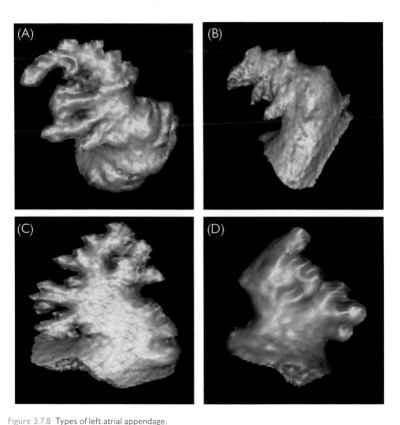

Figure 3.7.8 Types of left atrial appendage.
(A) Windsock. (B) Chicken wing. (C) Cactus. (D) Cauliflower.

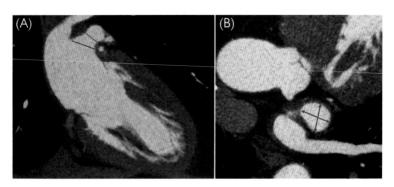

Figure 3.7.9 Left atrial appendage occluder sizing device.

(A) The ostium (red line) is defined as the line connecting the pulmonary vein ridge to the the circumflex artery. The landing zone (blue line) measurements is 10 mm inside the ostium. (B) Cross-section of the ostium.

- Cardiac CT provides high-resolution 3D data sets and is a useful tool to characterize precisely the anatomy of the LAA, the size of the occluder device, and to exclude the presence of thrombus before the LAA occlusion procedure.
- LAA shape, depth, and number, and the positioning of lobes are accurately depicted by cardiac CT (Figure 3.7.8). Cross-sectional orthogonal CT views for diameter measurements of the LAA ostium and landing zone are obtained using multiplane reconstruction images. Each device manufacturer has its own guidelines for determining which size to use (Figure 3.7.9); currently, device sizing is based on the maximum diameter of the landing zone, with 3–6-mm device oversizing. Moreover, an assessment of the atrial septal anatomy may facilitate a safe and optimal trans-septal crossing.
- The optimal C-arm angulation for intraprocedural guidance can readily be obtained from the postprocessing software.
- Cardiac CT is able to identify device malapposition, peridevice leaks, and device-related thrombus at follow-up.
- In follow-up, cardiac CT has a higher sensitivity than TOE in identifying peridevice leaks, especially during the venous phase (35–45 s) and is able to identify device-related thromboses.

Further reading

Calkins H, Hindricks G, Cappato R, Kim Y-H, Saad EB, Aguinaga L, et al. 2017 HRS/EHRA/ECAS/ APHRS/SOLAECE expert consensus statement on catheter and surgical ablation of atrial fibrillation. *Europace* 2018; 20: e1–160.

Guglielmo M, Baggiano A, Muscogiuri G, Fusini L, Andreini D, Mushtaq S, et al. Multimodality imaging of left atrium in patients with atrial fibrillation. *J Cardiovasc Comput Tomogr* 2019; 13: 340–6.

Korsholm K, Berti S, Iriart X, Saw J, Wang DD, Cochet H, et al. Expert recommendations on cardiac computed tomography for planning transcatheter left atrial appendage occlusion. *JACC Cardiovasc Interv* 2020; 13: 277–92.

Chapter 3.8

Infective endocarditis

Andrea Baggiano

Teaching points

- Benefits from CT angiography (CTA) in infective endocarditis (IE) and cardiac device-related IE (CDRIE) include the following:
  - the diagnosis of IE is a multimodality imaging effort as underlined by the 2015 European Society of Cardiology (ESC) guidelines (Figure 3.8.1);
  - CT or CTA (with or without radionuclide imaging) plays an important role in the diagnostic algorithm proposed by latest ESC Guidelines, for both native and prosthetic valves (Figure 3.8.2);
  - while transoesophageal echocardiography is superior for the assessment of vegetations and leaflet perforations, CTA allows for better evaluation of complications such as perivalvular involvement (abscesses, pseudoaneurysms) and embolic complications, and thus is useful for surgical planning (Table 3.8.1).

Why CT angiography in infective endocarditis and cardiac device-related infective endocarditis?

Echocardiography with a transoesophageal approach remains the first-line test in assessing patients with suspected or known infective endocarditis (IE) or cardiac device-related IE (CDRIE); however, CT angiography (CTA) could give additional or complementary information in many clinical settings:

- the identification of valvular/endocardial vegetations, especially in patients with poor acoustic windows;
- the assessment of the extension of perivalvular tissue involvement—a crucial point in planning surgical management;
- the identification of the extracardiac consequences of IE (i.e. septic embolization to other organs) with complete coverage of the thorax and abdomen.

Major criteria

1. Blood cultures positive for IE

a. Typical microorganisms consistent with IE from 2 separate blood cultures:
  - *Viridans streptococci, Streptococcus gallolyticus (Streptococcus bovis), HACEK group, Staphylococcus aureus*; or
  - Community-acquired enterococci, in the absence of a primary focus; or

b. Microorganisms consistent with IE from persistently positive blood cultures:
  - ≥ 2 positive blood cultures of blood samples drawn > 12 h apart; or
  - All of 3 or a majority of ≥ 4 separate cultures of blood (with first and last samples drawn ≥ 1 h apart); or

c. Single positive blood culture for *Coxiella burnetii* or phase I IgG antibody titre > 1:800.

2. Imaging positive for IE

a. Echocardiogram positive for IE:
  - Vegetation;
  - Abscess, pseudoaneurysm, intracardiac fistula;
  - Valvular perforation or aneurysm;
  - New partial dehiscence of prosthetic valve.

b. Abnormal activity around the site of prosthetic valve implantation detected by ^{18}F-FDG PET/CT (only if the prosthesis was implanted for > 3 months) or radiolabelled leukocytes SPECT/CT.

c. Definite paravalvular lesions by cardiac CT.

Minor criteria

1. Predisposition such as predisposing heart condition, or injection drug use.
2. Fever defined as temperature > 38°C.
3. Vascular phenomena (including those detected by imaging only): major arterial emboli, septic pulmonary infarcts, infectious (mycotic) aneurysm, intracranial haemorrhage, conjunctival haemorrhages, and Janeway's lesions.
4. Immunological phenomena: glomerulonephritis, Osler's nodes, Roth's spots, and rheumatoid factor.
5. Microbiological evidence: positive blood culture but does not meet a major criterion as noted above or serological evidence of active infection with organism consistent with IE.

Figure 3.8.1 Definitions of the terms used in the European Society of Cardiology (ESC) 2015 modified criteria for the diagnosis of infective endocarditis (IE), adapted from the 2015 ESC guidelines for the management of IE.

^{18}F-FDG PET: ^{18}F-fluorodeoxyglucose positron emission tomography; SPECT: single photon emission CT.

Habib G, Lancellotti P, Antunes MJ, et al; ESC Scientific Document Group. 2015 ESC guidelines for the management of infective endocarditis: The Task Force for the Management of Infective Endocarditis of the European Society of Cardiology (ESC). Endorsed by: European Association for Cardio-Thoracic Surgery (EACTS), the European Association of Nuclear Medicine (EANM). *Eur Heart J.* 2015;36(44):3075–3128. doi: 10.1093/eurheartj/ehv319.
© European Society of Cardiolgy. Published with permission by Oxford Univeristy Press.

Vegetations

Mobile masses:
- usually attached to a native valve or mural endocardium (Figures 3.8.3–3.8.5);
- usually in the trajectory of a regurgitant jet;

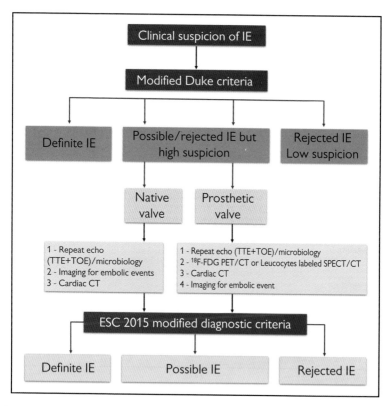

Figure 3.8.2 Algorithm for the diagnosis of infective endocarditis (IE), adapted from the 2015 European Society of Cardiology (ESC) guidelines for the management of IE.

TTE: transthoracic echocardiography; TOE: transoesophageal echocardiography; ^{18}F-FDG PET: ^{18}F-fluorodeoxyglucose; PET: positron emission tomography.

Habib G, Lancellotti P, Antunes MJ, et al; ESC Scientific Document Group. 2015 ESC guidelines for the management of infective endocarditis: The Task Force for the Management of Infective Endocarditis of the European Society of Cardiology (ESC). Endorsed by: European Association for Cardio-Thoracic Surgery (EACTS), the European Association of Nuclear Medicine (EANM). *Eur Heart J*. 2015;36(44):3075–3128. doi: 10.1093/eurheartj/ehv319. © European Society of Cardiolgy. Published with permission by Oxford Univeristy Press.

- no alternative anatomical explanation;
- potentially attached to prosthetic material (Figures 3.8.6 and 3.8.7);
- oscillating motion on four-dimensional CTA.

CT visualization:

- hypodense mass, usually with a Hounsfield unit (HU) below 145.

Table 3.8.1 How to optimize your scan protocol for assessment of patients with infective endocarditis (IE) or cardiac device-related IE

Medications	• Beta-blockers for heart rate control (clinical contraindications should be taken into consideration, such as second- or third-grade atrioventricular block, sick sinus syndrome, and decompensated heart failure)
Scan parameters	• Perform native ECG-gated scan • Use high-energy tube voltages (e.g. 120 kVp, or even 140 kVp in obese patients or when dense metallic artefacts are present) • Consider larger field of view to include the ascending aorta or parts of the chest (including pacemaker chest pocket) and/or abdomen (septic emboli)
Image reconstruction	• Use sharp reconstruction kernels in the presence of prosthetic valves or pacemakers • Prefer iterative reconstruction algorithms to reduce radiation exposure
ECG gating	• Consider retrospective ECG gating (or prospective ECG gating with large padding into systolic frames) for optimal evaluation of leaflet motion or prosthesis dysfunction (i.e. '4D-CTA') (e.g. rocking valve) • Consider disabling dose modulation
Contrast protocol	• For right-sided or interatrial devices, consider triphasic injection to opacify both the left and right heart chambers without streak artefacts of the superior vena cava

ECG: electrocardiogram.

Complications

Compared to other imaging techniques, CTA could be superior for the detection of perivalvular complications, particularly when prosthetic valves are affected.

Pseudoaneurysm

A pseudoaneurysm is a paravalvular cavity filled with contrast media, usually originating from prosthetic valve annulus (Figure 3.8.8).

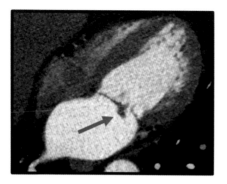

Figure 3.8.3 Infective endocarditis affecting the mitral anterior leaflet (red arrow).

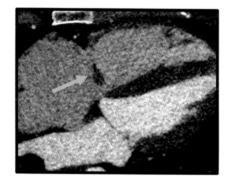

Figure 3.8.4 Infective endocarditis affecting the anterior leaflet of the tricuspid valve (yellow arrow).

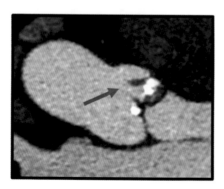

Figure 3.8.5 Infective endocarditis affecting the right coronary cusp of the aortic valve (red arrow).

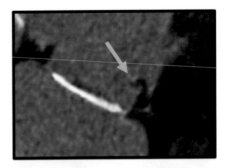

Figure 3.8.6 Infective endocarditis affecting the prosthetic ring of a mechanical mitral prosthesis (yellow arrow).

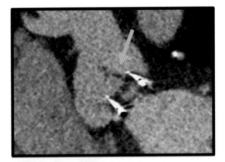

Figure 3.8.7 Infective endocarditis affecting the aortic bioprosthetic leaflets (yellow arrow).

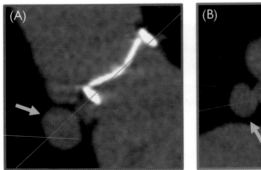
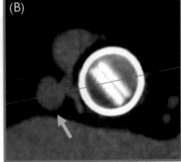

Figure 3.8.8 (A) Aortic long-axis and (B) short-axis view showing a pseudoaneurysm at a non-coronary sinus position in a patient with previous aortic valve replacement with mechanical valve after infective endocarditis (A and B, orange arrow).

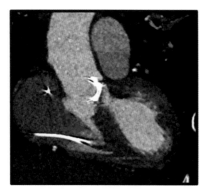

Figure 3.8.9 Fistula between the aortic root and right ventricle (red arrow) in a patient with a previous aortic valve replacement with a bioprosthesis complicated by infective endocarditis.

Intracardiac fistulae

Intracardiac fistulae are an acquired communication between the cardiac chambers, detected by contrast continuity (Figures 3.8.9 and 3.8.10).

Pacemaker/implantable cardioverter defibrillator lead infection

Pacemaker/implantable cardioverter defibrillator lead infection is an infection extending to the electrode leads, cardiac valve leaflets, or endocardial surface (Figures 3.8.11 and 3.8.12).

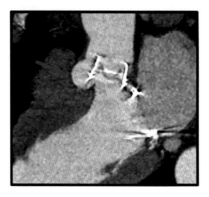

Figure 3.8.10 Aortic pseudoaneurysm (red arrow) in a patient with a previous aortic valve replacement with a bioprosthesis, complicated by fistulization with the left ventricle outflow tract (yellow arrow).

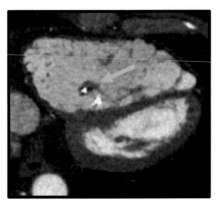

Figure 3.8.11 CT angiography showing infective endocarditis vegetation (yellow arrow) affecting the pacemaker lead in its right ventricular portion.

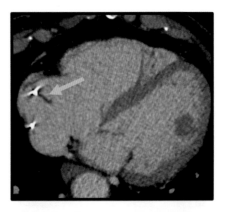

Figure 3.8.12 CT angiography showing infective endocarditis vegetation (yellow arrow) affecting the implantable cardiac defibrillator lead in its right atrial portion.

Abscess

An abscess is a dense paravalvular infiltration, usually with a surrounding layer of tissue with contrast uptake (Figures 3.8.13 and 3.8.14).

Partial dehiscence of prosthetic material

Partial dehiscence of prosthetic material involves loosening of the prosthesis anchor within the annulus/supporting structures (Figure 3.8.15).

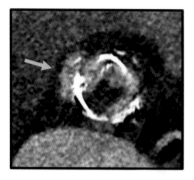

Figure 3.8.13 The presence of an abscess (yellow arrow) in a non-coronary sinus position as a consequence of infective endocarditis in an aortic bioprosthesis.

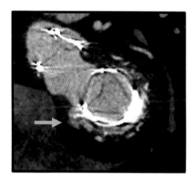

Figure 3.8.14 The presence of a septal abscess (yellow arrow) as a consequence of infective endocarditis in a mitral bioprosthesis.

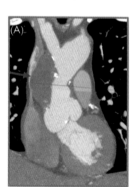
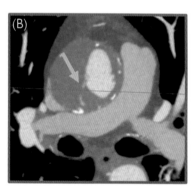

Figure 3.8.15 Termino-terminal ascending aorta prosthesis complicated, as a consequence of infective endocarditis, by (A, red arrow) almost circumferential aneurysmatic degeneration and (B, yellow arrow) 180° prosthesis dehiscence.

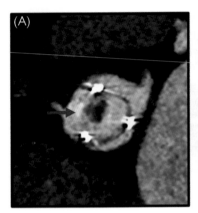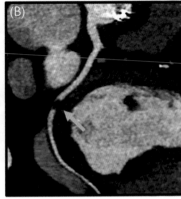

Figure 3.8.16 (A, red arrow) Infective endocarditis affecting an aortic bioprosthesis complicated by (B, yellow arrow) inferior myocardial infarction due to septic embolization of the dominant left circumflex artery.

Complications related to embolization

Complications related to embolization include septic or aseptic displacement from the origin site (usually valvular leaflets/cusps or prosthetic components) to other organs (Figure 3.8.16).

Further reading

Baumgartner H, Falk V, Bax JJ, De Bonis M, Hamm C, Holm PJ, et al. 2017 ESC/EACTS Guidelines for the management of valvular heart disease. *Eur Heart J* 2017; 38: 2739–91.

Habib G, Lancellotti P, Antunes MJ, Bongiorni MG, Casalta J-P, Del Zotti F, et al. 2015 ESC guidelines for the management of infective endocarditis: the Task Force for the Management of Infective Endocarditis of the European Society of Cardiology (ESC). Endorsed by: European Association for Cardio-Thoracic Surgery (EACTS), the European Association of Nuclear Medicine (EANM). *Eur Heart J* 2015; 36: 3075–128.

Schoepf UJ (ed.). *CT of the Heart—Contemporary Medical Imaging*. 2nd edn. New York: Humana Press, 2019.

Chapter 3.9

Thoracic great vessels

Michael Messerli

Teaching points

- The thoracic great vessels include the thoracic aorta and the pulmonary artery. Both arteries are visualized (at least their central portions) in a cardiac CT scan. Occasionally, the field of view of standard coronary CT angiography can be enlarged to include the entire thoracic aorta and all pulmonary branches (Table 3.9.1).

- The CT protocol should be tailored to the clinical problem and may include a non-contrast phase (e.g. intramural haematoma), an arterial phase (with an appropriate contrast injection protocol to visualize both the aorta and the pulmonary artery), and/or a venous phase (e.g. prior endovascular repair). ECG gating is mandatory for evaluation of the aortic root and ascending aorta.

- The main role of CT for the great vessels is to assess the integrity of the wall (dissection, haematoma, ulcers, inflammation), identify intravascular structures (thrombus, neoplasm), and/or quantify and track aneurysmal dilatation.

- CT plays an increasing role in pre- and postsurgical procedures involving the aorta (e.g. planning of aortic valve interventions, assessment of early complications, and follow-up after endovascular aortic repair).

Diseases of the thoracic aorta

The thoracic aorta includes the aortic root, an ascending part, the aortic arch, and a descending part (Figure 3.9.1).

Aortic aneurysm

- Permanent dilation of the aorta of at least 50% increase in diameter.
- Generally, the term aortic aneurysm is used when the axial diameter exceeds 5.0 cm for the ascending aorta and >4.0 cm for the descending aorta (Figure 3.9.2).
- The normal diameter of the aorta varies based on sex, age, and body surface area (for normal reference dimensions, see Chapter 3.2).

Table 3.9.1 Practical tips: how to set up your scanner for imaging the thoracic great vessels

Scan parameters	• Consider large field of view to cover the entire thoracic aorta and/or peripheral pulmonary vasculature • kVp and mA according to local protocol and scanner (see Chapter 1.5)
ECG gating	• ECG gating crucial to avoid pulsation artefacts in the aortic root and ascending aorta
Non-contrast gated CT scan	• Important for calcifications, surgical material, and IMH of the aorta
Contrast protocol	• Venous phase scan to assess for endoleaks after TEVAR • For pulmonary angiography, CT acquisition must be triggered for optimal opacification at the level of the pulmonary artery
Dose reduction	• Optimize protocol for dose reduction (see Chapter 1.7)

ECG: electrocardiogram; IMH: intramural haematoma; TEVAR: thoracic endovascular aortic repair.

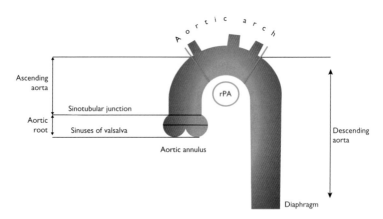

Figure 3.9.1 The normal anatomy of the thoracic aorta.

rPA: right pulmonary artery.

Source: Reproduced from Erbel R, Aboyans V, Boileau C, et al; ESC Committee for Practice Guidelines. 2014 ESC Guidelines on the diagnosis and treatment of aortic diseases: Document covering acute and chronic aortic diseases of the thoracic and abdominal aorta of the adult. The Task Force for the Diagnosis and Treatment of Aortic Diseases of the European Society of Cardiology (ESC). *Eur Heart J.* 2014;35(41):2873–926. doi: 10.1093/eurheartj/ehu281. Epub 2014 Aug 29. © European Society of Cardiolgy. Published with permission by Oxford University Press.

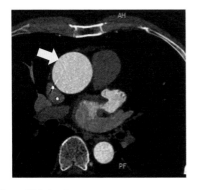 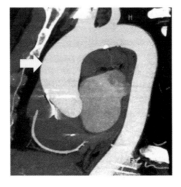

Figure 3.9.2 Aortic aneurysm.

A 65-year-old man with an incidentally detected aneurysm of the ascending aorta (arrow). Note the pacemaker leads in the superior vena cava.

Value of imaging and typical CT findings

- Measurement of aortic dimensions (size, shape, and length).
- Wall characteristics (calcifications, thrombus).
- Assessment of potential complications (e.g. leak, rupture, and fistula).
- Typical location of aortic aneurysm:
  - aortic root/ascending aorta—60%;
  - descending aorta—40%;
  - aortic arch—10%;
  - thoracoabdominal segment—10%.

Potential pitfall

Measuring the aorta on axial slices may result in inaccurate measurements in an aorta with a tortuous or oblique course (Figure 3.9.3; see also Chapter 3.2).

Aortic dissection

- Aortic dissection occurs when an intimal injury enables the blood to communicate with the media and propagate longitudinally along the course of the artery. Thereby, an intimal flap separates two compartments (i.e. the true and the false lumen).
- The dissection may extend into aortic branches (e.g. coronary arteries and supra-aortic vessels).

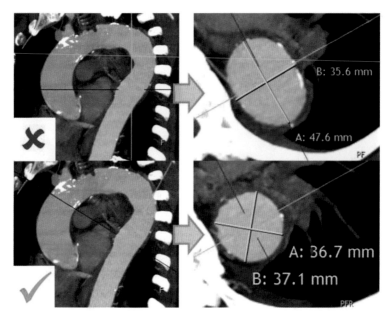

Figure 3.9.3 Potential pitfall: inaccurate measurements of the aorta in a tortuous vessel.

(Upper row) Aortic diameter measurements on axial slices overestimate the maximum aortic diameter by 1 cm due to tortuosity. (Lower row) Aortic dimensions should be obtained from double-oblique planes perpendicular to the central axis of the vessel.

- Obstruction of branches may occur through intimal flaps or compression from false lumen expansion.
- Aortic regurgitation and pericardial effusion may be seen on CT.

Value of imaging and typical CT findings
- Classification of aortic dissection (De Bakey and Stanford; Figure 3.9.4).
  - Stanford type A (60–70%): involvement of the ascending aorta with possible extension into the descending aorta (Figure 3.9.5).
  - Stanford type B (30–40%): limited to the descending aorta (conventional landmark dissection originating distally to left subclavian artery).
- Imaging clues that may help in differentiating between true and false lumen:
  - true lumen—smaller, fast enhancement, and may contain intimal calcifications;
  - false lumen—larger, slow enhancement, and may contain thrombus.

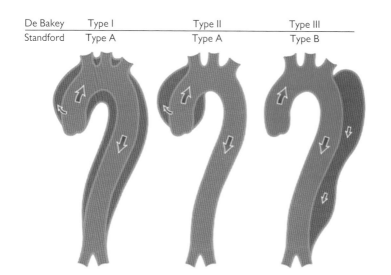

De Bakey	Type I	Type II	Type III
Standford	Type A	Type A	Type B

Figure 3.9.4 Classification of thoracic aortic dissection.

Schematic drawing of aortic dissections, subdivided into De Bakey types I, II, and III, and Stanford classes A and B.

Source: Reproduced from Erbel R, Aboyans V, Boileau C, et al; ESC Committee for Practice Guidelines. 2014 ESC Guidelines on the diagnosis and treatment of aortic diseases: Document covering acute and chronic aortic diseases of the thoracic and abdominal aorta of the adult. The Task Force for the Diagnosis and Treatment of Aortic Diseases of the European Society of Cardiology (ESC). *Eur Heart J*. 2014;35(41):2873–926. doi: 10.1093/eurheartj/ehu281. Epub 2014 Aug 29. © European Society of Cardiolgy. Published with permission by Oxford University Press.

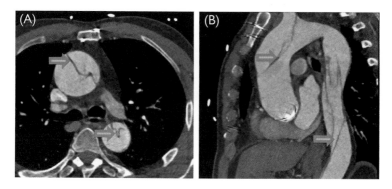

Figure 3.9.5 Type A aortic dissection.

(A) Axial contrast-enhanced CT images of a 55-year-old man with an aortic dissection; images show a dissection flap in the ascending and descending thoracic aorta (arrows). (B) CT oblique view of the same patient.

Potential pitfall

In untriggered images, pulsation artefacts from cardiac motion may mimic dissection flaps, particularly around the aortic root and ascending aorta (Figure 3.9.6). This can be overcome by ECG-gated image acquisition.

Intramural haematoma

- Intramural haematoma (IMH) is defined as a haemorrhage within the media of the aorta due to rupture of vasa vasorum.
- IMH weakens the integrity of the arterial wall and may therefore progress to a dissection, aneurysm, or aortic ulcer.
- IMH presents typically on non-contrast-enhanced CT as crescentic hyperattenuating thickening of the aortic wall (Figure 3.9.7).
- In contrary to aortic dissection and atherosclerotic ulcers, the intima remains intact in IMH.

Penetrating atherosclerotic ulcer

- Penetrating atherosclerotic ulcer (PAU) refers to a focal tear in the intima that extends into the media (Figure 3.9.8). PAUs are most frequently located in the descending thoracic aorta.
- PAU typically present as a small, focal outpouching defect of the aorta.

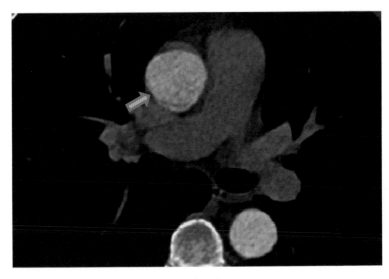

Figure 3.9.6 Potential pitfall: cardiac motion mimicking dissection.

Axial contrast-enhanced CT without electrocardiogram triggering shows typical pulsation artefacts in the ascending aorta that could be mistaken for an intimal flap.

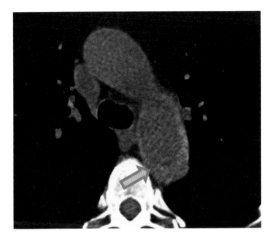

Figure 3.9.7 Intramural haematoma.

Electrocardiogram-triggered non-contrast-enhanced CT images of a 61-year-old woman with an acute intramural haematoma (IMH) of the descending aorta (arrow). Non-contrast-enhanced CT yields the highest sensitivity for detecting the classical appearance of an acute IMH as crescentic hyperattenuating thickening of the aortic wall.

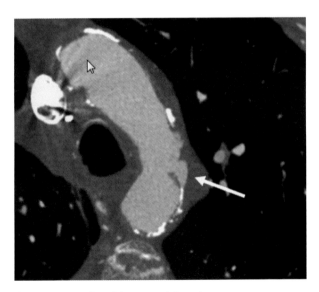

Figure 3.9.8 Penetrating aortic ulcer of the aortic arch (arrow).

- There may be difficulties in distinguishing PAU from:
  - dissection—longer abnormality with two lumens;
  - pseudoaneurysms—disruption of total arterial wall (PAU has preserved external wall);
  - ulcerated atherosclerotic plaques—affecting an intact intima, and have a lower risk of dissection than PAU.

PAU is typically associated with heavy atherosclerosis (unlike aortic dissection).

Aortic pseudoaneurysm

- Pseudoaneurysms represent a 'contained perforation' and result in a perfused cavity communicating with the lumen of the vessel (Figure 3.9.9), in some cases, the pseudoaneurysm is only covered by adventitia or perivascular soft tissue.
- Pseudoaneurysms may progress to complete rupture if untreated.
- Pseudoaneurysms may result from any insult to the aortic wall.
- Predisposing factors include PAU, atherosclerosis, trauma, inflammation/infection, and surgical/interventional injury.

Aortic thrombus

- Aortic thrombi are uncommon but can occur in patients with extensive atherosclerosis, indwelling catheters, slow-flow and hypercoagulable states,

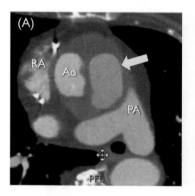 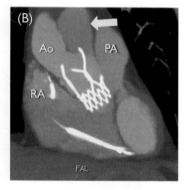

Figure 3.9.9 Aortic pseudoaneurysm.

(A) Axial source and (B) oblique coronal maximum intensity projections of a 73-year-old woman with S/p aortic repair after type A dissection 5 years previously and transcatheter aortic valve implantation for aortic root failure 3 years earlier with a Boston Scientific Accurate Neo prosthesis. CT shows para-aortic pseudoaneurysm (arrow) caused by a strut of the aortic prosthesis impinging on the aortic wall at the site of anastomosis with the supracoronary graft.

Ao: ascending aorta; PA: pulmonary artery; RA: right atrium (with implantable cardioverter defibrillator electrodes).

iatrogenic injury, and in the context of thromboemboli from a cardiac origin or right-to-left shunt.

- They appear as focal luminal perfusion defects on CT usually adjacent to the vessel wall and/or catheters.
- Acute thrombus can cause peripheral emboli, in which patients might present with signs of peripheral ischaemia.

Aortitis

- Aortitis refers to a non-infectious or infectious condition with inflammation (i.e. vasculitis) of the aortic wall.
- Most frequently, aortic wall thickening is the main (and relatively unspecific) imaging feature (Figure 3.9.10A).
- Aetiology:
  - non-infectious (e.g. giant cell arteritis, Takayasu arteritis, and other rheumatological disorders (such as rheumatoid arthritis, systemic lupus erythematosus, granulomatosis with polyangiitis, etc.));
  - infectious—syphilitic aortitis, tuberculous aortitis, aortitis in HIV, and infected (mycotic) aortic aneurysm.
- Aortic and branch vessel disease can manifest with aneurysm, stenosis, occlusion, ulceration, or rupture, depending on the degree of inflammatory response and associated wall destruction.
- Takayasu arteritis may affect the coronary arteries (mainly ostial segments; Figure 3.9.10B).
- CT may be combined with ^{18}F-fluorodeoxyglucose positron emission tomography to assess aortic wall inflammatory activity.

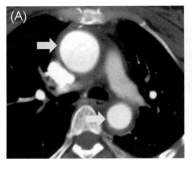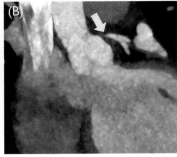

Figure 3.9.10 Takayasu arteritis.

(A) Axial CT angiography images of a 48-year-old man with thickening of the ascending and descending (arrows) aortas due to a Takayasu arteritis. (B) CT images of a 12-year-old girl with a stenosis of the left main coronary artery (arrow) due to a Takayasu arteritis.

Congenital conditions of the great vessels

Congenital conditions of the great vessels include transposition, coarctation, patent ductus arteriosus, etc. (see Chapter 3.10).

Imaging of the aorta after endovascular repair

Patients with aortic disease who have undergone aortic repair require life-long surveillance, including clinical evaluation, reassessment of medication, and imaging of the aorta.

Value of imaging and typical CT findings
- CT is the modality of choice for follow-up imaging after surgery or thoracic endovascular aortic repair (TEVAR).
- After TEVAR, regular CT follow-up should be performed at the following intervals:
  - at 1 month of treatment, to exclude the presence of early complications;
  - at 6 months of treatment, to assess for endoleaks (Figure 3.9.11);
  - and every 12 months thereafter.
- Imaging after aortic repair include a non-contrast phase (surgical material), an arterial phase (lumen of the aorta), and a venous phase (leakage of contrast media).

Diseases of the pulmonary artery

Pulmonary embolism

- Pulmonary embolism refers to embolic (usually thrombotic) obstruction/occlusion of the pulmonary arterial system.
- CT pulmonary angiography shows filling defects in the pulmonary vasculature (Figure 3.9.12).
- Signs for severe pulmonary embolism on CT are right ventricular dilatation, paradoxical movement of the septum into the left ventricle, and reflux of contrast into the azygos vein or inferior vena cava.
- Differential diagnosis: pulmonary sarcoma—extremely rare tumours originating from the intima of the pulmonary artery that can be mistaken for pulmonary embolism.

Differentiation of acute and chronic embolism with CT
- Acute pulmonary embolism:
  - filling defects within the pulmonary vasculature, with embolus having an *acute* angle with the vessel, as compared to chronic emboli.
- Chronic pulmonary embolism:
  - eccentric organized thrombi adherent to the pulmonary wall;
  - dilatation of proximal/central pulmonary arteries;

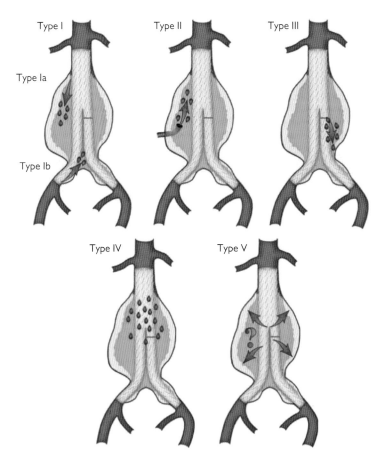

Figure 3.9.11 Classification of endoleaks.

Type I: leak at graft attachment site above, below, or between graft components (Ia: proximal attachment site; Ib: distal attachment site). Type II: aneurysm sac filling retrogradely via single (IIa) or multiple branch vessels (IIb). Type III: leak through mechanical defect in graft, mechanical failure of the stent graft by junctional separation of the modular components (IIIa), or fractures or holes in the endograft (IIIb). Type IV: leak through graft fabric as a result of graft porosity. Type V: continued expansion of aneurysm sac without demonstrable leak on imaging (endotension, controversial).

Source: Reproduced from Erbel R, Aboyans V, Boileau C, et al; ESC Committee for Practice Guidelines. 2014 ESC Guidelines on the diagnosis and treatment of aortic diseases: Document covering acute and chronic aortic diseases of the thoracic and abdominal aorta of the adult. The Task Force for the Diagnosis and Treatment of Aortic Diseases of the European Society of Cardiology (ESC). Eur Heart J. 2014;35(41): 2873–926. doi: 10.1093/eurheartj/ehu281. Epub 2014 Aug 29. © European Society of Cardiolgy. Published with permission by Oxford University Press.

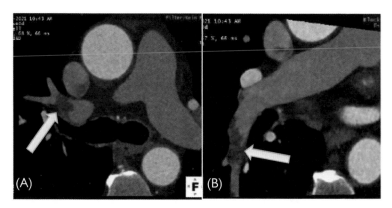

Figure 3.9.12 Pulmonary embolism with thrombus visible in the (A) right upper and (B) lower lobe of the pulmonary artery (arrows).

Note: despite biphasic contrast injection protocol triggered to the ascending aorta (standard coronary CT angiography protocol) the proximal pulmonary arteries remain evaluable in this case.

- stenoses of lobar and segmental vessels (irregularity of vessel calibre);
- intraluminal fibrous bands (webs);
- further imaging features—enlargement of the right ventricle, with thickening of the ventricle wall and mosaic perfusion of the lung.

Pulmonary infarction

- Occurs in a minority of patients with pulmonary embolism (around 10%).
- Imaging features:
  - typically wedge-shaped consolidations located subpleurally;
  - lower lobe > upper lobe;
  - signs of infarctions may remain for months and may leave a linear scar;
  - cavitation (in septic embolism).

Pulmonary hypertension

- Pulmonary hypertension is defined as an average resting mean pulmonary arterial pressure of 25 mmHg or higher on right heart catheterization.
- CT shows an enlarged pulmonary trunk (measured at the pulmonary bifurcation on axial slices vertical to the long axis):
  - >29 mm diameter is generally used as a cutoff and is considered the most specific sign on CT (Figure 3.9.13). Normal reference values for pulmonary artery diameter are provided in Chapter 3.2.
- Other signs on cardiac CT may include right ventricular hypertrophy, right ventricular dilatation, and dilatation of the hepatic veins and/or inferior vena cava.

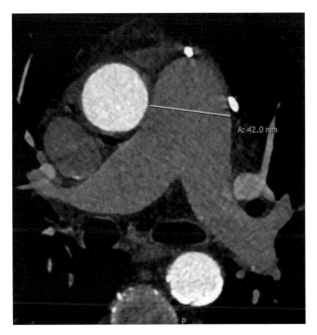

Figure 3.9.13 Pulmonary artery dilatation (42 mm) in a patient with pulmonary hypertension. Note the larger diameter of the main pulmonary artery compared to the ascending aorta.

Further reading

Berniker R, Mackey JE, Teytelboym OM. Intimal problems: a pictorial review of nontraumatic aortic disease at multidetector computed tomography. *Curr Probl Diagn Radiol* 2018; 47: 51–60.

Erbel R, Aboyans V, Boileau C, Bossone E, Di Bartolomeo R, Eggebrecht H, et al. 2014 ESC Guidelines on the diagnosis and treatment of aortic diseases: Document covering acute and chronic aortic diseases of the thoracic and abdominal aorta of the adult. The Task Force for the Diagnosis and Treatment of Aortic Diseases of the European Society of Cardiology (ESC). *Eur Heart J* 2014; 35: 2873–926.

Goldstein SA, Evangelista A, Abbara S, Arai A, Asch FM, Badano LP, et al. Multimodality imaging of diseases of the thoracic aorta in adults: from the American Society of Echocardiography and the European Association of Cardiovascular Imaging: endorsed by the Society of Cardiovascular Computed Tomography and Society for Cardiovascular Magnetic Resonance *J Am Soc Echocardiogr* 2015; 28: 119–82.

Restrepo R, Ocazionez D, Suri R, Vargas D. Aortitis: imaging spectrum of the infectious and inflammatory conditions of the aorta. *Radiographics* 2011; 31: 435–51.

Chapter 3.10

Adult congenital heart disease

Andreas A. Giannopoulos

Teaching points

- Adult congenital heart disease (ACHD) involves a great diversity of anatomical variations and prior correction(s).
- Cardiac CT provides high-resolution three-dimensional information on the complex anatomical relationship of cardiac structures in ACHD. It has an increasing role in guiding interventional or surgical corrective procedures, and assessing postoperative outcomes or complications.
- The CT exam must be tailored to each patient and to the specific clinical question, minimizing the risks and maximizing the diagnostic yield.
- Optimization of the injection protocol, the acquisition timing, and the application of radiation reduction techniques are critical.

Patients with congenital heart disease have seen a remarkable decrease in early and late mortality, mainly due to advances in screening and medical management, and the population of those with adult congenital heart disease (ACHD) is constantly increasing. Advanced imaging is critical for the morphological and functional follow-up of patients with ACHD surgically managed at a younger age and for the assessment of those not earlier diagnosed.

This chapter provides a quick and general introduction to cardiac CT in patients with ACHD (Figure 3.10.1). A complete and detailed compendium of ACHD and its individual imaging approaches exceeds the focus of this handbook. For more in-depth information, the interested reader is referred to more comprehensive literature exclusively dedicated to this topic.

Role of CT in adult congenital heart disease

- Echocardiography remains the workhorse for the initial evaluation and serial surveillance, while cardiac magnetic resonance (CMR) is increasingly being used for more detailed structural and functional assessment.
- Owing to its high isotropic spatial resolution, cardiac CT provides an excellent alternative to echocardiography/CMR to depict complex anatomical relationships and allows for exceptional three-dimensional reconstructions of patients with ACHD.

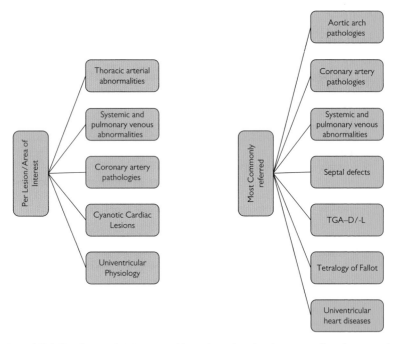

Figure 3.10.1 Classification of adult congenital heart disease based on the primary affected anatomical structures.
TGA: transposition of the great arteries (D: dextro; L: levo).

- CT is independent of acoustic windows, can have a large field of view, and provides excellent visualization of the tracheobronchial tree and the upper abdomen, which are commonly implicated in patients with ACHD.
- Motion artefacts are limited compared to CMR, and image quality is only marginally affected by implanted metallic devices (pacemakers, defibrillators, grafts, stents).
- In contrast, CT is less ideal for serial imaging owing to increased radiation and intravenous contrast exposure in these usually younger patients.
- As imaging patients with ACHD can be challenging, CT scanning should be performed by experienced cardiovascular imagers in close collaboration with ACHD cardiologists and/or cardiac surgeons.

Indications for cardiac CT imaging

- For diagnostic purposes as an adjunct to other modalities (or when echocardiography/CMR are non-diagnostic and/or contraindicated).
- Guidance of interventional or surgical treatment, and postoperative assessment of complications.
- Follow-up after surgical/interventional corrective procedures (e.g. stents, shunts, baffles, valve prostheses, and coils).
- Assessment of coronary artery anomalies and the presence of atherosclerosis in older patients.
- Functional evaluation of ventricular function, and assessment of native and prosthetic valves.
- Critically ill patients or patients of any age with learning difficulties.
- Evaluation of ventricular assist device or extracorporeal membrane oxygenation cannula positioning.
- Evaluation of extracardiac anatomy (e.g. lung parenchyma, airway, skeletal abnormality).

Cardiac CT protocol

The variant nature of the clinical questions and the highly variable anatomy of patients with ACHD makes selection of the appropriate CT protocol challenging. The scan parameters must be personalized and tailored to the individual patient's history, including original anatomical defects, prior correction(s), and the presence of any intracardiac shunts, as well as their anatomical trajectory and the current clinical question (see also Chapter 1.5). Table 3.10.1 provides a general approach to cardiac CT protocol.

Specific ACHD pathologies for cardiac CT imaging

Aortic arch pathologies

Aortic arch pathologies include aortic aneurysms/pseudoaneurysms, bicuspid aortic valve, patent ductus arteriosus, aortic coarctation, and vascular rings. (Figures 3.10.2 and 3.10.3; see also Chapter 3.9).

Specific indications for CT
- Planning of surgical or catheter-based intervention.
- Persistent ductus arteriosus size, length, and dimensions.
- Stent restenosis.
- Aortic aneurysm or pseudoaneurysm.
- Aortic dissection.

Table 3.10.1 General protocol recommendations for cardiac CT in patients with adult congenital heart disease (ACHD)	
Pressure monitoring	• Pressure should be measured on the correct arm (caution: patients with pressure difference between right and left arm)
IV line	• Extra care is needed to prevent air embolism through intracardiac shunting (e.g. ASD) • Choose IV access based on individual anatomy (right antecubital vein default access, left antecubital vein preferred with situs inversus or persistent left superior vena cava, simultaneous upper and lower extremity veins for Fontan patients, anomalous venous drainage)
Medication	• Beta-blockade and nitrates generally not needed (except for coronary assessment) (caution: patients in poor haemodynamic condition)
ECG gating	• Default: ECG-triggered axial scan mode • Retrospective ECG gating only for functional assessment (EF) or detailed coronary or valvular assessment (if HR is high/irregular or if leaflet motion should be assessed)
Scan triggering	• Consider prescan timing bolus in patients with ACHD due to variable transit time and complex anatomy • If a left-to-right shunt is suspected, opacify the left heart as in VSD and PDA • Opacify right heart for the assessment of Mustard baffle
Contrast injection protocol	• Biphasic injection protocol per default (see Chapter 1.10) • Triphasic injection for simultaneous opacification of the left and right heart structures • Venous two-phase injection protocol (two contrast boluses separated by a pause of 30–60 s) for simultaneous systemic arterial and venous opacification in a single acquisition • Consider slow and long contrast injections in patients with cyanotic ACHD
Radiation reduction	• Consider the young age of patients! Apply radiation reduction algorithms whenever possible and appropriate (e.g. prospective ECG triggering and low tube voltage)

IV: intravenous; ASD: atrial septal defect; ECG: electrocardiogram; EF: ejection fraction; HR: heart rate; VSD: ventricular septal defect; PDA: patent ductus arteriosus;

Specific protocol adjustments
• Intravenous (IV) placement in the upper extremities.
• Timing of contrast to the aorta.
• Consider larger field of view and include aortic arch in order to avoid missing coronary arteries with anomalous origin.
• For aortic valve evaluation, both systolic and diastolic phase acquisition.

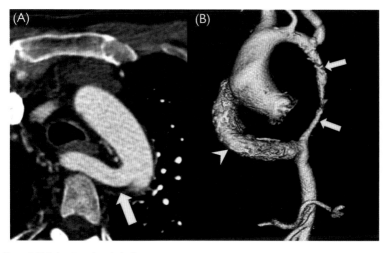

Figure 3.10.2 Aortic arch pathologies.

(A) A vascular ring in an aberrant left subclavian artery surrounding the trachea (arrow). (B) Volume rendering depicting a long aortic coarctation (arrow) and a hypoplastic aortic arch in a patient with Turner syndrome who underwent extra-anatomical bypass grafting of the descending aorta (arrowhead).

Coronary artery pathologies

Coronary artery pathologies include native origin, course, and termination anomalies, and aneurysms; postsurgery reimplantation, and unroofing (Figure 3.10.4).

For a more detailed discussion of coronary artery anomalies, see Chapter 2.8.

Specific indications for CT
- Assessment of the origin and course post-reimplantation.
- Coronary anomalies.
- Atherosclerosis.
- Prior to right ventricle (RV) reinterventions for the assessment of coronary relationship to RV outflow tract (RVOT)/sternum.

Specific protocol adjustments
- IV placement in the upper extremities.
- Timing of contrast to aorta.
- Use nitroglycerin ± beta-blockers.
- Delayed two-phase contrast injection.
- Both systolic and diastolic phase acquisition to assess dynamic compression.

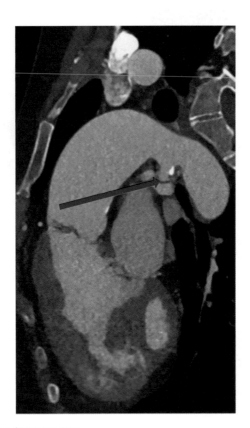

Figure 3.10.3 Patent ductus arteriosus.

Multiplanar reformatted CT images of a patient with a complex cyanotic congenital heart syndrome, including a double-outlet right ventricle and a hypoplastic left ventricle after Blalock–Taussig shunt. The scan was performed to assess the interventional closure of patent ductus arteriosus (red arrow)

Venous abnormalities

Venous abnormalities include systemic (bilateral superior vena cava (SVC), persistent left SVC, interrupted inferior vena cava (IVC)) and partial or total anomalous pulmonary venous return (Figures 3.10.5 and 3.10.6).

Specific indications for CT
Pulmonary veins

• Visualize partially or total anomalous pulmonary venous connections.

• Location and degree of pulmonary vein stenosis.

• Dilatation of RV/pulmonary artery.

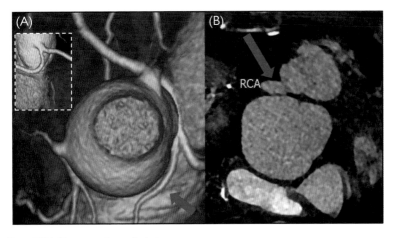

Figure 3.10.4 Coronary artery pathologies.

(A) Aberrant left circumflex artery arising from the right coronary artery (RCA). (B) Ostial RCA aneurysm in a patient after Fontan palliation.

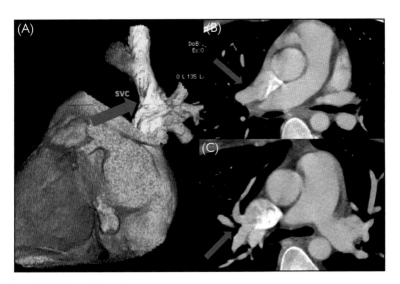

Figure 3.10.5 Venous abnormalities.

(A) Volume-rendered and (B, C) axial cardiac CT images of a right superior pulmonary vein connecting with the superior vena cava (SVC; red arrows).

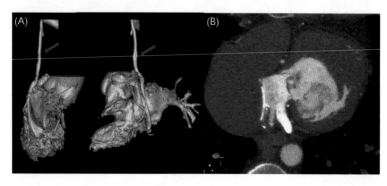

Figure 3.10.6 Persistent left superior vena cava (PLSVC).

A patient with a status post-repaired double inlet left with transposition of the great arteries. Coronary CT angiography with contrast injection from the left cubital vein demonstrating PLSVC (red arrows) draining in the coronary sinus (asterisk). (A) Volume-rendered images. (B) Axial images.

Systemic veins

• Visualize persistent left SVC.
• Assess communication with cardiac chambers.

Specific protocol adjustments
• Select appropriate arm for contrast injection.
• Delayed two-phase contrast injection.
• Longer injection and later image acquisition.
• Extend scan range to include the upper abdomen.
• Electrocardiogram (ECG) gating not required.

Septal defects

Septal defects include atrial, ventricular, and atrioventricular septal defects (Figure 3.10.7).

Specific indications for CT
• Device sizing for large atrial septal defect (ASD).
• Assess pulmonary vein anatomy and connections.
• Assess the retro-aortic course of anomalous left circumflex artery.
• Assess device protrusion or malposition after closure.

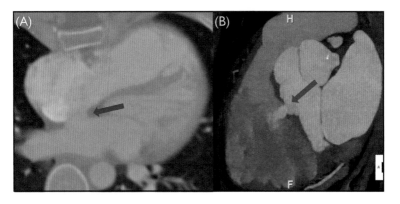

Figure 3.10.7 Septal defects.
Cardiac CT images in a patient with (A) atrial septal defect and (B) a perimembranous ventricular septal defect (red arrows).

Specific protocol adjustments
- IV placement in the upper extremities.
- Consider triphasic injection protocol to opacify both the right and left chambers.
- If a shunt is suspected (but not yet confirmed), a biphasic protocol may be preferred with differential opacification of chambers (to visualize positive or negative contrast jet).
- ECG gating is recommended.

Transposition of the great arteries

Transposition of the great arteries includes simple, complex, and congenitally corrected transposition (Figures 3.10.8 and 3.10.9).

Specific indications for CT
Postatrial switch

- Systemic and pulmonary venous baffle obstruction/leakage.
- Subpulmonary obstruction due to septal displacement into the left ventricular outflow tract.

Postarterial switch

- RVOT obstruction at the level of the neopulmonary valve or branch pulmonary arteries.

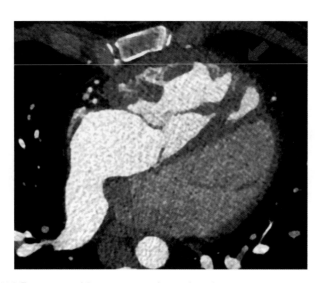

Figure 3.10.8 Transposition of the great arteries after atrial switch operation.
Axial cardiac CT images depicting the hypertrophic anatomical right (systemic) ventricle (red arrow).

- Ascending aorta stenosis at the neoaortic root anastomosis.
- Neoaortic root dilation.

Specific protocol adjustments
- IV placement in the upper extremities.
- Triphasic injection protocol when ASD/ventricular septal defect (VSD) is repaired.
- If a baffle leak is suspected, a biphasic protocol may be preferred with differential opacification of chambers (to visualize positive or negative contrast jet).
- Use nitroglycerin ± beta-blockers.
- Extend the scan range to include the proximal ascending aorta and branch pulmonary arteries.

Tetralogy of Fallot

Tetralogy of Fallot is a typical combination of ventricular septal defect, pulmonary or subpulmonary stenosis, over-riding aorta, and right ventricular hypertrophy. In adults, it is most commonly encountered after surgical correction (Figures 3.10.10 and 3.10.11).

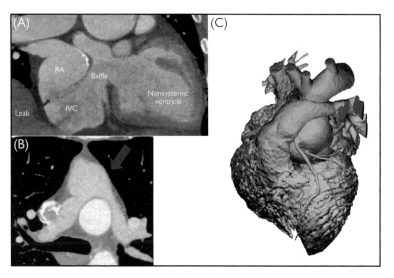

Figure 3.10.9 Transposition of the great arteries.

(A) An atrial baffle leak post-atrial switch. (B) Pulmonary trunk overriding the ascending aorta, showing a cardiac CT-derived three-dimensional reconstruction post-arterial switch (Lecompte procedure).

RA: right atrium; IVC: inferior vena cava.

Specific indications for CT
• Main and branch pulmonary artery or conduit (Blalock–Taussig shunt) stenosis.
• Right ventricular dilation.
• Aortic root dilation.
• Preprocedural planning for transcatheter interventions and coronary artery assessments.

Specific protocol adjustments
• Dual-injection protocol and timing of contrast to aorta when VSD not repaired and RVOT obstruction.
• Triphasic injection protocol when the VSD is repaired.
• Extend scan range to include ascending aorta and branch pulmonary arteries.

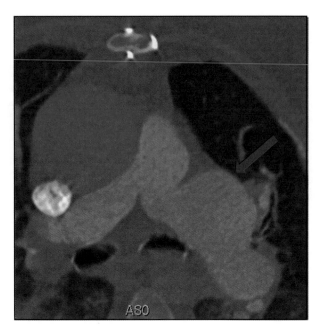

Figure 3.10.10 Tetralogy of Fallot.

Axial cardiac CT images with an aneurysm of the left main pulmonary artery (red arrow).

Univentricular heart disease

Univentricular heart diseases include tricuspid atresia and hypoplastic left heart syndrome. Commonly, there is post-Glenn or Fontan palliation (Figure 3.10.12).

Specific indications for CT
- Stenosis of the SVC, IVC, and pulmonary arteries.
- Baffle obstruction/leak.
- Thrombus in Fontan circulation or the pulmonary arteries (Table 3.10.2).
- Systemic vein occlusions.
- Aortic coarctation.
- Aortopulmonary collaterals.

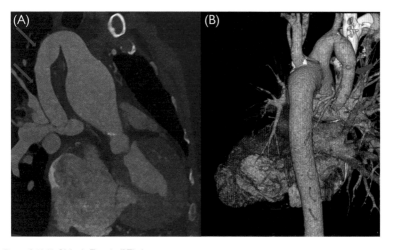

Figure 3.10.11 Blalock–Taussig (BT) shunt.
Cardiac CT images of a patient with complex congenital disease, including a hypoplastic left ventricle, criss-cross connection of the atrioventricular valves, and transposition of the great arteries. (A) Coronal images of the BT shunt between the right subclavian artery and the right pulmonary artery (red arrows). (B) Three-dimensional rendering of the cardiac CT images with the BT shunt indicated by the red arrow.

Specific protocol adjustments
• See Table 3.10.2.
• IV placement in upper extremities, and also in the lower extremities for Fontan patients.
• Delayed two-phase contrast injection.
• Use larger contrast volume.
• Extend the scan range to include the ascending aorta and branch pulmonary arteries.

Common surgical procedures in patients with adult congenital heart disease

Table 3.10.3 gives an overview of the most commonly encountered surgical procedures in ACHD and their anatomical presentation of CT.

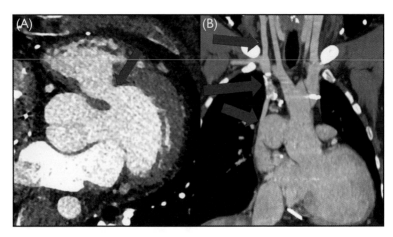

Figure 3.10.12 Cardiac CT post-Fontan palliation.

(A) Axial cardiac CT images with a ventricular septal defect (red arrow). (B) Coronal images with connection of the superior vena cava with the main pulmonary artery (red arrows).

Table 3.10.2 Cardiac CT in Fontan circulation	
Common challenges	<ul><li>Suboptimal anatomical opacification</li><li>Wrong contrast timing, not enough contrast</li><li>Pseudothrombus/pseudoembolism due to incomplete mixing of contrast medium</li></ul>
Optimizing the CT protocol	<ul><li>Consider simultaneous contrast injection from the upper and lower extremities (to improve mixing of contrast medium in the Fontan conduit) or in both upper extremities (in the case of bilateral Glenn)</li><li>Use a larger contrast volume (2.5–3 ml/kg, up to 150 ml)</li><li>Alternatively, consider single acquisition of delayed venous phase (80–100 s after contrast injection; for Fontan evaluation only)</li><li>A venous two-phase protocol (using 50% of the contrast for the first phase) allows simultaneous assessment of the aorta and coronary arteries, as well as Fontan circuit</li></ul>

Procedures	Description	Indication
Atrial redirection procedures	• Removal of atrial septum and redirection of the systemic venous pathways to the subpulmonary LV and pulmonary venous blood to the systemic RV • Rerouting of systemic venous blood by infolding the atrial walls (Senning) or by using synthetic or pericardial patch (Mustard)	TGA
Arterial switch	• PA bifurcation looped posteriorly (Lecompte manoeuvre) and anastomosed to the distal aorta (neoaorta) • Aorta anastomosed to branch pulmonary (neopulmonary trunk)	D-TGA
Rastelli	• VSD patching • Pulmonary valve is oversewn, the pulmonary trunk divided or ligated, and continuity between the PA and RV is established by a conduit	D-TGA with VSD and LVOT or pulmonary obstruction
Blalock–Taussig shunt	• Classical: distal ligation of subclavian artery and rerouting of proximal portion to the ipsilateral branch of the PA • Modified: Gortex™ graft between subclavian artery and PA	RVOT obstruction (i.e. tetralogy of Fallot) or initial staged repair of hypoplastic left heart syndrome
Glenn shunt	• Classical (unilateral): SVC anastomosis to right PA and right PA disconnected from PA trunk • Bidirectional (hemi-Fontan): SVC anastomosis to undivided right PA	• Cyanotic heart diseases with a single anatomical or functional ventricle • Hypoplastic left/right heart syndrome
Fontan palliation	• Staged procedure • Classical: atriopulmonary connection with RA connecting to PA • Modified: total cavopulmonary connection Glenn shunt with SVC connected via extracardiac conduit to PA	Cyanotic heart diseases with a single functional ventricle when a biventricular repair is not feasible (i.e. tricuspid/pulmonary atresia, double inlet ventricle, and hypoplastic left heart syndrome)

LV: left ventricle; RV: right ventricle; TGA: transposition of the great arteries; PA: pulmonary artery; D-TGA: dextro-transposition of the great arteries; VSD: ventricular septal defect; LVOT: left ventricular outflow tract; RVOT: right ventricular outflow tract; SVC: superior vena cava; RA: right atrium.

Specific ACHD pathologies

283

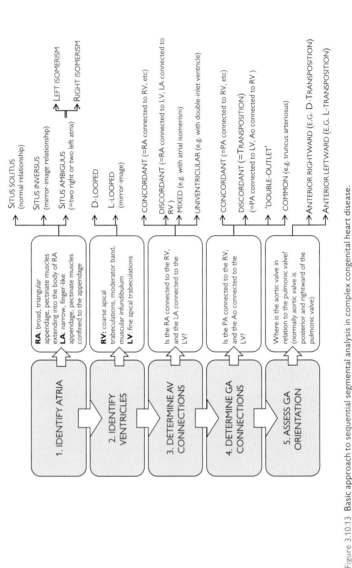

Figure 3.10.13 Basic approach to sequential segmental analysis in complex congenital heart disease.

AV: atrioventricular; GA: great arteries; RA: right atrium; LA: left atrium; RV: right ventricle; LV: left ventricle; PA: pulmonary arteries; Ao: aorta.

Advice on structured review/reporting of ACHD scans (sequential segmental analysis)

- Determine the cardiac position: levo-, meso-, and dextrocardia.
- Three segments within the heart: atria, ventricles, and great arteries.
- Each segment is defined by the morphology of its structures rather than the location or concordance within the chest.
- A simplified, basic approach to sequential segmental reporting in complex ACHD is given in Figure 3.10.13.

Further reading

Budoff MJ, Shinbane JS (eds). *Cardiac CT Imaging. Diagnosis of Cardiovascular Disease*. 3rd edn. New York: Springer International, 2016.

Han BK, Rigsby CK, Hlavacek A, Leipsic J, Nicol ED, Siegel MJ, et al. Computed tomography imaging in patients with congenital heart disease, part I and II: rationale and utility. An Expert Consensus Document of the Society of Cardiovascular Computed Tomography (SCCT): endorsed by the Society of Pediatric Radiology (SPR) and the North American Society of Cardiac Imaging (NASCI). *J Cardiovasc Comput Tomogr* 2015; 9: 472–92.

Schoepf UJ (ed.). *CT of the Heart—Contemporary Medical Imaging*. 2nd edn. New York: Humana Press, 2019.

Chapter 3.11

Cardiomyopathies

Dominik C. Benz

Teaching points

- Cardiomyopathies include a variety of heterogeneous disease entities affecting the cardiac muscle. The 2008 European Society of Cardiology classification of cardiomyopathies provides a classification scheme based on phenotypical presentation (see Figure 3.11.1).

- Echocardiography and cardiac magnetic resonance are often the first-line imaging modalities. However, there are a number of clinical scenarios where cardiac CT may be a useful alternative (e.g. imaging of patients with non-magnetic resonance conditional devices, critically ill patients, poor acoustic windows, and low patient compliance (such as adherence to breath hold or claustrophobia)).

- The main roles of CT in patients with cardiomyopathy include the assessment of underlying coronary and/or valvular disease, the characterization of the type of cardiomyopathy, the evaluation of volumes and function, and the planning of specific treatments (Table 3.11.1).

- CT perfusion and delayed contrast enhancement CT can assess the presence of perfusion abnormalities and irreversible myocardial fibrosis in certain patients with cardiomyopathies (see also Chapter 2.5).

Hypertrophic cardiomyopathy

Definition

Inappropriate left ventricular (LV) hypertrophy that is disproportionate to the degree of LV loading conditions and occurs in the absence of another cardiac or systemic disease, metabolic, or multiorgan syndrome associated with LV hypertrophy.

Value of cardiac CT

- Anatomical assessment of the epicardial coronary arteries (e.g. myocardial bridging, coronary artery disease, and prior to alcohol septal ablation).

- Evaluation of myocardial perfusion and quantification of myocardial fibrosis by delayed contrast enhancement CT.

- Excluding intracavitary thrombus (apex).

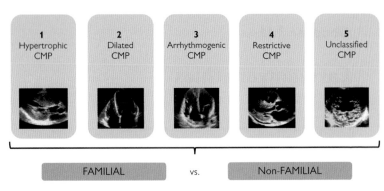

Figure 3.11.1 Simplified European Society of Cardiology classification of cardiomyopathies (CMP).
Source: Data from Elliott P, Andersson B, Arbustini E, et al. A classification of the cardiomyopathies: a position statement from the European Society Of Cardiology Working Group on Myocardial and Pericardial Diseases. *Eur Heart J.* 2008;29(2):270–6. doi: 10.1093/eurheartj/ehm342.

Table 3.11.1 Practical tips: how to set up your scanner for a cardiomyopathy scan	
Scan parameters	• Slice thickness, scan range, and field of view as per local protocol and scanner • kVp and mA according to local protocol and scanner (see Chapter 1.5) (For CT perfusion or scar imaging, see Chapter 2.5)
ECG gating	• Prospective if low HR and primary aim is to evaluate coronary arteries • Retrospective for functional information (volumes, EF, wall motion assessment) or if high HR
Medications	• Medications are only needed for assessment of coronary arteries • Beta-blockers for HR control (caution: very low EF or decompensated state) • Sublingual nitrates (caution: dynamic LVOT obstruction, severe RV dysfunction)
Contrast protocol	• Biphasic protocol for coronary arteries • Consider triphasic injection to opacify both left and right heart chambers without streak artefacts of the superior vena cava (e.g. arrhythmogenic right cardiomyopathy) • Consider venous phase scan for right-sided pathologies only
Dose reduction	• Optimize the protocol for dose reduction (see Chapter 1.7)

ECG: electrocardiogram; HR: heart rate; EF: ejection fraction; LVOT: left ventricular outflow tract; RV: right ventricle

- Other than that, cardiac CT is limited to scenarios where echocardiographic images are suboptimal and cardiac magnetic resonance (CMR) contraindicated.

Cardiac CT diagnostic finding (adapted from echocardiography/cardiac magnetic resonance)

- LV wall hypertrophy >15 mm, often asymmetrical (>13 mm in the presence of other features of hypertrophic cardiomyopathy; see Figure 3.11.2).
- Right ventricle (RV) wall hypertrophy >6 mm
- Systolic anterior motion of the anterior mitral valve leaflet.
- Decreased systolic wall thickening at the hypertrophic site compared to the non-hypertrophic site.
- Mid-wall delayed contrast enhancement (caution: extent of fibrosis underestimated by ~4%).

Dilated cardiomyopathy

Definition

LV or biventricular dilatation and systolic dysfunction (LV ejection fraction <45%) that are not explained by abnormal loading conditions (e.g. hypertension or valve

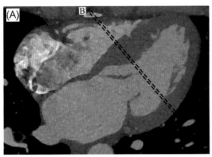 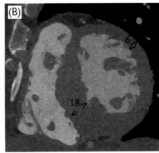

Figure 3.11.2 A 43-year-old woman with hypertrophic cardiomyopathy and left ventricular outflow tract obstruction was referred for coronary CT angiography due to typical angina.

(A) Horizontal long-axis and (B) short-axis views at the 75% phase of the RR interval illustrate a maximal wall thickness of 18 mm in the inferoseptal wall, extending to the inferior and anteroseptal walls. Coronary artery disease was excluded.

disease) or coronary artery disease (CAD; sufficient to cause global systolic impairment).

Value of cardiac CT

- Exclusion of CAD by coronary CT angiography (CCTA; see Figure 3.11.3).
- Assistance in heart failure interventions (e.g. cardiac resynchronization therapy, LV assist device, valve interventions).
- Exclusion of intracavitary thrombi.
- Other than that, limited to scenarios where echocardiographic images are suboptimal and CMR contraindicated.

Cardiac CT diagnostic finding

The findings are unspecific and include:

- Dilatation of the LV (and RV) volumes and reduced ejection fraction (see Figure 3.11.3).
- Thinning of LV wall thickness.

Arrhythmogenic cardiomyopathy

Definition

Arrhythmogenic cardiomyopathy is characterized by an acquired and progressive replacement of the ventricular myocardium by fibrous and fatty tissue.

Value of cardiac CT

- When echocardiographic images are suboptimal and CMR is contraindicated, cardiac CT is appropriate for the evaluation of structural remodelling in patients with arrhythmogenic cardiomyopathy (caution: ensure adequate opacification of the RV).
- Consider functional CT for RV functional assessment.

See Box 3.11.1.

Restrictive cardiomyopathy

Definition

Restrictive cardiomyopathy consists of a heterogeneous group of heart muscle diseases with a restrictive ventricular physiology. These include cardiac amyloidosis, haemochromatosis, Fabry cardiomyopathy, glycogen storage disease, cardiac sarcoidosis, and endomyocardial fibrosis (see Figure 3.11.5).

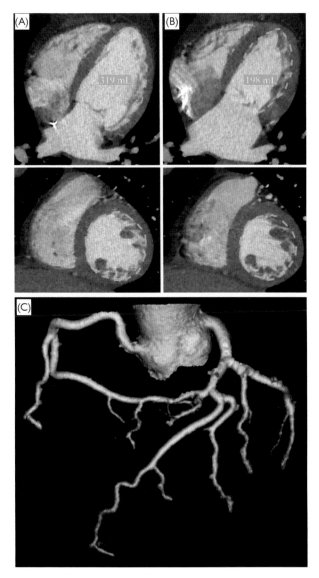

Figure 3.11.3 A 47-year-old woman with dilated cardiomyopathy and severe mitral regurgitation was referred for four-dimensional CT to evaluate suitability for percutaneous mitral annuloplasty.

Functional analysis revealed an (A) end diastolic volume of 319 ml (EDV index (EDVI) = 114 ml/m^2) and (B) an end systolic volume of 198 ml (EDVI = 71 ml/m^2), resulting in an ejection fraction of 38%. (C) Coronary CT angiography excluded coronary artery disease.

> **Box 3.11.1** Cardiac CT diagnostic findings (adapted from the 2010 modified arrhythmogenic cardiomyopathy Task Force Criteria)*
>
> Major criteria
> - Regional RV akinesia, dyskinesia, or dyssynchronous contraction *plus one of the following:*
>   - ratio of RV end diastolic volume to body surface area (BSA) ≥110 ml/m^2 (in males) or BSA ≥110 ml/m^2 (in females);
>   - RV ejection fraction (RVEF) ≤40%.
>
> Minor criteria
> - Regional RV akinesia, dyskinesia, or dyssynchronous contraction *plus one of the following:*
>   - ratio of RV end diastolic volume to BSA ≥100 to <110 ml/m^2 (in males) or ≥90 to <100 mL/m^2 (in females);
>   - RVEF >40 to ≤45%
>
> Other features of arrhythmogenic cardiomyopathy
> - Focal aneurysms of the myocardium (see Figure 3.11.4).
> - Increased trabeculations.
> - Fatty infiltrations (as areas of hypoattenuation between −120 and −60 Hounsfield units).
>
> *Marcus FI, McKenna WJ, Sherrill D, Basso C, Bauce B, Bluemke DA, et al. Diagnosis of cardiomyopathy/dysplasia: proposed modification of the Task Force Criteria. *Eur Heart J* 2010; 31: 806–14.

Value of cardiac CT

- Exclusion of constrictive pericarditis by pericardial thickening or calcifications.
- Visualization of extracardiac manifestations of the disease (see 'Cardiac CT diagnostic findings').
- Myocardial texture assessment with extracellular volume (ECV) quantification is feasible with dynamic equilibrium CT (e.g. ECV↑ in cardiac amyloidosis; see Figure 3.11.6).
- Other than that, limited to scenarios where echocardiographic images are suboptimal and CMR is contraindicated.

Cardiac CT diagnostic findings

The findings are non-specific and include:
- abnormal LV wall thickness and mass;
- dilatation of the atria and systemic veins;
- non-specific/patchy pattern of delayed contrast enhancement;
- pulmonary congestion and pleural effusions, and pericardial effusion.

Typical extracardiac manifestations of systemic diseases causing restrictive cardiomyopathy are:
- in sarcoidosis—pulmonary nodules, pulmonary fibrosis, or lymphadenopathy;
- in amyloidosis—inhomogeneous hepatomegaly or small kidneys.

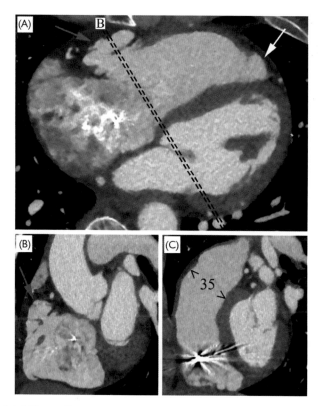

Figure 3.11.4 A 60-year-old woman with arrhythmogenic cardiomyopathy was referred to CT prior to ablation of recurrent right ventricular arrhythmia.

In (A) axial view, CT identified a dilated right atrium and right ventricle (RV) with prominent sacculation of the RV apex (white arrow). A large subtricuspid aneurysm is visualized on both the (A) axial and (B) oblique views (red arrow). (C) The RV outflow tract is dilated (35 mm).

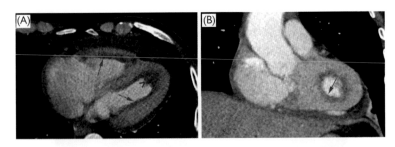

Figure 3.11.5 A 46-year-old man with endomyocardial fibrosis presented with heart failure with preserved ejection fraction.

The (A) axial and (B) coronal views of delayed enhanced cardiac CT demonstrate obliteration of the left ventricular apex (red arrowhead) and a low-attenuation endocardial rim in both the right and left ventricles (red arrows).

Source: Courtesy of Andreas A. Giannopoulos.

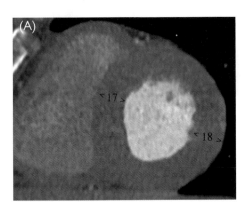
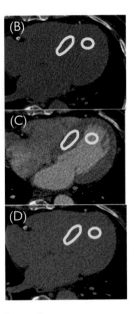

Figure 3.11.6 A 64-year-old man with dyspnoea and restrictive cardiomyopathy.

(A) Short-axis view of the left ventricle reveals symmetrical hypertrophy with a maximal wall thickness of 18 mm. Dynamic equilibrium CT (gated scan (B) before, (C) 1 min, and (D) 5 min after contrast administration) allows for calculation of the extracellular volume (ECV) according to the formula $ECV_{CT} = (1 - haematocrit) \times (\Delta HU_{tissue}/\Delta HU_{blood})$. A high ECV (>0.40) is characteristic of cardiac amyloidosis. HU: Hounsfield unit.

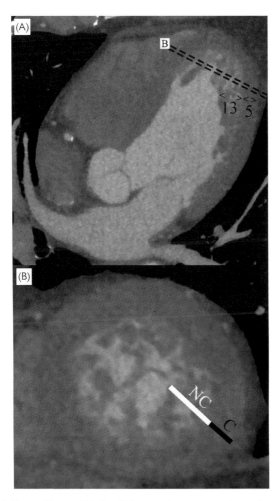

Figure 3.11.7 A 61-year-old man with isolated left ventricular non-compaction cardiomyopathy who underwent cardiac CT because of claustrophobia.

Horizontal (A) long- and (B) short-axis views demonstrate left ventricular dilatation and non-compaction of the apical myocardium extending to the midventricular segments. The thickness of the non-compacted (NC) and compacted (C) myocardium was 13 mm and 5 mm, respectively, resulting in an NC/C ratio of 2.6.

Unclassified cardiomyopathies: left ventricular non-compaction

Definition

LV non-compaction is characterized by a two-layered (thin compacted and thick non-compacted) myocardium, which presents as hypertrabeculations.

Value of cardiac CT

- Exclusion of CAD and coronary artery anomalies by CCTA.
- Detection of hypertrabeculations of the non-compacted myocardium and of thrombi within recesses.

Cardiac CT diagnostic findings

- Ratio of non-compacted to compacted myocardium >2.3 in the end diastolic long axis (see Figure 3.11.7)

Further reading

Cardim N, Galderisi M, Edvardsen T, Plein S, Popescu BA, D'Andrea A, et al. Role of multimodality cardiac imaging in the management of patients with hypertrophic cardiomyopathy: an expert consensus of the European Association of Cardiovascular Imaging Endorsed by the Saudi Heart Association. *Eur Heart J Cardiovasc Imaging* 2015; 16: 280.

Donal E, Delgado V, Bucciarelli-Ducci C, Galli E, Haugaa KH, Charron P, et al. Multimodality imaging in the diagnosis, risk stratification, and management of patients with dilated cardiomyopathies: an expert consensus document from the European Association of Cardiovascular Imaging. *Eur Heart J Cardiovasc Imaging* 2019; 20: 1075–93.

Haugaa KH, Basso C, Badano LP, Bucciarelli-Ducci C, Cardim N, Gaemperli O, et al. Comprehensive multi-modality imaging approach in arrhythmogenic cardiomyopathy-an expert consensus document of the European Association of Cardiovascular Imaging. *Eur Heart J Cardiovasc Imaging* 2017; 18: 237–53.

Habib G, Bucciarelli-Ducci C, Caforio ALP, Cardim, N, Charron P, Cosyns B, et al. Multimodality imaging in restrictive cardiomyopathies: an EACVI expert consensus document. In collaboration with the "Working Group on myocardial and pericardial diseases" of the European Society of Cardiology Endorsed by The Indian Academy of Echocardiography. *Eur Heart J Cardiovasc Imaging* 2017; 18: 1090–121.

Sidhu MS, Uthamalingam S, Ahmed W, Engel L-C, Vorasettakarnkij Y, Lee AM, et al. Defining left ventricular noncompaction using cardiac computed tomography. *J Thorac Imaging* 2014; 29: 60–6.

Chapter 3.12

Cardiac masses

Andreas A. Giannopoulos

Teaching points

- Cardiac masses include non-neoplastic cardiac masses, normal variants, and benign and malignant cardiac tumours.
- Multimodality imaging may be necessary for accurate evaluation, and an interdisciplinary approach is paramount for diagnosis and management. Interpretation of the imaging findings must always be performed in an individualized clinical context.
- Cardiac CT can provide accurate assessment of the location, the extent, and the morphological characteristics of the lesions, while allowing for non-invasive evaluation of the coronary anatomy in view of surgical resection.
- Knowledge of common CT artefacts and the localization of commonly encountered normal variants can improve the diagnostic accuracy. Thrombi, and benign and malignant tumours are characterized by specific CT features, enabling differential diagnosis.

Classification of cardiac masses

- Cardiac masses are rare findings (<1% in autopsy series).
- They can be divided into non-neoplastic cardiac masses/normal variants, benign cardiac tumours, and malignant cardiac tumours. (Figure 3.12.1)
- Non-neoplastic masses (e.g. thrombus and vegetation) are more common than neoplastic disease and should be ruled out before suspecting a cardiac tumour.
- Among malignant cardiac tumours, metastatic disease is approximately 20–40 times more common than primary cardiac malignancy.
- Among primary cardiac tumours, approximately three out of four are benign (by far the most common is cardiac myxoma; Table 3.12.1).

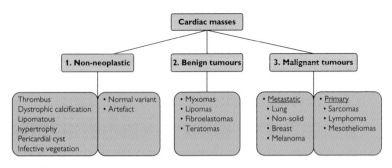

Figure 3.12.1 Classification of cardiac masses.

Localization of cardiac masses

Various cardiac masses have a particular predilection for specific sites (e.g. myxoma originating from the fossa ovalis or thrombus in the left atrial appendage (LAA)). Knowledge of these sites may help considerably in the correct identification of masses (Figure 3.12.2).

Cardiac CT evaluation

Image acquisition should be individualized in the case of a known mass that needs to be evaluated with cardiac CT, while additional scans might be necessary should the mass be an incidental finding. Table 3.12.2 provides a guide for the cardiac CT

Table 3.12.1 Relative frequencies of primary cardiac tumours			
Benign (~75%)	Frequency (%)	Malignant (~25%)	Frequency (%)
Myxoma	30	Angiosarcoma	9
Lipoma	10	Rhabdomyosarcoma	6
Fibroelastoma	10	Mesothelioma	4
Rhabdomyoma	8	Fibrosarcoma	3
Fibroma	4	Lymphoma	2
Haemangioma	3	Other sarcomas	3
Teratoma	3	Teratoma	<1
Others	5	Others	<1

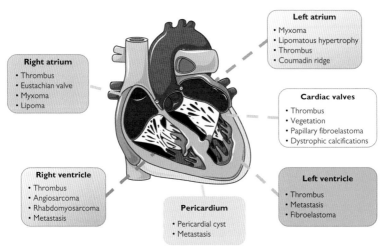

Right atrium
- Thrombus
- Eustachian valve
- Myxoma
- Lipoma

Left atrium
- Myxoma
- Lipomatous hypertrophy
- Thrombus
- Coumadin ridge

Cardiac valves
- Thrombus
- Vegetation
- Papillary fibroelastoma
- Dystrophic calcifications

Right ventricle
- Thrombus
- Angiosarcoma
- Rhabdomyosarcoma
- Metastasis

Pericardium
- Pericardial cyst
- Metastasis

Left ventricle
- Thrombus
- Metastasis
- Fibroelastoma

Figure 3.12.2 Localization of cardiac masses. Creative assistance for the preparation of the figure was provided by Servier Medical Art. (https://smart.servier.com)

protocol for the evaluation of cardiac masses. Table 3.12.3 summarizes classical sites and common CT features of the most frequent cardiac masses.

Non-neoplastic cardiac masses/normal variants

Thrombi

- Most frequently in the left cardiac chambers (LAA and left ventricle (LV)).
- Generally, not contrast-enhanced and of low attenuation (~65 Hounsfield units (HU)). Chronic LV thrombi may develop spotty calcifications.
- Cardiac CT is highly sensitive for excluding LAA thrombi, delayed imaging further increases the positive predictive value for thrombus detection from 41% to 92% (distinguishing slow-flow phenomenon from true thrombus; Figure 3.12.3). (See also Chapter 3.7.)

Lipomatous hypertrophy

- Non-encapsulated mass of fatty tissue that infiltrates the atrial septum.
- Hourglass-shaped structure with typically sparing of the fossa ovalis.
- CT attenuation of fatty tissue (<0 HU) with an homogenous appearance, sharp margins, and no or minimal contrast enhancement (Figure 3.12.4).

Table 3.12.2 Tips on how to set up your scanner for imaging cardiac masses	
Scan parameter	• Tube voltage and current according to local protocol (lower kVp for better tissue differentiation) • Consider larger field of view (in case of tumours spreading to adjacent structures)
ECG gating	• Prospective ECG triggering default mode (low radiation) • Consider retrospective ECG gating to assess motion of structures (vegetations, intracavitary tumours like myxoma/ fibroelastoma)
Medication	• No need for beta blockade or nitrates (except for evaluation of coronary arteries)
Non-contrast-enhanced cardiac CT acquisition	• Essential for identification of high attenuation regions, primarily calcifications pertinent to the mass, or for the differentiation of fat and thrombus

Contrast injection	• For right-sided masses consider triphasic contrast protocols to reduce streak artefacts in the superior vena cava
	• Delayed imaging may be useful for:
	  • discrimination between slow-flow phenomenon vs. cardiac thrombi, particularly in the LAA (see also Chapter 3.7)
	  • assessment of contrast enhancement of masses

ECG: electrocardiogram; LAA: left atrial appendage

Dystrophic calcification of the mitral annulus

• Deposition of calcium along the myocardial tissue, with the atrioventricular valves being particularly prone.

• Native cardiac CT can provide accurate assessment of the localization and extent (focal vs. diffuse) of calcifications.

• May progress to caseous calcification: typically located within the posterior portion of the mitral annulus, characterized by a necrotic centre with a typically low attenuation (~50 HU), and with no contrast enhancement (Figure 3.12.5).

Vegetation

• Irregular- or round-shaped hypoattenuating mass attached to a cardiac valve.

• More frequently on the upstream side of the valves (as opposed to fibroelastoma).

• Look for: paravalvular abscesses and pseudoaneurysms, as well as septic emboli.

• Cine images can show oscillating movement of the vegetation and/or dysfunction of prosthetic valves due to vegetation (Figure 3.12.6; see also Chapter 3.8).

Table 3.12.3 Common location and CT characteristics of most common cardiac masses

	Common location	Cardiac CT characteristics
Thrombi	LAA, LV, LA	Low HU (~65 HU), no CE, late scans are helpful
Lipomatous hypertrophy	Interatrial septum, RA, LA	Hourglass shape, low attenuation values (<0 HU)
Myxoma	LA septum (80%), RA, LV, RV	Solitary, intracavitary, lobulated, coarse calcifications, heterogeneous CE
Lipoma	Intracavitary or pericardial	Homogeneous, fat attenuation, no CE
Dystrophic calcification	Mitral valve annulus	Peripheral calcification with hypoattenuating centre (50 HU), no CE
Fibroelastoma	Valves, left chambers, papillary muscles	No CE, endocardial origin
Sarcoma	RV, RA, myocardium, pericardium	Low-attenuation focal, irregular, broad base or diffuse myo- and pericardial infiltration, heterogeneous CE
Metastasis	Pericardium, myocardium	Iso- or hypoattenuating, various degree of CE
Pericardial cyst	Right anterior cardiophrenic angle	Smooth border, homogenous low attenuation (−10 to 10 HU)

CE: contrast enhancement; LAA: left atrial appendage; LV: left ventricle; LA: left atrium; HU: Hounsfield unit; RA: right atrium; RV: right ventricle.

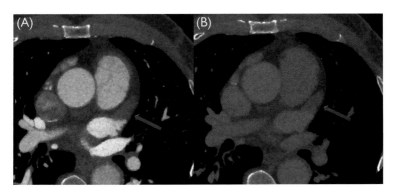

Figure 3.12.3 LAA thrombus.

(A) Axial cardiac CT images with the presence of thrombus in the LAA (red arrow), confirmed in (B) the late scan, showing persistence of low attenuation at repeat scan 60 s later.

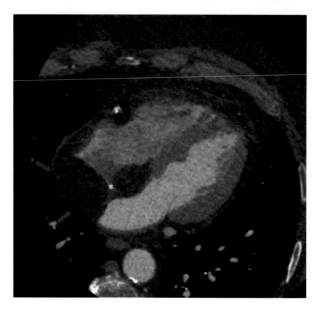

Figure 3.12.4 Lipomatous hypertrophy of the interatrial septum.

Cardiac CT images demonstrating a mass with fat attenuation (average −101 HU) that spares the fossa ovalis (*). Note that the mass also extends to involve the posterior wall of the right atrium (arrow), which may be seen in cases of more extensive lipomatous hypertrophy.

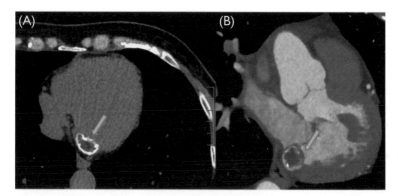

Figure 3.12.5 Caseous calcification of the mitral annulus.

(A) Native cardiac CT images demonstrating oval formed calcification at the posterior side of the left ventricle (yellow arrow). (B) Sagittal view of contrast-enhanced CT with no signs of enhancement of the calcified mass, localized at the mitral valve annulus.

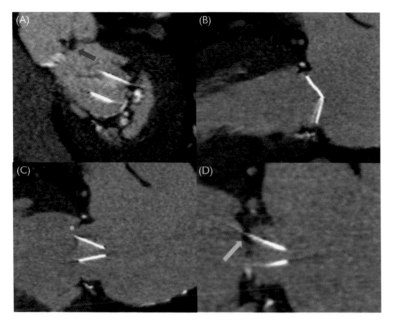

Figure 3.12.6 Cardiac CT of infective endocarditis of native aortic valve, and mechanical mitral prosthesis intermittent dysfunction.

(A) demonstrates an infective vegetation affecting the upstream side of the aortic valve (red arrow). (B) shows correct leaflets closure of the mechanical mitral prosthesis; (C) depicts reduced motility of anterior disk of the mechanical mitral prosthesis (yellow asterisk). (D) demonstrates endocarditic vegetations attached to the prosthetic ring interfering with anterior disk (yellow arrow).

Source: Courtesy of Dr. Andrea Baggiano.

Pericardial cyst

- Frequently located at the right cardiophrenic angle (~80%).
- Homogeneous, with a smooth border and water intensity (−10 to 10 HU) with no contrast enhancement (Figure 3.12.7).
- Cardiac CT offers help with differential diagnosis from pleural effusion or extracardiac cyst.

Persistent eustachian valve

- Remnant of the embryonic valve of the sinus venosus, frequently associated with patent foramen ovale.
- Located at the junction between the inferior vena cava and the right atrium (RA), and can be mistaken for a mass.
- In cardiac CT, it appears as a rigid, elongated membrane in the RA (Figure 3.12.8).

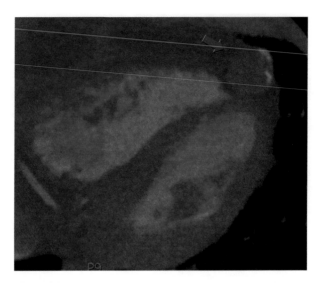

Figure 3.12.7 **Pericardial cyst.**

Axial CT image depicting a pericardial mass (red arrow) with homogeneous attenuation and peripheral calcifications.

Coumadin (left lateral) ridge

- Can mimic floating structures (thrombus, tumour; Figure 3.12.9).
- Low attenuation ridge between the LAA and the left superior pulmonary vein.

Benign cardiac tumours

Myxomas

- Most common primary cardiac tumour (up to 50% of all benign cardiac tumours).
- Most often located in the left atrium, typically in connection with the fossa ovalis.
- Usually solitary, intracavitary masses with a lobulated appearance and coarse calcifications.
- In native CT images, they typically have low attenuation values, while in contrast-enhanced images, they are ovoid with a smooth or lobular shape, and with heterogeneous enhancement (Figure 3.12.10).

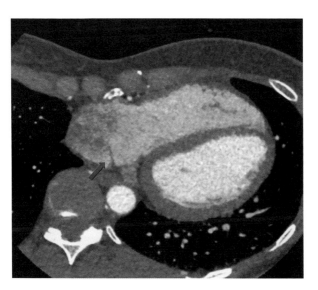

Figure 3.12.8 Persistent eustachian valve.

Axial CT images depicting persistent eustachian valve (red arrow) and the mixture of contrast agent with non-opacified blood from the inferior vena cava.

Lipomas

- Second most common benign cardiac tumour.
- Located either intracavitary or in the pericardium.
- Homogeneous mass in native CT images with fat attenuation (−60 to −120 HU) and with smooth contouring and no contrast enhancement.

(Papillary) Fibroelastoma

- Most common benign valvular tumour.
- Usually located at the aortic and mitral valve (less often on right-sided valves), as well as the papillary muscles.
- Typically, on the downstream side of the valves, and usually no destruction or relevant dysfunction of the valve (as opposed to vegetations).
- In native CT images, they appear as hypoattenuating small masses with microlobules.
- Avascular structures without contrast enhancement (Figure 3.12.11).

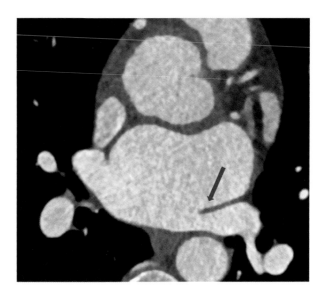

Figure 3.12.9 Coumadin ridge.

Axial CT images demonstrating the prominent ridge (red arrow).

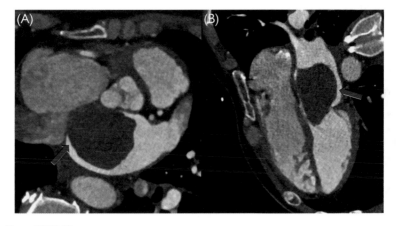

Figure 3.12.10 Myxoma.

(A) Axial and (B) sagittal CT images showing a large left atrial myxoma (red arrow) with diastolic prolapse into the left ventricle. Note the typical origin of the tumour at the fossa ovalis.

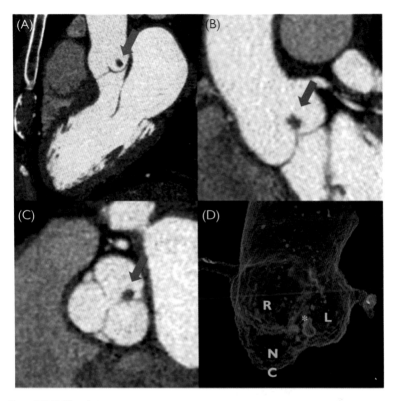

Figure 3.12.11 Fibroelastoma.

Cardiac CT images demonstrating a small, homogeneous (average 85 HU), non-contrast-enhanced mass at the aortic side of the left coronary cusp (red arrows in A–C; orange asterisk in D). (A) Three-chamber long-axis view. (B) Aortic long-axis view. (C) Aortic valve short-axis view. (D) Three-dimensional view of the aortic valve and ascending aorta with fibroelastoma in transparency.

R: right coronary cusp; L: left coronary cusp; NC: non-coronary cusp.

Source: Courtesy of Dr. Andrea Baggiano.

Malignant cardiac tumours

Metastatic tumours

- Twenty to forty times more frequent than primary cardiac malignancies.
- Spread via haematogenic (in myocardium) and lymphatic (in pericardium) routes, direct infiltration, or through venous extension (Table 3.12.4).
- Primaries usually include lung, non-solid tumours, breast, and melanoma.

Table 3.12.4 Most common primary malignancies with cardiac metastasis and spread route

Per continuity	Via venous extension	Hematogenic spread	Lymphatic spread
• Breast • Lung • Oesophagus • Mediastinal	• Renal cell • Adrenal • Thyroid • Lung • Hepatic	• Melanoma • Breast • Lung • Genitourinary • Gastrointestinal	• Lymphoma • Leukaemia

- Usually located in myocardium and rarely intracavitary (with a broad base).
- Appear as iso- or hypoattenuating in native CT images, while contrast enhancement depends on the stage of angiogenesis (Figure 3.12.12).
- Most metastases enhance less than the myocardium initially. After contrast administration, they accumulate and retain contrast gradually.

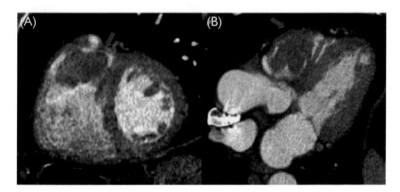

Figure 3.12.12 Metastatic cardiac tumours.

Cardiac CT images showing a lobulated mass (red arrows) attached to the right ventricular outflow tract in a patient with known hepatocellular carcinoma. (A) Left ventricle (LV) short-axis view. (B) A modified LV three-chamber long-axis view.

Source: Courtesy of Dr. Andrea Baggiano.

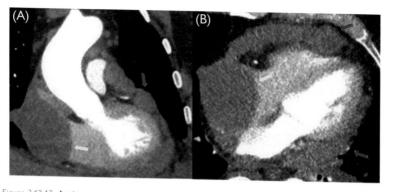

Figure 3.12.13 Angiosarcoma.

(A) Sagittal cardiac and (B) axial cardiac CT images of the same patient demonstrating a circular, smooth right atrial mass with no contrast enhancement and heterogeneous density (yellow arrows), as well as pericardial thickening (red arrows).

Primary cardiac sarcomas

- Most common (~95%) primary malignant cardiac tumour, followed by lymphoma.
- In native CT low-attenuation focal, irregular masses, frequently originating from the right atrium with a broad base.
- Can also present as diffuse myo- and pericardial infiltration.
- Contrast enhancement is heterogeneous with areas of necrosis; late phase acquisition might be useful (Figure 3.12.13).

Differential diagnosis of cardiac masses using CT

See Table 3.12.5 for help with the differentiation of cardiac masses.

Table 3.12.5 CT characteristics of benign versus malignant cardiac masses

	Benign	Malignant
Origin and localization of the mass	Intracavitary (pedunculated, narrow attachment)	Intramyocardial or epicardial; adjacent to the heart or extracardiac; pericardial/pleural effusion
	More often left-sided chambers	More often right-sided chambers
Number of masses	Solitary	Non-solitary
Form and texture	Smooth, homogenous, discreet (except: myxoma may be heterogenous/calcified)	Lobulated, irregular borders, non-homogenous, calcified, infiltrative
Size (cm)	<5	≥5
CT attenuation	Fat-rich tumours less than −10 to −100 HU (e.g. lipoma and lipomatous hypertrophy)	Calcifications >130 HU: common in myxoma, chronic thrombi, metastasis
	Cystic masses −10 to 10 HU	
Contrast enhancement	Typically lack of enhancement (exception: myxomas may show minimal/mild postcontrast enhancement)	Arterial phase enhancement = vascularized tumours; late phase enhancement = suggestive of malignant tumours, inflammation, intratumour necrosis

Further reading

Budoff MJ, Shinbane JS (eds). *Cardiac CT Imaging. Diagnosis of Cardiovascular Disease*. 3rd edn. New York: Springer International Publishing, 2010.

Bruce CJ. Cardiac tumours: diagnosis and management. *Heart* 2011; 97: 151–60.

Lim TH (ed.). *Practical Textbook of Cardiac CT and MRI*. 1st edn. New York: Springer, 2015.

Chapter 3.13

Pericardial disease

Sarah Moharem-Elgamal

Teaching points

- Cardiac CT offers excellent spatial and temporal resolution for visualization of normal or pathological pericardium. While echocardiography remains the first-line imaging technique for the evaluation of pericardial disease, CT may provide complementary information to echocardiography and/or cardiac magnetic resonance.

- Pericardial effusion is readily visible by cardiac CT, and differentiation of fluid composition is feasible based on attenuation values.

- Pathological thickening and/or pericardial calcifications are often seen in pericarditis. However, confirmation of constrictive or tamponade physiology requires further haemodynamic assessment by echocardiography and invasive catheterization.

Normal anatomy and function of the pericardium

The pericardium is an avascular double-walled sac that contains the heart and roots of the great vessels. It is comprised of an external fibrous layer surrounding the inner serous pericardium. The inner layer also consists of two layers—an outer parietal layer and an inner visceral layer—which are separated by a potential space, the pericardial cavity. The pericardial cavity normally contains 15–50 ml clear serous fluid. The pericardium acts as a barrier to inflammation and infection from adjacent mediastinal structures. It also limits the friction from cardiac motion within the mediastinum.

On CT, the normal pericardium:

- appears as a thin dense line of ≤2 mm thickness where the visceral layer cannot be seen (Figure 3.13.1);
- is best visualized during systole and over the right ventricle (RV);
- can be difficult to depict over the lateral and posterior aspect of the left ventricle (LV);
- contains little pericardial fluid with an attenuation value similar to water (~ 0 Hounsfield units).

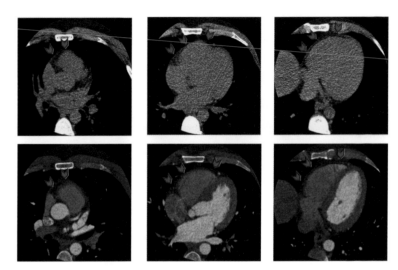

Figure 3.13.1 Normal pericardium.

Pericardium (arrows) can be seen as a thin line in CT with and without contrast.

Pericardial recesses

- The transverse sinus is located superior to the left atrium (LA) and posterior to the ascending aorta and pulmonary artery (PA); superior and inferior aortic and right and left pulmonary recesses arise from it (Figure 3.13.2).
- Normal superior pericardial recesses can mimic acute aortic syndromes and enlarged lymph nodes to the untrained eye.
- The oblique sinus is a space that lies behind the LA and inferior to the transverse sinus, from which it is separated by pericardial reflections.
- The posterior pericardial recess arises from the oblique sinus. It extends superiorly behind the right PA and medial to the bronchus intermedius.

Congenital absence of pericardium

- Absence of the pericardium can be congenital or the result of surgery or trauma.
- Congenital absence of the pericardium is usually partial but can be complete.
- Partial absence is due to premature atrophy of the left common cardinal vein and thus poor blood supply to the left pleuropericardial membrane that forms the left pericardium (Figure 3.13.3).

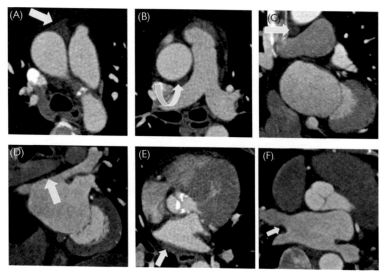

Figure 3.13.2 Pericardial recesses.

(A) Axial image shows anterior superior aortic recesses (arrow). (B) Axial image shows posterior superior aortic recesses (curved arrow). (C) Coronal image shows lateral superior aortic recess (arrow). (D) Coronal image shows a right pulmonary artery recess inferior to the right pulmonary artery (arrow). (E) Axial image shows the oblique sinus (arrow). (F) Axial image shows the right pulmonic vein recess.

- Partial absence of the right pericardium is less common (17%) as the right common cardinal vein forms the superior vena cava and usually has an adequate blood supply during development.
- Total absence is rare.

Congenital heart defects that are usually associated with the absence of pericardium are:

- atrial septal defect;
- patent ductus arteriosus;
- tetralogy of Fallot;
- mitral stenosis;
- malformations of the lungs, chest wall, and diaphragm.

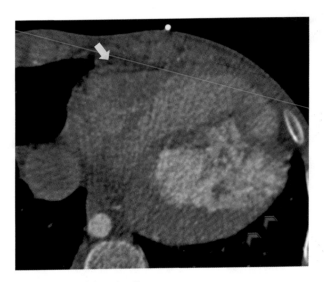

Figure 3.13.3 Partial absence of the pericardium.
The absence of the pericardium is usually difficult to visualize. The heart shows marked left-sided rotation and displacement in the anterior portion of left hemithorax in the absence of any other condition. The pericardium is depicted over the right ventricular free wall (yellow arrow) but not elsewhere (blue arrowheads).

Signs of total or partial pericardial absence on CT are:

- interposition of the lung tissue between the aorta and main PA on axial images, or between left hemi-diaphragm and the heart on coronal images;
- the heart axis is shifted leftward or posterior;
- it is usually an incidental finding, but complications include an increased risk of traumatic aortic dissection, herniation, and entrapment of a cardiac chamber.

Pericardial effusion

Pericardial effusion appears as a low attenuation, non-enhancing fluid accumulation in the pericardial cavity. This accumulation of fluid occurs with heart failure, renal and liver insufficiency, inflammation, infection, malignancy, trauma, and myocardial infarction (Figure 3.13.4).

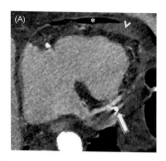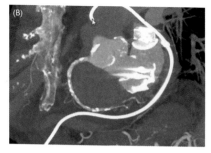

Figure 3.13.4 Pericardial effusion after pericardial drainage.

(A) Residual mild effusion with pneumopericardium (arrow points to the drain; the asterisk indicates the pneumopericardium; the arrowhead points to residual effusion). (B) A thick-slap maximum intensity projection demonstrating the entire course of the 8 F pericardial drain.

CT can confirm the presence, severity, and extent of fluid; characterize the nature of fluid by its attenuation values; and detect pericardial inflammation. Usually, cardiac tamponade is diagnosed clinically and by echocardiography. However, CT may offer additional clues to confirm the haemodynamic relevance of pericardial effusion:

- flattening, impinging, or compression of the right atrium and/or RV wall;
- flattening of the interventricular septum;
- distention of the venae cavae;
- reflux of contrast into the inferior vena cava.

Pericardial fluid in excess of 50 ml is considered abnormal, and this will generally correspond to a pericardial width in excess of 4 mm. A pericardial width >5 mm usually corresponds to a moderate effusion of 100–500 ml fluid. Table 3.13.1 shows typical CT attenuation values for the different components of pericardial fluid.

Pericarditis

Pericarditis may be seen with or without constriction; its aetiology includes infectious disease, autoimmune disease, post-myocardial infarction, post-cardiotomy syndrome, haemopericardium, haemorrhagic effusion, irradiation and idiopathic. The CT appearance includes pericardial enhancement on post-contrast imaging, smooth pericardial thickening, a variable amount of effusion with or without protuberance of epicardial fat in the acute phase, and calcification with chronic pericarditis.

Table 3.13.1 Different components of pericardial fluid and their characteristic CT attenuation values

	Transudate	Exudate	Haemopericardium	Chylopericardium	Pneumopericardium
CT attenuation (HU)	<10	20–60	>60*	−60 to −80	−1000

Note: values are approximate; significant overlap may exist between transudate, exudate, and haemopericardium. *Value decreases with time. HU: Hounsfield units.

Constrictive pericarditis

Constrictive pericarditis can be caused by thickened or normal-thickness fibrotic pericardium.

The aetiology of constrictive pericarditis includes infectious disease, autoimmune disease, post-myocardial infarction, post-cardiotomy syndrome, haemopericardium, haemorrhagic effusion of any origin, irradiation and idiopathic.

CT findings that suggest constrictive pericarditis include:

• increased thickness of >4 mm, and in 50% of patients there is calcified pericardium (Figure 3.13.5).

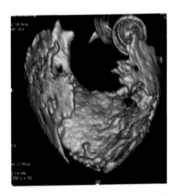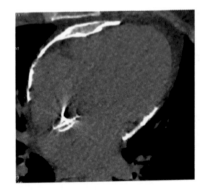

Figure 3.13.5 Constrictive pericarditis with extensive calcifications.

Note the presence of an Amplatzer left atrial appendage and septal occluder *in situ*.

- Other secondary findings (indicative of constrictive physiology) include:
  - enlarged atria;
  - dilated venae cavae, hepatic veins, and coronary sinus;
  - the presence of pleural effusion;
  - hepatic congestion and ascites.

However, constrictive physiology needs to be confirmed by diagnostic catherization by the simultaneous measurement of left and right ventricular diastolic pressure.

Pericardial calcification

Pericardial calcification can be present in the absence of pericardial constriction. CT can accurately depict calcification, which on magnetic resonance imaging has a low signal intensity similar to fibrosis.

Pericardial masses

Primary pericardial tumours are rare; most pericardial neoplasms are metastases. Benign pericardial tumours include lipoma, fibroma, teratoma, and haemangioma. Pericardial cysts are usually an incidental CT finding that is most

Table 3.13.2 Practical tips: how to set up your scanner for imaging pericardial pathologies	
Scan parameters	• Wide field of view may be indicated to identify associated chest pathology • kVp and mA according to local protocol and scanner (see Chapter 1.5)
ECG gating	• In case of high HR consider retrospective ECG gating or padding into systolic frames • Consider retrospective ECG gating (with or without dose modulation) to assess systolic and diastolic signs for tamponade (RV indentation, septal bounce, etc.)
Medications	• Beta-blockers and nitrates only needed for the assessment of coronary arteries (caution: nitrates and beta-blockers should be avoided in haemodynamically unstable patients with tamponade)
Scan protocol	• Native ECG-triggered scan recommended (calcifications, CT density of pericardial fluid) • Usually arterial phase only • Consider delayed venous phase to assess for pericardial contrast enhancement
Contrast protocol	• Biphasic protocol
Dose reduction	• Optimize protocol for dose reduction (see Chapter 1.7)
ECG: electrocardiogram; HR: heart rate; RV: right ventricle.	

commonly found in the right cardiophrenic angle and has thin, smooth walls without internal septations.

Malignant tumours include sarcoma and mesothelioma. Metastases involving the pericardium include lung, breast, and oesophageal cancers, melanoma, lymphoma, and leukaemia.

CT allows localization, characterization of the tumour and effusion, and extension of the mass. An irregular, thickened nodular pericardium is suggestive of malignancy, but this can also be present with inflammation.

For more information on pericardial masses see Chapter 3.12. Table 3.13.2 provides tips on how to set up your scanner to image pericardial pathologies.

Chapter 3.14

Implanted cardiac devices and how to recognize them on CT

Dominik C. Benz

Teaching points

- As implanted cardiac devices (see Figure 3.14.1) are more commonly used in clinical practice, cardiovascular imagers should be familiar with normal imaging features and also be aware of potential complications.
- While cardiac CT is not performed routinely to assess procedural success, it has emerged as a complementary tool when device dysfunction or other complications are suspected.
- Cardiac CT allows the acquisition of three-dimensional datasets over time (i.e. '4D-CT') with the assessment of devices in double-oblique planes. Further advantages include the high sensitivity for thrombus and calcifications, as well as assessment of cardiac and extracardiac interventional complications.
- The assessment of implanted cardiac devices can be improved by optimizing scan protocols (e.g. late scan, triphasic contrast injection protocol, or beam-hardening reduction algorithms).

This chapter provides an overview of the most common implanted cardiac devices (Tables 3.14.1–3.14.8). It focuses on the recognition of the device type.

The list of devices below may be incomplete. It focuses on the most prevalent commercially available cardiac devices used in Europe and the USA. For more in-depth information the reader is referred to the respective manufacturer's product descriptions.

Valvular devices

For more in-depth information about pathological findings after valve surgery/intervention, see Chapter 3.6.

For more in-depth information on prosthetic valve design, product information, dimensions, and sizes consult the following reference guide: www.valveguide.ch.

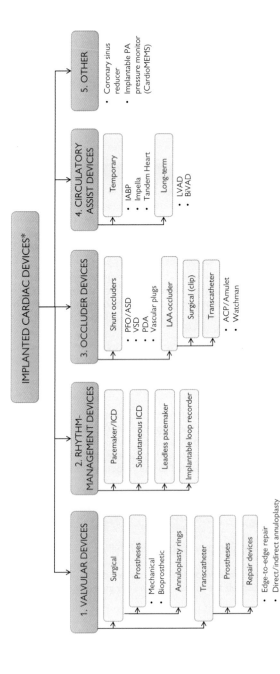

Figure 3.14.1 Overview of the most common cardiac implanted devices (CE-marked and commercially available).

*Excluded from this overview are stents (which are discussed separately in Chapter 2.7). ICD: implantable cardioverter defibrillator; PFO: patent foramen ovale; ASD: atrial septal defect; VSD: ventricular septal defect; PDA: patent ductus arteriosus; IABP: intra-aortic balloon pump; LVAD: left ventricular assist device; BiVAD: biventricular assist device; PA: pulmonary artery.

Table 3.14.1 Prostheses

Category	Device	Characteristics
Surgical prostheses		
Mechanical prostheses		
Bi-leaflet valves	Masters/Regent® (St. Jude Medical), ATS Open Pivot™ (Medtronic), Anatomic (On-X®), Carbomedics (Sorin)	Radiopaque ring-like valve housing, visibility of leaflets (as semilunar discs; see Figure 3.14.2)
Single tilting disc valves	Hall (Medtronic), Björk-Shiley Monostrut (Shiley), OmniScience/ OmniCarbon (Medical Inc.), Allcarbon (Sorin)	• Radiopaque housing and disc (see Figure 3.14.3) • Strong metallic artefacts (more than bi-leaflet valves)
Caged-ball valves	Starr-Edwards (see Figure 3.14.4)	Four-strut cage with a hollow silicone ball
Bioprostheses		
Stented bioprostheses	Hancock™ and Mosaic™ (Medtronic)	Three floating radiopaque markers at the distal end of the radiolucent stent posts, radiopaque (Hancock) or radiolucent (Mosaic) base ring
	CE Standard; CE PERIMOUNT (Edwards)	Radiopaque thin frame with three posts and three valleys (asymmetric frame thickening; = non-continuous base) at the post (Perimount) or valley (Standard)
	CE Perimount Magna (Edwards; Figure 3.14.5)	Radiopaque, undulating basal ring with regular indentations; radiopaque thin frame above basal ring with three posts
	INSPIRIS RESILIA (Edwards)	Similar to Magna, undulating basal ring with visible size markers and expansion zones for future valve-in-valve
	Mitroflow (Sorin)	Radiopaque undulating sewing ring; radiolucent stent posts
	Biocor® and Epic™ (St. Jude Medical)	Thin radiopaque undulating basal ring
	Trifecta™ (St. Jude Medical; see Figure 3.14.6)	Radiopaque stent frame forming three-pronged coronet
Stentless bioprostheses	Freestyle™ (Medtronic), Toronto SPV® (SJM), Prima (Edwards)	Radiolucent

Valvular devices

321

(continued)

Table 3.14.1 Continued		
Category	Device	Characteristics
Sutureless bioprostheses	3f Enable (Medtronic)	Three-level frame with three commissural posts
	Perceval® (Sorin)	Three-level frame with three straight commissural and six sinusoidal struts
	INTUITY (Edwards)	Similar design to CE Perimount Magna (with additional radiopaque skirt)
Transcatheter prostheses		
Balloon-expandable prostheses (see Figure 3.14.7)	SAPIEN (Edwards)	Four-level frame with three commissural posts
	SAPIEN XT (Edwards)	Three-level frame with three commissural posts
	SAPIEN 3 and SAPIEN 3 Ultra (Edwards)	Five-level frame with larger cells between the fourth and fifth level, without commissural posts
Self-expandable prostheses	CoreValve Evolut™ and Evolut™ PRO (Medtronic; see Figure 3.14.8)	Hourglass shape extending into ascending aorta
	Engager™ (Medtronic)	Control arms to capture the native leaflets
	Portico/Navitor™ (Abbott; see Figure 3.14.9)	Hourglass shape extending into ascending aorta, with large cell area in the aortic segments
	LOTUS™ (Boston Scientific; see Figure 3.14.10)	Radiopaque marker in the centre of the stent frame causing beam-hardening artefacts
	Accurate™ (Boston Scientific)	Three stabilization arches, radiopaque stent commissures
	ALLEGRA™ (NVT; see Figure 3.14.10)	Tube shape extending into ascending aorta, T-shaped connecting bars, radiopaque gold markers

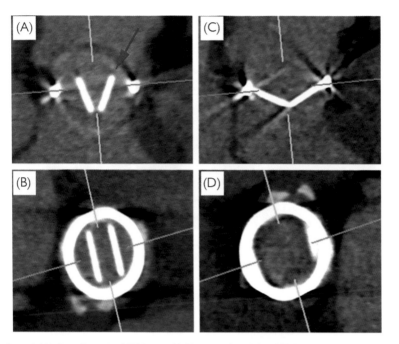

Figure 3.14.2 Four-dimensional CT showing (A, B) opening (systole) and (C, D) closing motion (diastole) of an aortic bi-leaflet mechanical prosthesis (SJM Regent® 25 mm).

Note that the anterior semi-disc shows a slightly restricted opening motion (red arrow).

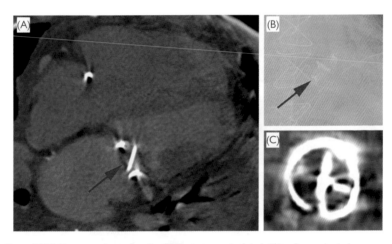

Figure 3.14.3 Contrast-enhanced cardiac CT illustrates a mitral single tilting disc mechanical prosthesis (Medtronic Hall 28 mm, red arrows) in the (A) horizontal long axis and (B) in the chest radiograph. (C) In the double-oblique view of the cardiac CT (transverse section), the disc and the single strut are identified.

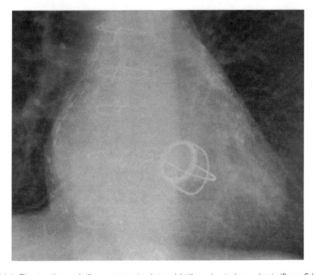

Figure 3.14.4 Chest radiograph illustrates a mitral caged-ball mechanical prosthesis (Starr-Edwards).

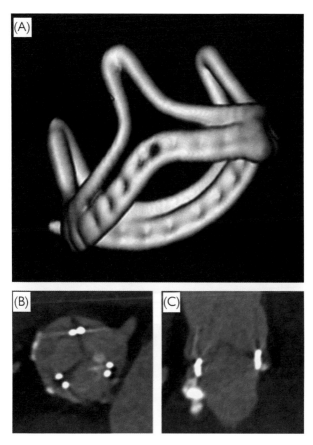

Figure 3.14.5 (A) Contrast-enhanced cardiac CT visualizes an aortic stented bioprosthesis (CE Perimount Magna 19 mm) as a volume-rendered image. Nine years after implantation, there are signs of degeneration in the (B) transverse and (C) longitudinal section.

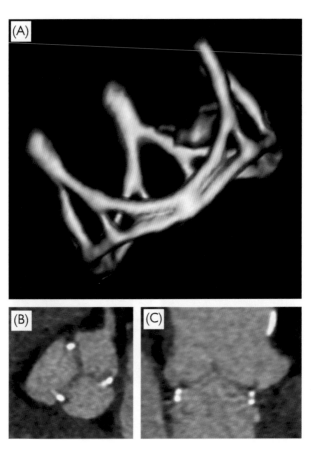

Figure 3.14.6 (A) Contrast-enhanced cardiac CT visualizes an aortic stented bioprosthises (St. Jude Medical Trifecta™ 21 mm) as a volume-rendered image. Eight years after implantation, there are signs of degeneration in the (B) transverse and (C) longitudinal section.

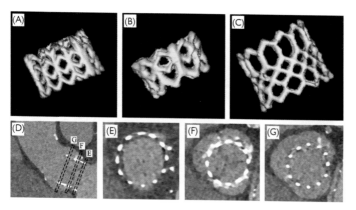

Figure 3.14.7 The three generations of Edwards transcatheter valves.

(A) Sapien (26 mm); (B) Sapien XT (23 mm); and (C) Sapien 3 (29 mm) are illustrated as volume-rendered images. (D) The Sapien 3 transcatheter valve is visualized as an oblique coronal view of the contrast-enhanced cardiac CT, and as transverse sections at the (E) annulus, (F) sinus of Valsalva, and (F) aortic root (F).

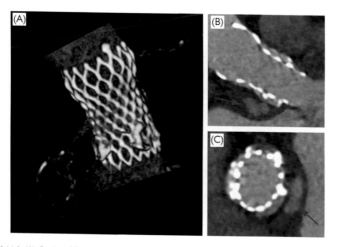

Figure 3.14.8 (A) Cardiac CT angiography, 1 day after implantation, illustrates the volume-rendered image of a CoreValve Evolut™ (29 mm) transcatheter aortic valve. The red arrowhead indicates a large calcification. In the (B) longitudinal and (C) transverse section a small pseudoaneurysm (red arrow) originating from the non-coronary cusp can be seen—a complication from the postdilation after implantation that caused laceration of the aortic root. Note the oval shape of the self-expandable nitinol frame.

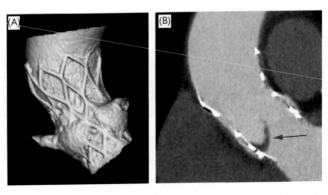

Figure 3.14.9 The contrast-enhanced cardiac CT demonstrates (A) a volume-rendered image and (B) an oblique coronal image of the hourglass-shaped Portico transcatheter aortic valve (27 mm) extending into the ascending aorta. Note the hypoattenuated leaflet thickening with near-complete leaflet involvement (>75%; red arrow).

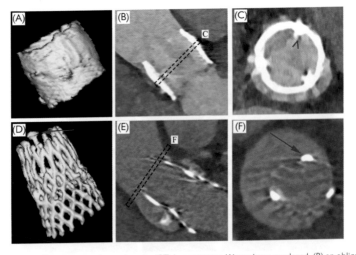

Figure 3.14.10 The contrast-enhanced cardiac CT demonstrates (A) a volume-rendered, (B) an oblique coronal, and (C) a double-oblique image of the Lotus transcatheter aortic valve (23 mm). Note the characteristic beam-hardening artefacts by the radiopaque marker in the centre of the stent frame (red arrowhead). The tube-shaped ALLEGRA™ transcatheter aortic valve (31 mm) extending into the ascending aorta is visualized as (D) a volume-rendered, (E) an oblique coronal, and (F) a double-oblique image. Note the characteristic T-shaped connecting bars at the very top of the stent frame (red arrow).

Category	Device	Characteristics
Table 3.14.2 Repair devices		
Surgical repair devices		
Valve annuloplasty ring (see Figure 3.14.11)	Various	Complete or incomplete radiopaque ring around mitral or tricuspid annulus
Transcatheter repair devices		
Edge-to-edge repair devices (see Figure 3.14.12)	MitraClip™ (Abbott)	Two-armed clip between anterior and posterior mitral valve leaflets
	PASCAL (Edwards)	Clip with two paddles and central spacer
Direct annuloplasty devices	Cardioband (Edwards; see Figure 3.14.11)	Single anchors around the mitral annulus but not Cardioband itself are visualized
	Millipede Annular Ring (Boston Scientific)	Stent frame with eight anchors and eight collars
Indirect annuloplasty devices	Carillon Mitral Contour System® (Cardiac Dimensions)	Proximal anchor at the ostium of the coronary sinus, connected over a 6–8 cm segment to a distal anchor in the great cardiac vein
	MONARC Coronary Sinus Device (Edwards)	Proximal anchor at the ostium of the coronary sinus, connected over a 12–16 cm segment to a distal anchor in the anterior interventricular vein

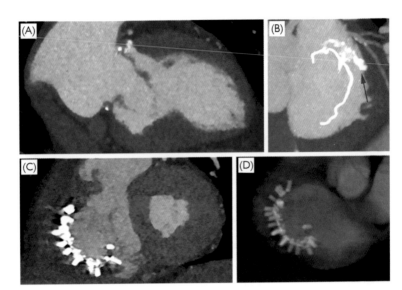

Figure 3.14.11 A surgical valve annuloplasty ring (St. Jude Medical Tailor ring, 35 mm) around the mitral annulus is visualized in (A) the vertical long axis and (B) maximal intensity projection of the contrast-enhanced cardiac CT. Note the calcifications at the anterior mitral annulus (red arrow). (C, D) Similarly, a transcatheter direct annuloplasty device (Cardioband, size F) around the tricuspid annulus is illustrated.

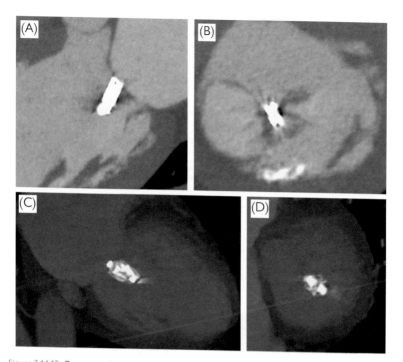

Figure 3.14.12 Contrast-enhanced cardiac CT visualizes a MitraClip™ NTR in the (A) long and (B) transverse section. In addition, a PASCAL transcatheter valve repair system is illustrated in (C) the vertical long and (D) short axis of the heart.

Source: Panels (C) and (D) by courtesy of Christoph Gräni, MD, PhD.

Table 3.14.3 Rhythm-management devices

Category	Device	Characteristics
Transvenous pacemaker/ICD (see Figures 3.14.13, 3.14.20, and 3.14.21)	Various vendors	Electrodes in the right atrium, right and/or left ventricle
Subcutaneous ICD (see Figure 3.14.14)	EMBLEM™ S-ICD (Boston Scientific)	Battery and electrodes in the subcutaneous tissue, on the left side of the chest
Leadless pacemakers (see Figure 3.14.15)	Micra™ (Medtronic)	Battery-shaped density of 26 × 7 mm, localized in the right ventricle
Implantable loop recorder	Reveal LINQ™ (Medtronic; see Figure 3.14.16)	Rectangular density of 45 × 7 × 4 mm in the subcutaneous tissue over the left pectoral muscle
	Confirm™ (St. Jude Medical)	Rectangular density of 56 × 19 × 8 mm in the subcutaneous tissue over the left pectoral muscle

ICD: implantable cardioverter defibrillator.

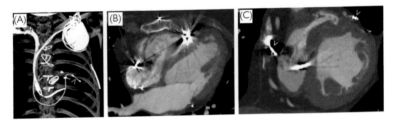

Figure 3.14.13 CT reveals multiple implanted cardiac devices in a patient with congenital heart disease (transposition of the great arteries).

(A) In the three-dimensional overview, an aortic bi-leaflet mechanical prosthesis (St. Jude Medical Regent 23 mm, red asterisk) and a cardiac resynchronization therapy device system (Medtronic Claria magnetic resonance imaging) are visualized. Note the right atrial (blue arrowhead), right ventricular (orange arrowhead), and left ventricular electrode (green arrowhead). In the (B) axial and (C) coronal images, the characteristic beam-hardening artefact of the right atrial electrode impedes assessment of the right coronary artery (red arrow).

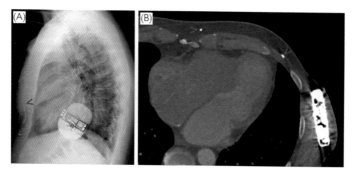

Figure 3.14.14 A subcutaneous implantable cardioverter defibrillator (ICD; Boston Scientific EMBLEM™ MRI S-ICD) is visualized on (A) chest radiograph and (B) axial cardiac CT. The course of the S-ICD is indicated by red arrowheads.

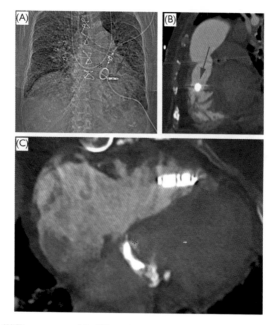

Figure 3.14.15 (A) The topogram of the CT reveals a mitral bi-leaflet mechanical prosthesis (ATS Open Pivot™ 27 mm (Medtronic), red asterisk) and a leadless pacemaker (Micra™ (Medtronic), red arrow). In the (B) sagittal and (C) axial view, the location of the devices is further visualized.

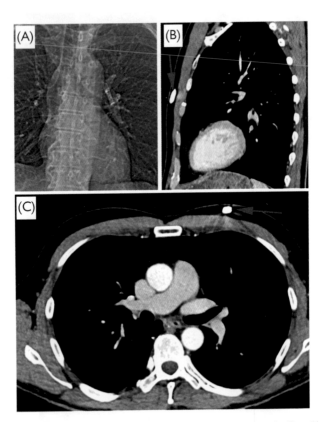

Figure 3.14.16 (A) The topogram of the CT illustrates an implantable loop recorder (Reveal LINQ (Medtronic), red arrow). In the (B) sagittal and (C) axial view, the location of the devices is further visualized.

Table 3.14.4 Occluder devices

Category	Device	Characteristics
Shunt occluders	AMPLATZER™ PFO Occluder (St. Jude Medical; see Figure 3.14.17)	Umbrella-like device with two discs (right > left atrial disc), connected by small waist (in multifenestrated 'cribriform' septal occluder: left = right atrial disc)
	AMPLATZER™ atrial septal occluder (St. Jude Medical)	Umbrella-like device with two discs (left > right atrial disc), connected by large waist
	AMPLATZER™ Duct Occluder or AMPLATZER™ Duct Occluder II (St. Jude Medical)	Asymmetric with larger diameter at the aortic side than pulmonary end, or two symmetrical retention discs (AMPLATZER™ Duct Occluder II)
	AMPLATZER™ VSD occluders (St. Jude Medical)	Umbrella-like device with two discs, connected by large waist and variable designs (membranous, muscular, P.I. Muscular VSD occluder)
	AMPLATZER™ Vascular Plugs 1 to 4 (St. Jude Medical)	Variety of differently shaped vascular plugs to close venovenous or aortopulmonary collaterals, pulmonary arteriovenous malformations, or perivalvular leaks
	CARDIOFORM Septal or ASD Occluder (Gore Medical)	Radiopaque circular wire frame forming two discs in the right and left atrium
LAA occluders	WATCHMAN™ (Boston Scientific; see Figure 3.14.18)	Single disc with umbrella-like shape
	AMPLATZER™ Cardiac Plug (St. Jude Medical)	Two discs with occlusive disc and anchoring lobe, connected by short waist, with six pairs of stabilizing wires
	AMPLATZER™ Amulet (St. Jude Medical; see Figure 3.14.17)	Same design as AMPLATZER™ Cardiac Plug, but with 6–10 pairs of stabilizing wires and larger lobe
	AtriClip® (AtriCure)	Radiopaque linear clip along the ostium of the LAA

LAA: left atrial appendage.

Valvular devices

335

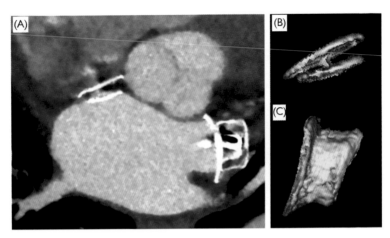

Figure 3.14.17 Axial view on (A) the left atrium illustrates (B) an AMPLATZER™ PFO Occluder between the right and left atria, and (C) an AMPLATZER™ Amulet occluding the left atrial appendage.

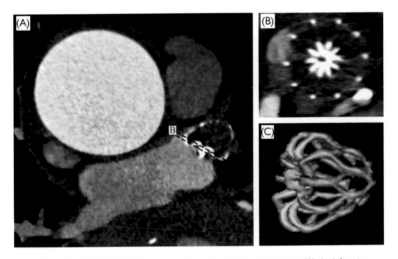

Figure 3.14.18 The WATCHMAN™ occluder is illustrated in the axial view on (A) the left atrium, (B) transverse section, and (C) volume-rendered image. As an incidental finding, there is an aneurysm of the thoracic aorta.

Table 3.14.5 Circulatory assist devices

Category	Device	Characteristics
Surgically implanted VAD	HeartWare™ HVAD™ (HeartWare International; see Figure 3.14.19)	Circular impeller unit, in the pericardial space, central inflow cannula, straighter outflow cannula
	HeartMate III™ (Abbott)	Circular impeller unit, in the pericardial space, central inflow cannula, angled outflow cannula
	INCOR® (Berlin Heart)	Tube-shaped impeller unit, in the pericardial space, between inflow and outflow cannula
Percutaneous VAD	TandemHeart® (Cardiac Assist)	Trans-septal cannula, connected to an extracorporeal impeller unit
	Impella® (Abiomed; see Figure 3.14.20)	10 × 0.7 cm device between radiopaque inflow area (next to the catheter tip in the LV) and radiopaque outflow area with pump motor (in the aortic arch)
Intra-aortic balloon pump	For example, Arrow AC3 Optimus™ (Teleflex) or Cardiosave (Getinge)	Radiopaque marker of the distal catheter (positioned at the level of the carina), 25-cm-long balloon visualized during diastole as a tubular lucency

VAD: ventricular assist device; LV: left ventricle.

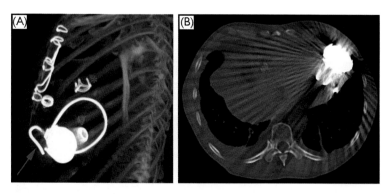

Figure 3.14.19 The lateral view on (A) the three-dimensional image and (B) the axial image of the CT illustrates a surgically implanted ventricular assist device (HeartWare™ HVAD™) with the driveline (red arrow) and inflow cannula (red arrowhead). Note the aortic stented bioprosthesis (CE Perimount Magna (Edwards), red asterisk).

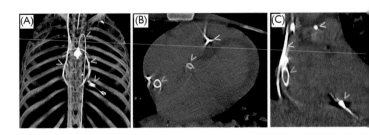

Figure 3.14.20 Three-dimensional illustration of (A) the CT reveals multiple cardiac device: an Impella® (Abiomed) in the left ventricle (blue arrowhead), the catheter tip of extracorporeal membrane oxygenation in the right atrium (green arrowhead), a pulmonary artery catheter (ye arrowhead), and a central venous catheter (orange arrowhead). In the (B) axial and (C) corona the location of the devices is further visualized.

Table 3.14.6 Other		
Category	Device	Characteristics
Coronary sinus reducer	Neovasc ReducerTM (Neovasc Medical; see Figure 3.14.21)	Hourglass-shaped stent in the coronary sinus
Implantable PA pressure monitor	CardioMEMS (St. Jude Medical)	Radiopaque, 4-mm-long linear de in the lower lobe region of the let

PA: pulmonary artery.

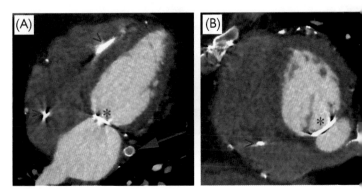

Figure 3.14.21 In the (A) axial and (B) oblique views, contrast-enhanced cardiac CT illustrates a coronary sinus reducer (Neovasc Reducer™; Neovasc Medical) in the coronary sinus (red arro Note the mitral valve annuloplasty ring (CE Physio Annuloplasty Ring Mitral (Edwards), red ast and right ventricular electrode (Siello S60 (Boston Scientific); red arrowhead) of a transvenous pacemaker (Altrua™ 60; Boston Scientific).

Table 3.14.7 Practical tips: how to optimize your scan protocol for device imaging

Scan parameters	• Use high-energy tube voltages (e.g. 120 kVp, or even 140 kVp in obese patients or when dense metallic artefacts are present) to reduce beam hardening artefacts • Consider larger field of view to include ascending aorta (particularly after TAVR or in patients with circulatory assist devices) • Repeat focused imaging of the LAA about 60 s after the initial contrast bolus to exclude pseudothrombus (particularly for LAA occluders)
Image reconstruction	• Use sharp reconstruction kernels • Prefer iterative reconstruction algorithms to reduce radiation exposure
ECG gating	• Consider retrospective ECG gating (or prospective ECG gating with large padding into systolic frames) for optimal evaluation of leaflet motion (i.e. '4D-CT'; particularly for valvular imaging) • Consider disabling dose modulation
Medications	• Beta-blockers for HR control (caution: clinical contraindications include severe aortic regurgitation or decompensated heart failure)
Contrast protocol	• For right-sided or interatrial devices, consider triphasic injection to opacify both left and right heart chambers without streak artefacts of the superior vena cava • Consider delayed scan to assess peridevice leak through LAA occluder

ECG: electrocardiogram; TAVR: transcatheter aortic valve replacement; LAA: left atrial appendage; HR: heart rate;

Table 3.14.8 Practical tips: implanted cardiac device—what should the CT report include

Valvular devices	• Device: type, position, expansion, valve leaflet thickening and calcification, thrombus • Prostheses: leaflet/cusp motion • Surroundings: origins of coronary arteries, wall thickening or dissection of aorta, pseudoaneurysm
Rhythm-management devices	• Device: type, position • Surroundings: access vein complications, perforation of myocardium, pericardial effusion
Occluders	• Device: type, position, peridevice leaks, residual shunts, thrombosis • Surroundings: interference with aorta or mitral valve, compromise of pulmonary venous return
Haemodynamic assist devices	• Device: type, position and integrity of pump, as well as inflow and outflow cannula, anastomosis, thrombosis • Surroundings: pericardial effusion, gas or fluid collections, cardiac valve and chamber function
Others	• Device: type, position • Surroundings: Vascular complications (e.g. pleural or pericardial effusion)

Further reading

Conyers JM, Rajiah P, Ahn R, Abbara S, Saboo SS. Imaging features of leadless cardiovascular devices. *Diagn Interv Radiol* 2018; 24: 203–8.

Ginat D, Massey HT, Bhatt S, Dogra VS. Imaging of mechanical cardiac assist devices. *J Clin Imaging Sci* 2011; 1: 21.

Ismail TF, Panikker S, Markides V, Foran JP, Padley S, Rubens MB, et al. CT imaging for left atrial appendage closure: a review and pictorial essay. *J Cardiovasc Comput Tomogr* 2015; 9: 89–102.

Salgado RA, Budde RPJ, Leiner T, Shivalkar B, Van Herck PL, Op de Beeck BJ, et al. Transcatheter aortic valve replacement: postoperative CT findings of Sapien and CoreValve transcatheter heart valves. *Radiographics* 2014; 34: 1517–36.

Valve Guide. Reference website for prosthetic heart valves and annuloplasty rings. Available at: www.valveguide.ch (accessed 30 June 2022).

Chapter 3.15

Extracardiac findings

Michael Messerli

Teaching points

- Extracardiac findings (ECF) are categorized into clinically significant (with therapeutic consequences) and non-significant findings.
- The overall prevalence of ECFs is approximately 40%; significant ECFs are found in about 15% of all coronary CT angiographies; acutely life-threatening conditions and/or malignant ECFs may be found in up to 2.5% of cases.
- The prevalence of ECFs is even higher (up to 70%) on CTs for transcatheter aortic valve implantation work-up due to the larger field of view and elderly population.
- Of clinically significant ECFs, by far the most common are pulmonary nodules (approximately 25% of all clinically significant ECFs), followed by hiatal hernia, pulmonary consolidation, and pleural effusion.
- Appropriate detection and interpretation of ECFs requires close collaboration between cardiologists and radiologists

Neighbouring organs (lungs, mediastinum, aorta, skeletal structures, and upper abdominal organs) are included in every coronary CT angiography (CCTA). With wider coverage (e.g. transcatheter aortic valve implantation (TAVI) CT) an entire thoracic and abdominal scan may be obtained. Appropriate detection and interpretation of pathological findings in extracardiac organs is crucial and may have important implications for patient management. Extracardiac findings (ECFs) may be categorized based on their clinical relevance into:

- significant findings—with immediate therapeutic consequences, or even acutely life-threatening (e.g. malignancy or aortic dissection);
- non-significant findings—without any immediate consequences for the patient (e.g. degenerative skeletal changes).

Prevalence and distribution of extracardiac findings

- Overall, ECFs are found in 27–56% of CCTAs; significant ECFs are found in 9–24% (Table 3.15.1).
- The most common anatomical territory with ECFs is the lung, followed by the abdomen, vessels, mediastinum, and others.

Table 3.15.1 Distribution and prevalence of clinically significant extracardiac findings (ECFs)	
ECF	Prevalence (%)
Suspicious pulmonary nodule	0.4–16.5
Hiatal hernia	0.2–6.4
Pulmonary consolidation	0.4–6.2
Pleural effusion	0.1–4.0
Cholelithiasis	0.1–3.6
Mediastinal lymphadenopathy	0.1–2.3
Indeterminate hepatic nodule	0.0–2.3
Pulmonary embolism	0.0–1.9
Aortic aneurysm	0.3–1.6

- Acutely life-threatening or malignant ECFs may be found in up to 2.5% of CC (Table 3.15.2).

Table 3.15.2 Prevalence of severe (acutely life-threatening or malignant) extracardiac findings (ECFs)	
ECF	Approximate prevalence (%)
Aortic aneurysm/dissection	1.9
Pulmonary embolism	0.2
Other vascular*	0.1
Lung cancer/metastasis	0.1
Bone metastasis	0.06
Other malignancy†	0.1

*Aortic thrombus, splenic artery aneurysm, superior vena cava thrombosis, and pulmonary thrombus. †Mesothelioma, hepatic metastasis, kidney tumour, oesophageal carcinoma, breast cancer, and lymphoma

Lung

- Incidental pulmonary nodules are the most common ECF (Figure 3.15.1).
- Approximately half of pulmonary nodules need further follow-up or work-u malignancy (Table 3.15.3).

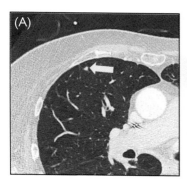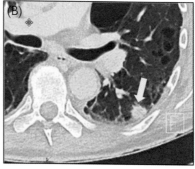

Figure 3.15.1 (A) A 4-mm nodule (arrow) in the right upper lobe of an 89-year-old non-smoking woman. No further follow-up was needed. (B) A 15-mm irregular, spiculated nodule in the left lower lobe abutting the pleura (arrow), highly suspicious for malignancy, in a 57-year-old smoker with emphysema. Further specialist management needed (CT-guided puncture, etc.).

Table 3.15.3 Fleischner Society guidelines for the managements of incidental solid* pulmonary nodules†

Single nodule		
Nodule size (mm)	Low-risk patient	High-risk patient‡
<6	No follow-up	• Optional CT at 12 months • If no change, no further follow-up
6–8	CT at 6–12 months, then *consider* CT at 18–24 months	CT at 6–12 months, then at 18–24 months
>8	Consider CT at 3 months, PET/CT, or tissue sampling	
Multiple nodules		
<6	No follow-up	• Optional CT at 12 months • If no change, no further follow-up
6–8	CT at 3–6 months, then *consider* CT at 18–24 months	CT at 3–6 months, then at 18–24 months
>8		

PET: positron emission tomography. *This table applies only to *solid* nodules. Subsolid nodules (ground glass, partly solid) typically have longer doubling times and therefore warrant longer follow-up periods (up to 5 years). †In patients >35 years of age. ‡Criteria for high risk: tobacco smoking, family history of lung cancer, spiculation, upper lobe location, rapid growth rate, emphysema, and fibrosis.

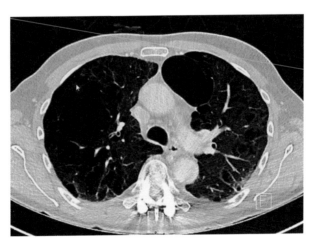

Figure 3.15.2 Advanced bilateral bullous pulmonary emphysema.

- A CT attenuation of −50 Hounsfield units or lower on non-contrast images indicates a predominantly fat density, most likely hamartoma.
- Central, diffuse, or lamellated calcification (e.g. old tuberculosis) or popcorn-shape (hamartoma) calcification are most likely benign; however, eccentric calcification may be found in malignancy.
- Other common pulmonary ECFs are pulmonary consolidation, emphysema (Figure 3.15.2), interstitial lung disease, pleural effusion, and bronchiectasis

Mediastinum

- The most common mediastinal ECFs are enlarged lymph nodes (≥10 mm in short diameter).
- The presence of a central fatty hilus and/or calcifications, or concomitant presence of pneumonia is often a sign of a benign aetiology.
- In hiatal hernia, the gastro-oesophageal junction is located above the diaphragmatic hiatus (may explain chest pain symptoms if gastro-oesophageal reflux is suspected; Figure 3.15.3).
- Anterior mediastinal masses may include thyroid masses (goitre), thymic tumours, lymphadenopathy, or germ-cell tumours.

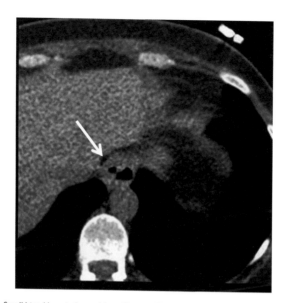

Figure 3.15.3 Small hiatal hernia (arrow) in a 49-year-old woman with atypical chest pain. Several weeks after treatement with a proton pump inhibitor, the symptoms resolved.

Vessels

- Symptoms of aortic dissection and acute coronary syndrome may be very similar (Figure 3.15.4).
- Aortic dilatation and aneurysm are frequent ECFs on CCTA; aortic dissection, intramural haematoma, or penetrating ulcers are life-threatening conditions that require immediate action (see Chapter 3.9 for more details).
- Standard contrast injection protocols for CCTA target optimal contrast of the left-sided chambers; therefore, opacification of the pulmonary arteries may be poor and embolism (particularly small or peripheral) may be overlooked. However, a large central pulmonary embolism may be visible even on a small field of view CCTA (see Chapter 3.9).

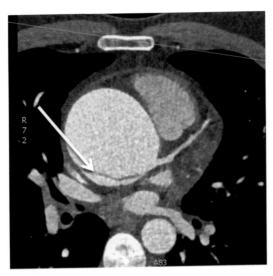

Figure 3.15.4 Incidental finding of ascending aortic aneurysm with a small posterior dissection in a 36-year-old man with recent-onset chest pain referred for coronary CT angiography.

Abdomen

- A standard CCTA allows for evaluation of the upper subdiaphragmatic abdominal organs only; however, a transcatheter aortic valve implantation CT allows for assessment of the entire abdominal territory.
- The most common abdominal ECFs are cysts (renal, hepatic; Figure 3.15.5), haemangiomas, adrenal masses, and gall bladder (Figure 3.15.6) or renal stones.
- Most hepatic nodules <10 mm are benign. Peripheral nodular enhancement on arterial phase is typical for hamartoma.
- The liver is the second most common site for metastases after the lung. They appear as solid, low-attenuation, irregular nodules.

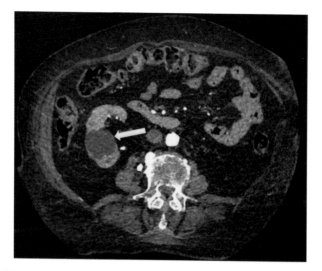

Figure 3.15.5 Renal cyst in the right kidney (arrow) in an 80-year-old woman with advanced renal failure (hypertensive, vascular, diabetic).

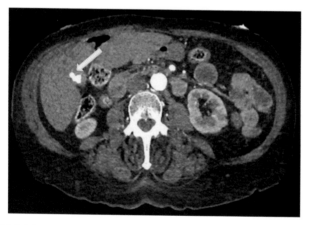

Figure 3.15.6 Calcified gall bladder concrements (arrow).

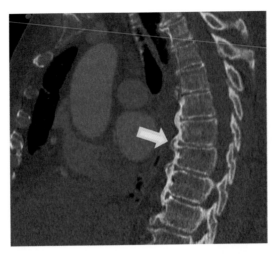

Figure 3.15.7 Advanced spondylosis of the lower thoracic spine: extensive spondylophytes with partial calcification of the anterior longitudinal ligament (arrow).

Skeleton

- Degenerative skeletal abnormalities are common ECFs, particularly in elderly patients (spondylarthrosis, spondylophytes, osteochondrosis; Figure 3.15.7).
- Rip fractures or osteoporotic vertebral fractures may be an alternative cause of chest pain.

Breasts

- The prevalence of breast nodules on CCTA is up to 0.6%. Of these, up to 50% may be malignant.
- Patients with pathological findings in breast tissue should be referred to a specialist for further investigations/management.

Further reading

Karius P, Schuetz GM, Schlattmann P, Dewey M. Extracardiac findings on coronary CT angiography: a systematic review. *J Cardiovasc Comput Tomogr* 2014; 8: 174–82.

MacMahon H, Naidich DP, Goo JM, Lee KS, Leung ANC, Mayo JR, et al. Guidelines for management of incidental pulmonary nodules detected on CT images: from the Fleischner Society 2017. *Radiology* 2017; 284: 228–43.

Schoepf UJ (ed.). *CT of the Heart—Contemporary Medical Imaging.* 2nd edn. New York: Humana Press, 2019.

Chapter 3.16

Artificial intelligence in cardiac CT

Márton Kolossváry

> **Teaching points**
>
> - Artificial intelligence is a general term used to describe computational processes that mimic or surpass human intelligence.
> - These algorithms may potentially provide better image quality, automate labour-intensive processes, and also help patient prognostication.
> - These techniques have yet to prove their additive value in general clinical practice.

Conventional clinical assessment relies on expert domain-specific knowledge and is often based-on visual subjective descriptors of pathologies. The problem with conventional image interpretation and analysis is that these qualitative imaging markers have bad reproducibility, even among experts. Also, they only capture a minimal part of the information present on images. Much attention has been paid to the possible implementations of artificial intelligence (AI) in medicine, as it may provide a more automated and objective methodology for the assessment of medical data.

Overview of artificial intelligence

AI is a general term used to describe computational processes that mimic or surpass human intelligence (Figure 3.16.1). The main part of these processes is machine learning (ML), which takes inputs and, using novel analytical and statistical techniques, maps them to given outputs. These ML algorithms are very good at finding patterns in the data and are capable of modelling non-linear relationships, which allows them to solve complex problems that conventional analytical and statistical techniques might not be capable of. However, this is also one of the Achilles' heel of AI, as it requires vast amounts of data and is prone to overfitting.

Generation of new forms of data from images

However, before we can utilize AI, first we need data. Conventional parameters may also be inputs to these models, but in past years much effort has been put into the generation of new imaging features using radiomics. Radiomics extracts a vast amount of quantitative imaging biomarkers from radiological images that describe the spatial pattern of the voxels in the given volume of interest (Figure 3.16.2). This

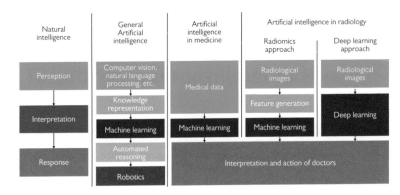

Figure 3.16.1 Flow diagram showing the possible implementations of artificial intelligence to medical data and showing the similarities and differences between radiomics, machine learning, and deep learning.

Source: Reproduced from Kolossváry M, De Cecco CN, Feuchtner G, Maurovich-Horvat P. Advanced atherosclerosis imaging by CT: Radiomics, machine learning and deep learning. *J Cardiovasc Comput Tomogr.* 2019 Sep–Oct; 13(5): 274–280. doi: 10.1016/j.jcct.2019.04.007 with permission from Elsevier.

methodology generates big data from single lesions and therefore allows for precision phenotyping of diseases.

Machine learning models

There are over 100 different ML algorithms. Some of these can be considered evolutions of the regression algorithm (i.e. LASSO regression). However, many are

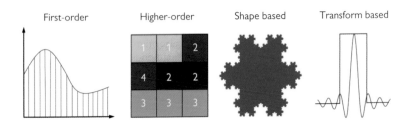

Figure 3.16.2 Pictograms of classes of radiomic parameters. First-order parameters calculate statistics based on the Hounsfield distribution of the voxel values and discard all spatial information. Higher-order metrics calculate statistics based on the spatial co-occurrence of specific voxel values. Shape-based statistics quantify the spatial complexity and self-symmetry of the lesion. Transform-based methods convert the spatial information into another domain, such as the frequency domain to calculate radiomic statistics.

Source: Reproduced from Kolossváry M, De Cecco CN, Feuchtner G, Maurovich-Horvat P. Advanced atherosclerosis imaging by CT: Radiomics, machine learning and deep learning. *J Cardiovasc Comput Tomogr.* 2019 Sep–Oct; 13(5): 274–280. doi: 10.1016/j.jcct.2019.04.007 with permission from Elsevier.

based on different ideas, such as decision trees, where the classification is made by splitting our data based on a sequence of criteria until we reach a given desired accuracy. While simple regression always results in the same answer, these models have so-called hyperparameters. Changing these predefined hyperparameters usually results in a different answer and therefore these need to be tuned to their ideal values during training. However, this increases the chances of overfitting; therefore, the fitted model should be evaluated on a separate data set to assess its diagnostic accuracy.

Tasks for machine learning

ML tasks can be categorized in to two main groups:

- *Supervised learning*: the process of taking inputs and defining which category they belong to or what value they have. For this, we need a labelled data set, where the ML algorithm learns what inputs correspond to a given output.

- *Unsupervised learning*: does not require a labelled data set. Instead of figuring out which class a given instance belongs to, it tries to find patterns in the data and assigns a case to a given cluster of other observations.

Deep learning

Deep learning (DL) is a subdivision of ML that does not rely on hand-crafted features; instead, it uses the raw data as input to the model. These raw data can be the raw data of the CT machine to create DL-based reconstruction algorithms or they can be the voxels themselves to create segmentations or classification of lesions. DL is the most flexible ML architecture and therefore is the most promising new methodology to create and analyse medical images. However, owing to this flexibility, it requires a vast number of images to be trained on and is very prone to overfitting.

Applications of artificial intelligence

As previously discussed, AI is just a new methodology to analyse and interpret data. It can be applied to all fields where conventional analyses can also be done.

- *Image reconstruction*: DL-based algorithms are faster than iterative techniques with similar noise reduction. Furthermore, they can provide different settings to different tissues and therefore different filter settings are not needed.

- *Image segmentation*: DL-based algorithms are showing promising results regarding the segmentation of heart chambers and coronary calcium scores. This would allow for more precise, objective, and automatic evaluation of cardiac diseases.

- *Plaque characterization*: AI implementations may expand our knowledge of cardiovascular diseases and provide more personalized care. Implementation of radiomic analysis to coronary plaques has shown that risk factors make a unique contribution to plaque morphology.

- *Pericoronary fat evaluation*: attenuation patterns in the pericoronary fat represent the inflammatory status of the tissue, which, in turn, has an effect on plaque development, progression, and rupture.
- *Myocardial tissue characterization*: radiomic analysis has shown that the texture of the myocardium may allow for the identification of myocardial infarction, even on non-contrast scans.
- *Prosthetic heart valve evaluation*: radiomics may identify the underlying pathology behind periprostatic masses and therefore may aid clinical evaluation and treatment.

In the future we will see which applications will actually make it into clinical software and be used to help with patient care. Currently, we only have limited data from controlled environments. These techniques are very promising and have the potential to transform medical imaging as we know it, but time will tell how useful they will actually be in everyday clinical practice.

Further reading

Chen C, Qin C, Qiu H, Tarroni G, Duan J, Bai W, Rueckert D. Deep learning for cardiac image segmentation: a review. *Front Cardiovasc Med* 2020; 7: 25.

Géron A. *Hands-on Machine Learning with Scikit-Learn, Keras, and TensorFlow: Concepts, Tools, and Techniques to Build Intelligent Systems.* Newton, MA: O'Reilly Media, 2019.

Kolossvary M, Kellermayer M, Merkely B, Maurovich-Horvat P. Cardiac computed tomography radiomics: a comprehensive review on radiomic techniques. *J Thorac Imaging* 2018; 33, 26–34.

Kolossvary M, Gerstenblith G, Bluemke DA, Fishman EK, Mandler RN, Kickler TS, et al. Contribution of risk factors to the development of coronary atherosclerosis as confirmed via coronary CT angiography: a longitudinal radiomics-based study. *Radiology* 2021; 299: 97–106.

Mannil M, von Spiczak J, Manka R, Alkadhi H. Texture analysis and machine learning for detecting myocardial infarction in noncontrast low-dose computed tomography: unveiling the invisible. *Invest Radiol* 2018; 53: 338–43.

Maroules CD, Hamilton-Craig C, Branch K, Lee J, Cury RC, Maurovich-Horvat P, et al. Coronary artery disease reporting and data system (CAD-RADS™): inter-observer agreement for assessment categories and modifiers. *J Cardiovasc Comput Tomogr* 2018; 12: 125–30.

Nam K, Suh YJ, Han K, Park SJ, Kim YJ, Choi BW. Value of computed tomography radiomic features for differentiation of periprosthetic mass in patients with suspected prosthetic valve obstruction. *Circ Cardiovasc Imaging* 2019; 12: e009496.

Oikonomou EK, Williams MC, Kotanidis CP, Desai MY, Marwan M, Antonopoulos AS, et al. A novel machine learning-derived radiotranscriptomic signature of perivascular fat improves cardiac risk prediction using coronary CT angiography. *Eur Heart J* 2019; 40: 3529–43.

European Association of Cardiovascular Imaging certification standards in cardiac CT

Andrea Baggiano

Teaching points

- The benefits of European Association of Cardiovascular Imaging cardiac CT certification include:
  - ensuring the physician performing the scan has the necessary expertise in cardiac CT, ensuring patient welfare;
  - providing cardiac CT trainees with the opportunity to benchmark their knowledge against a common European standard;
  - the professional credibility of any individual practicing cardiac CT.

Competency levels

- *Level 1:* an understanding of the basic principles, indications, applications, and technical limitations of cardiac CT. Level 1 competency does not qualify a trainee to perform or interpret cardiac CT studies independently.
- *Level 2:* a minimum requirement to report cardiac CT studies individually. Fulfils the requirement of subspecialty training in cardiac imaging, as set out in the European Society of Cardiology curricula.
- *Level 3:* practitioners can independently acquire and interpret scans, review pre-reported exams, and train others.

Level 2 and 3 prerequisites

The applying candidate must:
- be a physician;
- have sat and passed the European cardiac CT exam;

- have completed the training and competency for levels 2 or 3, or have completed a comparable certification within an internationally recognized certification programme;
- have completed 30 credits (level 2) and 50 credits (level 3) of continuing medical education specifically related to cardiac CT.

European Association of Cardiovascular Imaging cardiac CT core syllabus

- The European Association of Cardiovascular Imaging (EACVI) cardiac CT core syllabus contains the educational requirements for individuals who wish to practice cardiac CT.
- It helps trainees prepare for knowledge-based assessments and European certification.
- The content of the EACVI cardiac CT certification exam is based on the current EACVI cardiac CT syllabus.

General standards of training

All trainees, irrespective of their subspecialty and level of competency, must:
- know the indications and contraindications for appropriate cardiac CT patient referral;
- understand the principles of cardiac CT scan acquisition techniques, electrocardiogram synchronization, and dose-saving algorithms;
- display and interpret cardiac CT images in the clinical context;
- be aware of the side effects of contrast media and radiation risks to patients and personnel.

European cardiac CT exam

- It is an electronic exam based on multiple choice questions (MCQs)
- There are two parts to the exam:
  1. One hundred MCQs to test the candidate's theoretical knowledge, covering all items included in the syllabus.
  2. Several clinical cases to assess the candidate's practical experience.
- Candidates are required to pass both parts of the examination to be successful.

Training recommendations

- Structured didactic lectures and/or courses covering all the basic aspects of cardiac CT as defined in the core cardiac CT syllabus.
- Reading material and viewing of case files covering the physics, technical considerations, and clinical applications of cardiac CT.
- Educational programmes must provide a good understanding and knowledge of:
  - quality parameters and optimization techniques;
  - artefact recognition and management;
  - patient selection, preparation, and specific protocol modifications;
  - radiation dose, its determinants and techniques, and strategies to minimize it;
  - basic knowledge on iodine contrast media characteristics and adverse reactions.
- Practical experience through direct training under a level 3 supervisor or, in case of a lack of sufficient case load or case mix, through online cases available with virtual acquisition and workstations.

Requirements for cardiac CT competency levels

Level 1

- Onsite training at a cardiac CT facility, through EACVI-endorsed level 1 courses, EACVI case collections, the European Society of Cardiology's ESCeL platform, multimodality conferences, and/or online resources.
- Level 1 competency is not sufficient for the practice or independent clinical interpretation of cardiac CT.
- An EACVI cardiac CT theoretical exam is not required.
- No formal certification process is provided by the EACVI for level 1 competency.

Levels 2 and 3

There are three steps:
1. Knowledge assessment: passed the European cardiac CT theoretical exam.
2. Practical training and skills assessment.
3. Lectures and courses (with documentation confirming participation).

Caseload requirements

For levels 2 and 3, 150 non-contrast enhanced cardiac CT cases and 150 (level 2)/ 300 (level 3) contrast-enhanced CCT cases:
- live scanning acquisition of 50 (level 2)/150 (level 3) cases;
- interactive manipulation of reconstructed data sets using a three-dimensional imaging workstation, in the reporting and clinical interpretation of:

- 150 cases for level 2 (at least 30 cases assessment of structural and/or congenital heart disease, 50 cases of revascularized patients, and 50 cases compared to invasive angiography and/or myocardial perfusion imaging);
- 300 cases for level 3 (at least 60 cases assessment of structural and/or congenital heart disease, 100 cases of revascularized patients, and 150 cases compared to invasive angiography and/or myocardial perfusion imaging).

A maximum of 50 (level 2)/100 (level 3) cases from the EACVI virtual three-dimensional imaging workstation, which contains clinical information, cardiac CT data, analysis capabilities, and appropriate correlative data, need to be viewed.

Further reading

Gillebert TC, Brooks N, Fontes-Carvalho R, Fras Z, Gueret P, Lopez-Sendon J, et al. ESC core curriculum for the general cardiologist (2013). *Eur Heart J* 2013; 34: 2381–411.

Nieman K, Achenbach S, Pugliese F, Cosyns B, Lancellotti P, Kitsiou A. Cardiac computed tomography core syllabus of the European Association of Cardiovascular Imaging (EACVI). *Eur Heart J Cardiovasc Imaging* 2015; 16: 351–2.

Pontone G, Moharem-Elgamal S, Maurovich-Horvat P, Gaemperli O, Pugliese F. Training in cardiac computed tomography: EACVI certification process. *Eur Heart J Cardiovasc Imaging* 2018; 19: 123–6.

Index

357